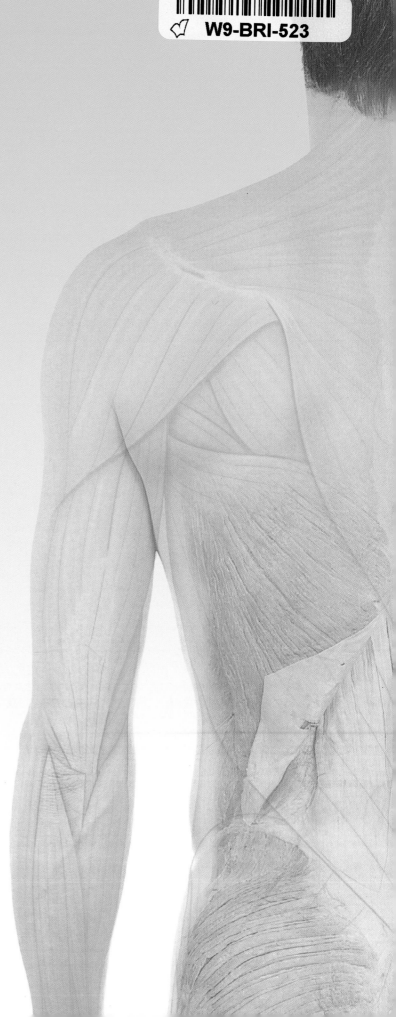

# McMINN'S
# Clinical
## ATLAS OF
# Human
# Anatomy

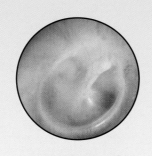

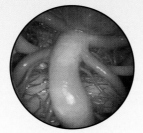

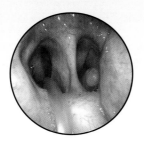

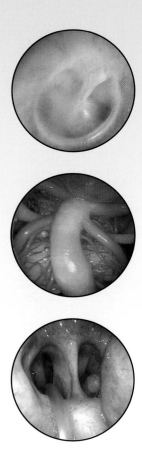

*For Elsevier*

*Commissioning Editor:* Madelene Hyde
*Development Editor:* Louise Cook
*Project Manager:* Gemma Lawson
*Design:* George Ajayi
*Illustration Manager:* Bruce Hogarth
*Illustrator:* Richard Tibbetts and Kim Knoper
*Marketing Manager(s) (UK/USA):* Ian Jordan/Allan McKeown

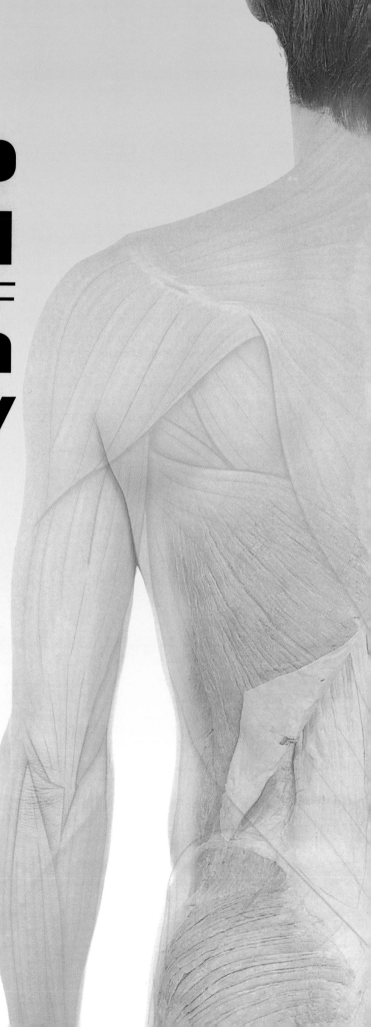

SIXTH EDITION

# McMINN'S

# Clinical
# ATLAS OF
# Human
# Anatomy

**Peter H. Abrahams**, MB BS, FRCS (Ed), FRCR, DO (Hon)
Professor of Clinical Anatomy, Warwick Medical School, UK
Professor of Clinical Anatomy, St Georges University, Grenada, W.I.
Extraordinary Professor, Department of Anatomy,
University of Pretoria, South Africa
Fellow, Girton College, Cambridge, UK
Examiner, MRCS, Royal Colleges of Surgeons (UK)
Family Practitioner, Brent, London, UK

**Johannes M. Boon**, MBChB, MMed (Fam Med), PhD
Formerly Professor of Clinical Anatomy, University of Pretoria, South Africa

**Jonathan D. Spratt**, MA (Cantab), FRCS (Eng),
FRCS (Glasg), FRCR
Consultant Clinical Radiologist, University Hospital of North Durham, UK
Examiner in Anatomy, Royal College of Surgeons of England
Visiting Professor of Radiology, University of Wisconsin, Madison, USA

*Photography by*

**Ralph T. Hutchings**
Photographer for Imagingbody.com
Formerly Chief Medical Laboratory Scientific Officer, Royal College of
Surgeons of England, London, UK

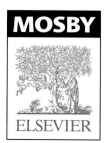

MOSBY

ELSEVIER

**MOSBY**
ELSEVIER

MOSBY An imprint of Elsevier Limited
© 2008, Elsevier Limited. All rights reserved.

First published 2008
First edition 1977 by Wolfe Publishing
Second edition 1988 by Wolfe Publishing
Third edition 1993 by Mosby-Wolfe, and imprint of Times Mirror International Publishers Ltd
Fourth edition 1998 by Mosby, an imprint of Mosby International Ltd
Fifth edition 2003 by Elsevier Science Ltd

All photographs taken by Ralph Hutchings remain in his sole copyright.

The right of Peter Abrahams, Johannes Boon, Jonathan Spratt and Ralph Hutchings to be identified as author of this work has been asserted by them in accordance with the Copyright, Designs and Patents Act 1988.

**Main edition ISBN:** *978-0-323-03605-4*
**International edition ISBN:** *978-0-8089-2318-3*

**British Library Cataloguing in Publication Data**
A catalogue record for this book is available from the British Library

**Library of Congress Cataloging in Publication Data**
A catalog record for this book is available from the Library of Congress

**Notice**
Medical knowledge is constantly changing. Standard safety precautions must be followed, but as new research and clinical experience broaden our knowledge, changes in treatment and drug therapy may become necessary or appropriate. Readers are advised to check the most current product information provided by the manufacturer of each drug to be administered to verify the recommended dose, the method and duration of administration, and contraindications. It is the responsibility of the practitioner, relying on experience and knowledge of the patient, to determine dosages and the best treatment for each individual patient. Neither the Publisher nor the author assume any liability for any injury and/or damage to persons or property arising from this publication.
**The Publisher**

Printed in China
Last digit is the print number: 9 8 7 6 5 4 3 2 1

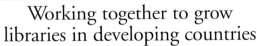

# Contents

## Systemic review    1

## Head, neck and brain    2

## Vertebral column and spinal cord    3

## Upper limb    4

# Dedication

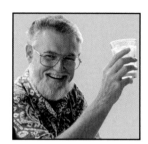

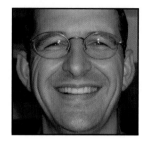

The preparation of this 6th edition of the McMinn Atlas has in many ways been a challenge made more difficult by two tragedies. First, not long after the appearance of the 5th edition, Sandy Marks Jr was suddenly taken from us. His untimely death robbed *Clinical Anatomy* of an Editor, the AACA of its Past President and Honoured Member, and I of my 'anatomical older brother', who had assisted and guided the 4th and 5th editions. His international respect and worldwide friendships are reflected in a collection of memories to be found on the DVD. None of these worthy documents replace anything of the warm-hearted family man who was a Colossus in the world of international clinical anatomy.

So the task of filling such big shoes was not an easy one. After much searching, the world over, I found at last a young medical anatomist who not only was a former PhD student of mine but truly had the potential to fill those shoes. Hanno Boon, clinical anatomist from Pretoria University, joined me with Jonathan Spratt, another former student of surgical anatomy, who is a Radiologist at the University Hospital of North Durham. This young but multi-talented team now started in earnest, with various meetings on three continents, in the preparation for this 6th edition.

Most of the major decisions of our future plans were made when a second tragedy struck. This time it was the senseless murder of Hanno in an armed robbery just 3 miles from his home in Mamelodi, where every week he did emergency medicine to complement his full-time day job as Professor of Clinical Anatomy in Pretoria University. This disgusting event robbed his young family of a caring father, me of an 'academic son' and academic clinical anatomy of one of its brightest rising stars. He had already, at the tender age of 34, been recognised and honoured by the BACA, AACA and EACA and was to be the new African editor of the journal *Clinical Anatomy*.

This most untimely death was recorded not only in his own medical school and South Africa publications but in journals as far apart as Turkey, USA and the Caribbean, where he had been a popular visiting professor (see DVD). All who knew him will never forget the boyish smile, quiet charm and sharp intellect of a devoted religious family man whose humble nature belied his passion and focus for medical academia in all its aspects.

Thus the preparation of this new atlas lost a most important member. However, to honour Hanno's contribution to clinical anatomy, a Hanno Boon Dissection Master Class attracted teachers and students from all over South Africa as well as the USA and Europe (see acknowledgements) and most of the new dissections in this edition were performed during that master class.

He would, I am sure, be proud to see this new edition with nearly all his suggestions of new content, dissections, and the wide-reaching DVD illustrating so many aspects of anatomy within clinical practice. These clinical cases were prompted by the landmark publication of the AACA, 'A clinical anatomy curriculum for the medical student of the 21st century', *Clinical Anatomy* 9: 71–99, 1996. We all felt that both teachers and students of the human body would welcome this extensive teaching resource. It consists of clinical cases, operative photographs, endoscopic shots, dissections of procedures and a library of imaging pathology as a practical way of integrating anatomy into all the health sciences and general medical education.

This edition, with its many clinical cross-references, new dissections, related endoscopies and a complete new section on lymphatics, as well as the one thousand photographs for personal study available on the enclosed DVD will, we hope, stand as a memorial and proud memory in years to come for Hanno's young children.

# Preface

In preparing the 6th edition of *McMinn's Clinical Atlas of Human Anatomy*, we have concentrated on making its use as intuitive as possible to the wide audience that the book enjoys, particularly to students of medicine, physical and occupational therapy, radiography, surgery and dentistry. Towards that end we have:

- Prepared 200 new dissections that provide an improved view of the anatomy of each region and include the lymphatics
- Added 50 new surface anatomy illustrations on real people throughout all the regions of the body
- Adopted a completely redesigned, integrated page layout to make the book more intuitively user-friendly
- Increased the use of endoscopy with over 50 new images from almost every cavity within the body systems
- Used sequential dissections of the same specimen (e.g. see infratemporal fossa, popliteal fossa, and sole of foot) to enhance the presentation of spatial relationships
- Improved the clarity of each page by reducing the amount of text – citing the popular clinical correlations at the foot of the page and showing their thumbnails at the end of each chapter
- Self-test facility is by means of MCQs along the USMLE format as well as problem solving tutorial questions with a clinical bias that are often used in short answer and oral examinations. Answers to all of these clinical anatomy problems are also provided.

Another unique educational feature of this edition is the inclusion of a DVD expanding both the information and over 1000 clinical anatomy digital images for students worldwide to make their own collections of relevant anatomical information. The text and numerous related images are arranged in regions and alphabetical order within each region. Some topics such as ophthalmoscopy have as many as 10 images illustrating all the common clinical conditions. These images have been especially collected from all over the world and grateful thanks go to all those colleagues who kindly gave their material and are acknowledged below.

Given the increasing significance of real clinical anatomy information in medical education and clinical practice, use of this DVD will provide the student with the earliest possible experience of 'the real world of medicine'.

DVD

The general order of presentation in the 6th edition follows that used in the 5th, except that the new section on lymphatics has been gathered at the end of the book, Chapter 8. Our aim has been to make each page as self-explanatory as possible with respect to location and orientation. Most of the new dissections replace previous images, thus improving the overall quality of the presentations. We have also added 300 new radiographic and laparoscopic images on the DVD to illustrate the anatomical foundation of contemporary health sciences.

P H Abrahams and J D Spratt
2008

# Acknowledgements

An atlas of this kind is not only the work of the authors but of numerous technical, scientific and clinical friends and colleagues who have been so generous of their knowledge and given permission for the inclusion of their original photographs of clinical cases. Hopefully, like the Carlsberg advert, this book and DVD are 'probably the greatest image collection of clinical anatomy cases in the world'. However, this dissection atlas would not be possible were it not for the talents of a special group of people – the prosectors and dissectors listed below.

**Dissections** Hanno Boon Masterclass, June 2005, Pretoria.

The following professors, doctors and students worked closely together as a team to honour the name of Professor Hanno Boon who had been their student, friend, mentor and an inspiration (see Dedication).

Donal Shanahan (UK); Stephen Carmichael, Rob Spinner (USA); Jan Meiring, Marius Bosman, Linda Greyling, Japie v Tonder, Andrea da Silva, Corrie Jacobs, Nanette Lizamore, Anna Oettle, Nadia Navsa, Albert van Schoor (Pretoria); Helena de Villiers, Daleen Raubenheimer, Francis Klopper (UFS); Nirusha Lachman (DIT).

*Post-graduate students*: Johan Aikman, Quenton Wessels, Carl Holt, Dawie Kruger, Stephen Lambert, Desire Schabort, Renee Botha, Maira du Plessis, Claire Robinson (Pretoria). *Support team in Pretoria*: Gert Lewis, Marius Loots, Marinda Pretorius, Coen Nienaber, Alet van Heerden, Tshepo Lelaka.

During the past 5 years, the following worldwide contributions have also produced some magnificent dissections, which appear for the first time in this 6th edition.

Mr Bari Logan, formerly The University Prosector, Department of Anatomy, University of Cambridge, England; Dr Marios Loukas, Associate Professor of Anatomy, St George's University, Grenada, West Indies and medical students Lynsey Stewart and B. Hallner from the American University of the Caribbean, St Maarten, West Indies; Ms Lynette Nearn-Forest, Department of Anatomy and Cell Biology, University of Illinois at Chicago (UIC), Illinois, USA; Dr Donal Shanahan, Prosector, Department of Anatomy and Clinical Skills, School of Medical Education Development, University of Newcastle-Upon-Tyne, UK; Ms Sue Standley, Department of Anatomy, University of East Anglia, Norwich, UK.

**Clinical cases**
The authors and publishers thank the following individuals and their institutions for kindly supplying various clinical, operative, endoscopic and imaging photographs for both the book and especially the DVD.

Dr Solomon Abrahams, Consultant Physiotherapist – Clinical Director, 'Anatomie Physiotherapy Plus', Harrow, Middlesex; Dr Tania Abrahams, Paediatrician, Great Ormond Street Hospital, London; Dr Rosalind Ambrose, Consultant Radiologist, St Vincent, West Indies; Ms Louise Anning, medical student, Girton College, Cambridge; Mr Chris Anderson, Consultant Urologist, Cromwell Hospital, London; Dr Ray Armstrong, Rheumatologist, Southampton General Hospital, Southampton and 'Arthritis Research Campaign (ARC)'; Ms Sally Barnett, Australian athlete, London; Private Johnson Gideon Beharry VC of 1st Battalion Prince of Wales' Royal Regiment and Grenada, West Indies; Professor Paul Boulos, Institute of Surgical Studies, UCL, Medical School, London; Mr John Bridger, Surgeon Anatomist, Department of Anatomy, University of Cambridge; Professor Norman Browse, Emeritus Professor of Surgery – and Hodder Arnold Publishers to use illustrations from *Symptoms and Signs of Surgical Disease* 4th edn. 2005; Mr Carl Chow, Obstetrician and Gynaecologist, Kingston Hospital NHS Trust, Surrey; Professor Bruce Connolly, Hand Surgeon, Sydney Hospital, Sydney, Australia; Mr John Craven, formerly Consultant Surgeon, York District Hospital, York; Mr Paddy Cullen, Consultant Vascular Surgeon, University Hospital of North Durham, Durham; Mr D Dandy, Orthopaedic Consultant and Churchill Livingstone for permission to use illustrations from 'Arthroscopic

Management of the Knee'; Mr Alan Davis, Optometrist, Ashdown & Collins, Kensal Rise, London; Dr Marc Davison, Anaesthetist, Stoke Mandeville Hospital, Aylesbury, Bucks; Mr Simon Dexter, Consultant Surgeon, Leeds Infirmary, Leeds; Mr Michael Dinneen, Consultant Urologist, Chelsea and Westminster and Charing Cross Hospitals, London; Professors Enrico Divitiis and Paolo Cappabianca, Neurosurgeons – and Karl Storz Endo-press TM, Tuttlingen, Germany for permission to reproduce pictures from *Endoscopic Pituitary Surgery – Anatomy and Surgery of the Transsphenoidal Approach to the Sellar Region* 2004; Professor J.F. Dumon, France; Ms Brenda Ernst, medical student, SGU, Grenada West Indies; Ms Oghenekome Gbinigie, medical student, Girton College, Cambridge; Professor Francis Nichols, Cardiothoracic Surgeon, Mayo Clinic, Rochester, Minnesota, USA; Professor Ralph Ger, Surgeon and Prof Todd Olson, Anatomist, Albert Einstein College of Medicine New York – and Parthenon Publishers to use illustrations from *Essentials of Clinical Anatomy* 2nd edn. 1996; Professor J. Gielecki, Chairman, Department of Anatomy, Silesian Medical University, Poland; Ms Natalie Gounaris-Shannon, medical student, Girton College, Cambridge; Mr Nadim Gulamhuseinwala, Department of Plastic Surgery, Guy's and St Thomas' Hospitals, London; Mr Fares Haddad, Consultant Orthopaedic and Trauma Surgeon, UCLH, London; Mr I. C. Hargreaves, Hand and Wrist Surgeon, St Luke's Hospital, Sydney, Australia; Dr David Heylings, Senior Lecturer in Anatomy, School of Medicine Health Policy and Practice, UEA, Norwich; Professor Michael Hobsley, formerly Head of Dept of Surgical Studies, The Middlesex Hospital Medical School, London; Dr Mike Jones, Consultant in Infectious Diseases, Director Edinburgh International Health Centre, Edinburgh, Scotland; Ms Megan Kaminskyj, medical student, SGU, Grenada West Indies; Mr Umraz Khan, Plastic Surgeon, Charing Cross Hospital, London; Mr Stephen Kriss, Podiatrist, Hospital of St John and St Elizabeth, London; Dr Suzanne Krone, Anaesthetist, Queen Victoria Hospital, East Grinstead; Professor Stefan Kubik, Anatomist, formerly Zurich University, Switzerland; Dr Lahiri, Cardiologist and the 'Wellington Hospital Cardiac Imaging and Research Centre', London; Professor John Lumley, Director Vascular Surgery Unit, St Bartholomew's and Great Ormond Street Hospitals, London; Mr Alberto Martinez-Isla, Laparoscopic Surgeon, Charing Cross and Ealing Hospitals, London; Mr Nick Dawe and Medtronic medical equipment company; Professor Jan Meiring, Chairman and Clinical Anatomist, University of Pretoria, South Africa; Ms Kathryn Mitchell, medical student, Bristol University, Bristol; Professor Antony Narula, Head and Neck Surgeon, St Mary's Hospital, London; Dr Barry Nicholls, Anaesthetist and Ultrasonographer, Musgrove Park Hospital, Taunton, Somerset and B. Harris, K. Hill and S. Moss from Toshiba Medical Systems; Dr Nkem Onyeador, Paediatrician and Arochukwu Medical Mission, Nigeria; Mr David Peek, medical student, SGU, Grenada, West Indies; Mr Rob Pollock, Orthopaedic Surgeon, RNOH, Stanmore, Middlesex; Professor Stephen Porter, Oral Medicine, UCL Eastman Dental Institute, London; Dr Lonie Salkowski, Associate Professor of Radiology, University of Wisconsin School of Medicine and Public Health, Madison, WI, USA; Mr Ertan Saridogan, Gynaecologist, The Portland Hospital, London; Mr Peter Scougall, Hand Surgeon, Sydney, Australia; Mr Julian Shah, Senior Lecturer in Urology, Institute of Urology UCL, London; Smith and Nephew Healthcare, Cambridge – Arthroscopic diagrams of limb joints; Mr Rajeev Sharma, Consultant Orthopaedic Surgeon, QE2 Hospital, Welwyn Garden City, Herts; Mr Spencer Quick, medical student, Bristol University Medical School, Bristol; Professor Rob Spinner, Neurosurgeon, Mayo Clinic, Rochester, Minnesota, USA; Professor M. Stoller, Department of Urology, UCSF, San Francisco, USA; Dr William Torreggiani, Radiologist, The Adelaide and Meath Hospital, Tallaght, Dublin, Ireland; Miss Gilli Vafidis, Ophthalmologist, Central Middlesex Hospital, London; Mr Peter Valentine, ENT Consultant, Royal Surrey County Hospital Guilford, Surrey; Mr Joseph Venditto, medical student, SGU, St Vincent, West Indies; Mr Richard Villars, Orthopaedic Consultant and Butterworth Heinemann for permission to reproduce illustrations from 'Hip Arthroscopy'; Mr Peter Webb, Consultant Surgeon, Mayday Maritime Hospital, Kent; Mr Theo Welch, Surgeon, Fellow Commoner Queens' College, Cambridge; Professor Jamie Weir, Department of Clinical Radiology, Grampian University Hospitals Trust, Aberdeen, Scotland – and Imaging Atlas of Human Anatomy 3rd edn,, Elsevier 2003; Mr Heikki Whittet, ENT Surgeon, Singleton Hospital , Swansea, Wales; Professor Tony Wright, Director Ear Institute, UCL Hospitals, London; Dr C. B. Williams, Colonoscopist, The London Clinic Endoscopy Unit, London.

**Art, photographic and technical assistance**
I would also like to thank Erica Saville, Elizabeth Hawker, Valerie Newman, David Robinson, Marius Loots, Adrian Newman, Richard Tibbetts at Antbits and Kim Knoper, for their secretarial, photographic and artistic skills.

A big thank you to Inta Ozols, Madelene Hyde, Louise Cook, Tim Kimber, Katie Sotiris, Thom Gulseven and Gemma Lawson for their editorial and production talents, coping with my many questions and demands, and for providing a constant plate of tuna sandwiches.

All the mistakes, though hopefully very few, are ours but the following individuals have kept the errors to a minimum with their proof reading skills and expert knowledge: David Choi MA, MB ChB, FRCS, PhD; Elanor Clarke MB ChB, MD; Andrew Fletcher MA, MRCS, PhD; David J. Heylings MB BCh, FHEA; Vishy Mahadevan PhD, FRCS (Ed), FRCS; Michael Message MA, MB, BChir, PhD, MD (Hon. Kigezi); Mike Stansbie MA, BM, FRCS Eng. (Otol); Donal Shanahan BSc, PhD; Theo P. Welch MBBS, FRCS. Finally we would like to thank Marios Loukas MD, PhD and Stephen Carmichael PhD, DSc for their assistance with the multiple choice questions.

## User Guide

This book is arranged in the general order 'head to toe'. The Head and Neck section (including the brain) is followed by the Vertebral column and Spinal cord, then Thorax, Upper limb, Abdomen and Pelvis, Lower extremity and finally lymphatics. In each section, skeletal elements are shown first followed by dissections, with surface views included for orientation. All structures are labelled by numbers, and these are identified in lists beside each image. An arrowhead at the end of a leader indicates that the structure labelled is just out of view beyond the tip of the arrow. Text has been limited to that needed to understand how the preparation was made, and is not intended to be comprehensive.

The clinical links at the bottom of pages point to the thumbnail images at the end of each chapter. Searching under these titles on the DVD will lead to further clinical information and many more images, all of which can be downloaded for both teaching and personal study.

# Orientation

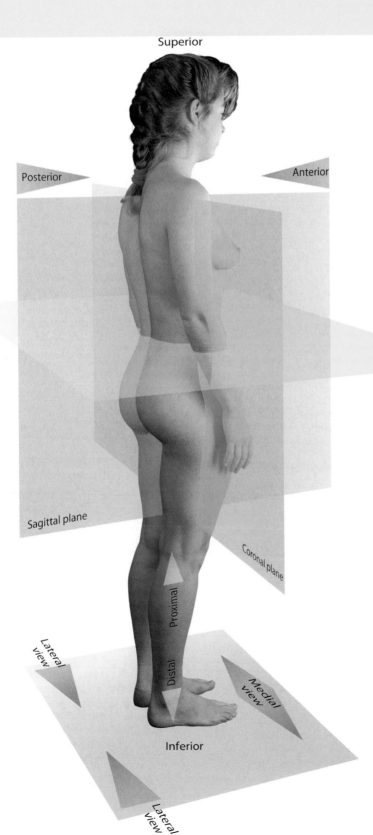

Superior

Posterior

Anterior

Transverse plane

Sagittal plane

Coronal plane

Proximal

Distal

Lateral view

Medial view

Inferior

Lateral view

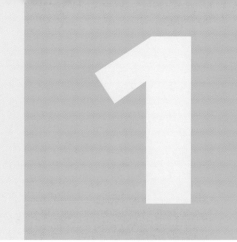
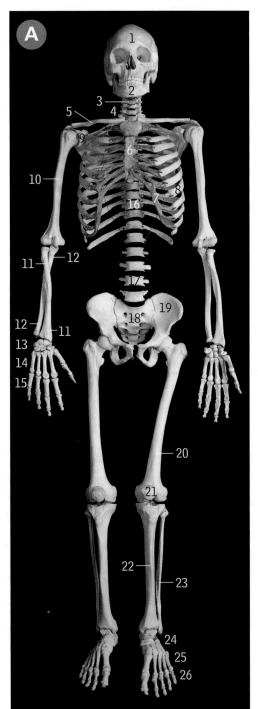

## Skeleton

**A** *from the front*

**B** *from behind*

**The left forearm is in the position of supination, the right in pronation in A.**

1 Skull
2 Mandible
3 Hyoid bone
4 Cervical vertebrae
5 Clavicle
6 Sternum
7 Costal arch cartilages
8 Ribs
9 Scapula
10 Humerus
11 Radius
12 Ulna
13 Carpal bones
14 Metacarpal bones
15 Phalanges of thumb and fingers
16 Thoracic vertebrae
17 Lumbar vertebrae
18 Sacrum
19 Hip bone
20 Femur
21 Patella
22 Tibia
23 Fibula
24 Tarsal bones
25 Metatarsal bones
26 Phalanges of toes
27 Coccyx

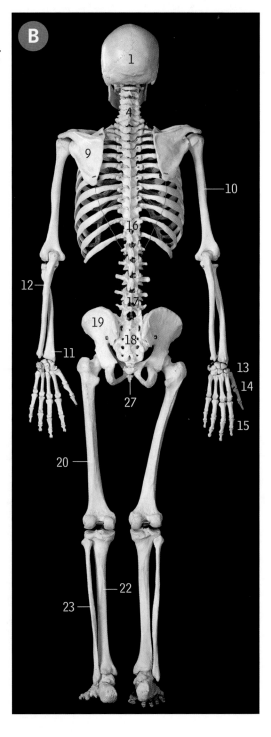

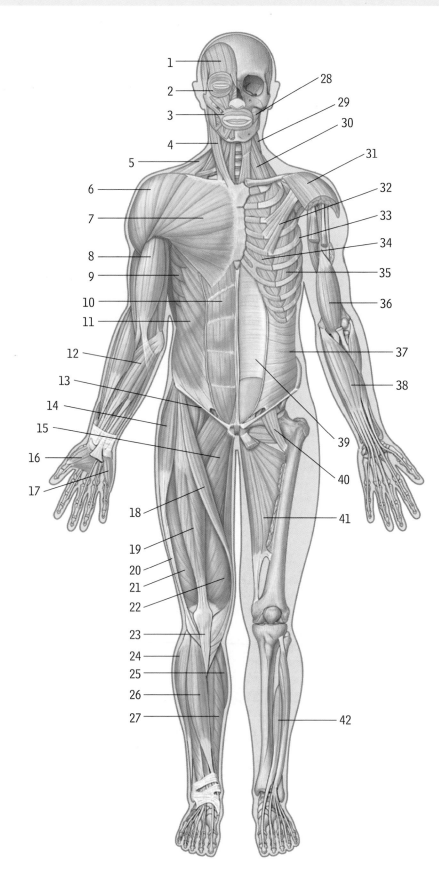

## Muscles *from the front*

**Superficial muscles on the right side the body, deep muscles on the left side.**

1 Frontalis part of occipitofrontalis
2 Orbicularis oculi
3 Orbicularis oris
4 Sternocleidomastoid
5 Trapezius
6 Deltoid
7 Pectoralis major
8 Biceps brachii
9 Serratus anterior
10 Rectus abdominis
11 External oblique
12 Superficial flexor muscles of forearm
13 Inguinal ligament
14 Tensor fasciae latae
15 Adductor muscles of hip
16 Thenar muscles
17 Hypothenar muscles
18 Sartorius
19 Rectus femoris
20 Iliotibial tract
21 Vastus lateralis
22 Vastus medialis
23 Patellar ligament
24 Peroneal (fibular) muscles
25 Gastrocnemius
26 Extensor compartment muscles of leg
27 Soleus
28 Buccinator
29 Levator scapulae
30 Scalenus anterior
31 Deltoid
32 Pectoralis minor
33 Serratus anterior, rib insertion
34 Internal intercostal
35 External intercostal
36 Brachialis
37 Internal oblique
38 Deep flexor muscles of forearm
39 Rectus sheath (posterior wall)
40 Psoas major and iliacus
41 Adductor magnus
42 Extensor hallucis longus

# Muscles *from behind*

**Superficial muscles on the left side of the body, deep muscles on the right side.**

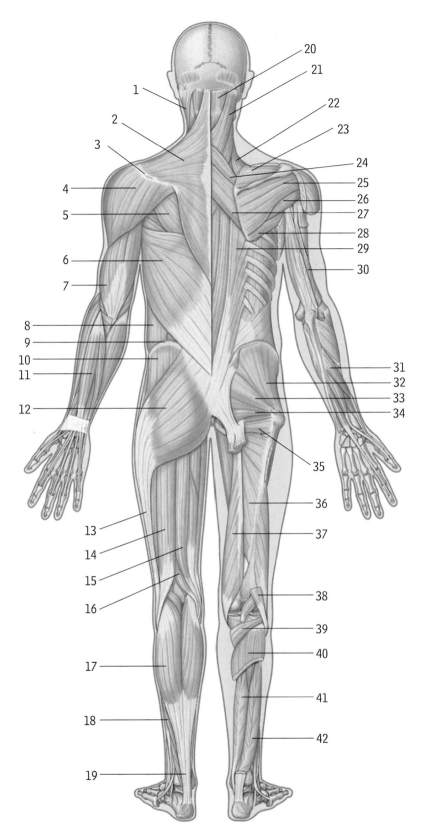

**1** Sternocleidomastoid
**2** Trapezius
**3** Spine of scapula
**4** Deltoid
**5** Infraspinatus
**6** Latissimus dorsi
**7** Triceps
**8** External oblique
**9** Iliac crest
**10** Gluteus medius
**11** Superficial extensor muscles of forearm
**12** Gluteus maximus
**13** Iliotibial tract
**14** Biceps femoris
**15** Semimembranosus
**16** Semitendinosus
**17** Gastrocnemius
**18** Soleus
**19** Tendocalcaneus (Achilles tendon)
**20** Semispinalis capitis
**21** Splenius
**22** Levator scapulae
**23** Supraspinatus
**24** Rhomboid minor
**25** Infraspinatus
**26** Teres minor
**27** Rhomboid major
**28** Teres major
**29** Erector spinae
**30** Triceps
**31** Deep extensor muscles of forearm
**32** Gluteus medius
**33** Piriformis
**34** Obturator internus
**35** Quadratus femoris
**36** Adductor magnus
**37** Semimembranosus
**38** Biceps femoris
**39** Popliteus
**40** Soleus
**41** Flexor digitorum longus
**42** Flexor hallucis longus

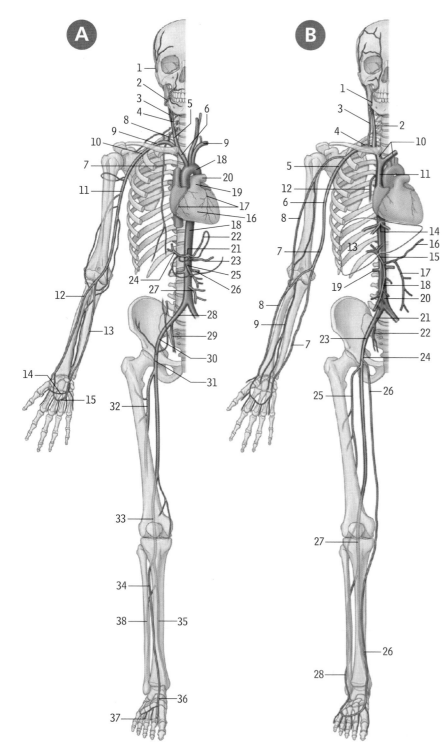

## A   Arteries

### *major arteries (a.), from the front*

| | | | |
|---|---|---|---|
| **1** | Superficial temporal a. | **20** | Pulmonary a. |
| **2** | Facial a. | **21** | Coeliac trunk |
| **3** | Internal carotid a. | **22** | Left gastric a. |
| **4** | External carotid a. | **23** | Splenic a. |
| **5** | Common carotid a. | **24** | Common hepatic a. |
| **6** | Brachiocephalic trunk | **25** | Superior mesenteric a. |
| **7** | Internal thoracic a. | **26** | Renal a. |
| **8** | Vertebral a. | **27** | Inferior mesenteric a. |
| **9** | Subclavian a. | **28** | Common iliac a. |
| **10** | Axillary a. | **29** | Internal iliac a. |
| **11** | Brachial a. | **30** | External iliac a. |
| **12** | Radial a. | **31** | Common femoral a. |
| **13** | Ulnar a. | **32** | Profunda femoris a. |
| **14** | Deep palmar arch | **33** | Popliteal a. |
| **15** | Superficial palmar arch | **34** | Anterior tibial a. |
| | | **35** | Posterior tibial a. |
| **16** | Heart | **36** | Dorsalis pedis a. |
| **17** | Coronary aa. | **37** | Plantar arch |
| **18** | Aorta | **38** | Peroneal (fibular) a. |
| **19** | Pulmonary trunk | | |

## B   Veins

### *major veins (v.), from the front*

**(The pulmonary veins enter the left atrium at the back of the heart and are not shown.)**

| | | | |
|---|---|---|---|
| **1** | Facial v. | **15** | Portal v. |
| **2** | Internal jugular v. | **16** | Splenic v. |
| **3** | External jugular v. | **17** | Inferior mesenteric v. |
| **4** | Subclavian v. | **18** | Superior mesenteric v. |
| **5** | Axillary v. | **19** | Renal v. |
| **6** | Brachial v. | **20** | Inferior vena cava |
| **7** | Basilic v. | **21** | Common iliac v. |
| **8** | Cephalic v. | **22** | Internal iliac v. |
| **9** | Median forearm v. | **23** | External iliac v. |
| **10** | Brachiocephalic vv. | **24** | Common femoral v. |
| **11** | Superior vena cava | **25** | Profunda femoris v. |
| **12** | Azygos v. | **26** | Great saphenous v. |
| **13** | Liver | **27** | Popliteal v. |
| **14** | Hepatic vv. | **28** | Small saphenous v. |

# Nerves

*main nerves (n.) including the facial nerve and major branches of the brachial, lumbar and sacral plexi*

**A** from the front

**B** from the back

1 Facial n.
2 Brachial plexus (divisions)
3 Musculocutaneous n.
4 Median n.
5 Ulnar n.
6 Lumbar plexus
7 Obturator n.
8 Femoral n.
9 Saphenous n.
10 Common peroneal (fibular) n.
11 Superficial peroneal (fibular) n.
12 Deep peroneal (fibular) n.
13 Axillary n.
14 Radial n.
15 Sacral plexus
16 Superior gluteal n.
17 Inferior gluteal n.
18 Pudendal n.
19 Posterior femoral cutaneous n.
20 Sciatic n.
21 Tibial n.
22 Sural n.

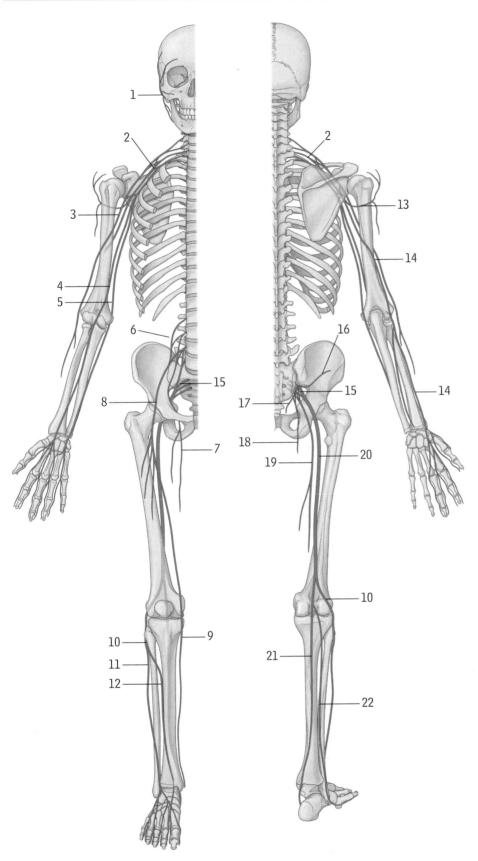

# Dermatomes of cranial, spinal and peripheral nerves

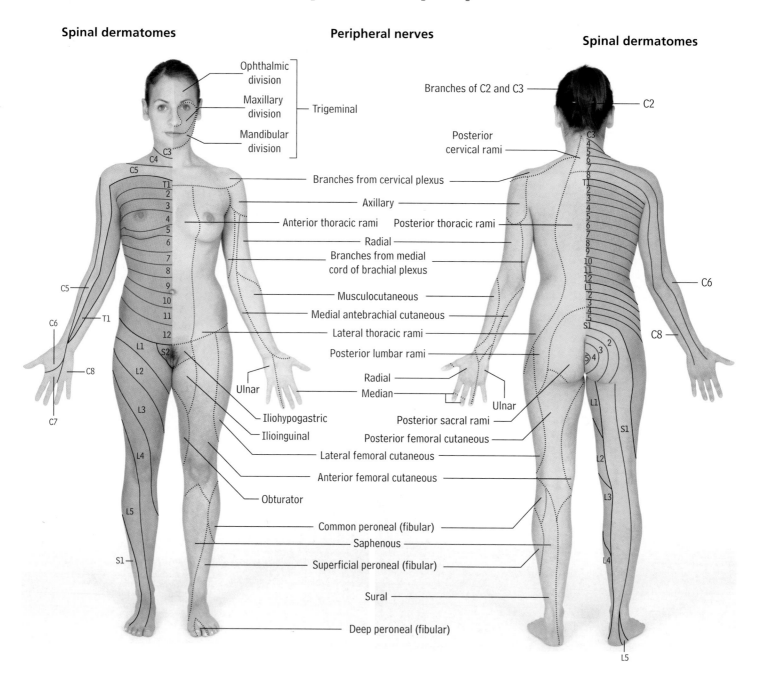

Spinal dermatomes

Peripheral nerves

Spinal dermatomes

Ophthalmic division

Maxillary division

Trigeminal

Mandibular division

Branches of C2 and C3

Posterior cervical rami

Branches from cervical plexus

Axillary

Anterior thoracic rami  Posterior thoracic rami

Radial

Branches from medial cord of brachial plexus

Musculocutaneous

Medial antebrachial cutaneous

Lateral thoracic rami

Posterior lumbar rami

Radial

Ulnar  Median

Iliohypogastric  Ulnar

Ilioinguinal  Posterior sacral rami

Posterior femoral cutaneous

Lateral femoral cutaneous

Anterior femoral cutaneous

Obturator

Common peroneal (fibular)

Saphenous

Superficial peroneal (fibular)

Sural

Deep peroneal (fibular)

**After Keegan et al. 1948 Anatomical Record 102; 409–437. There is great personal variation; see Foerster 1933 Brain 56; 1–39. Overlap of dermatomes occurs over 2–3 spinal root levels.**

# Cross-sections of the human body

## Head and neck *cross-sections*

**A** section at level of optic chiasma

**B** section at level of vocal cords

**1** Arytenoid cartilage
**2** Claustrum
**3** Common carotid artery
**4** Ethmoidal air cells
**5** Head of caudate nucleus
**6** Internal capsule of cerebrum
**7** Internal jugular vein
**8** Lamina of vertebra
**9** Lateral rectus muscle
**10** Lens
**11** Lentiform nucleus
**12** Levator scapulae muscle
**13** Ligamentum nuchae
**14** Longus colli muscle
**15** Medial rectus muscle
**16** Nasal cavity
**17** Optic canal
**18** Optic chiasma
**19** Optic nerve
**20** Optic radiation
**21** Orbital fat
**22** Piriform fossa, pharynx
**23** Platysma muscle
**24** Scalenus anterior muscle
**25** Scalenus medius and scalenus posterior
**26** Semispinalis capitis muscle
**27** Spinal cord
**28** Spinalis muscle
**29** Splenius capitis muscle
**30** Sternocleidomastoid muscle
**31** Superior sagittal sinus
**32** Temporal lobe, cerebrum
**33** Temporalis muscle
**34** Thalamus
**35** Thyroid cartilage
**36** Thyroid gland, lateral lobe
**37** Trapezius muscle
**38** Vertebral artery in transverse foramen
**39** Vertebral body
**40** Vertebral canal
**41** Vocal cord
**42** Zygomatic bone

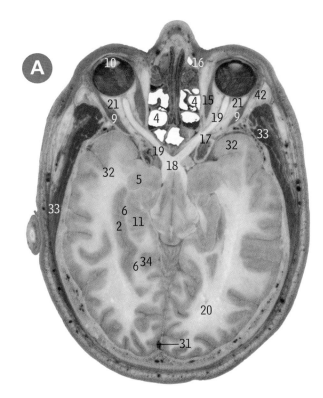

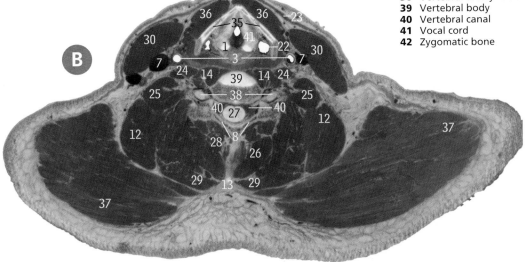

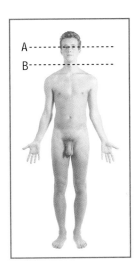

Images on pages 7–10 inclusive are from the National Library of Medicine (USA), Visible Human Data Set.

# Thorax *cross-sections*

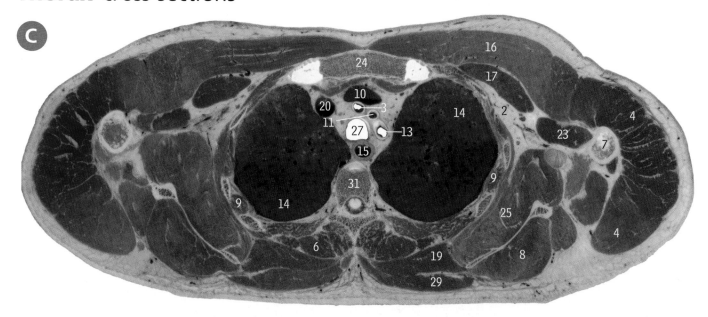

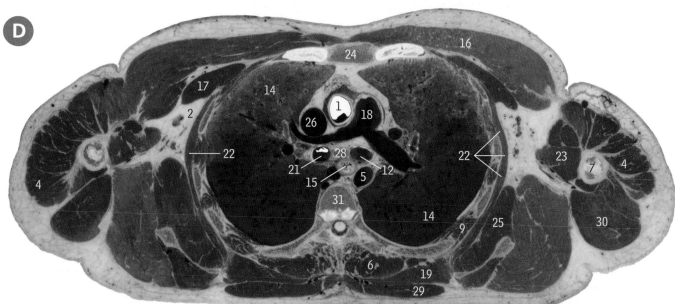

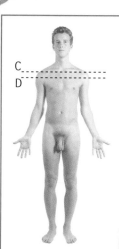

**C**   **section at T2 vertebral level**

**D**   **section at T4/5 vertebral level**

1   Ascending aorta
2   Axillary fat with brachial plexus
3   Brachiocephalic artery
4   Deltoid muscle
5   Descending aorta
6   Erector spinae muscle
7   Humerus

8   Infraspinatus muscle
9   Intercostal muscles
10   Left brachiocephalic vein
11   Left common carotid artery
12   Left main bronchus
13   Left subclavian artery
14   Lung
15   Oesophagus
16   Pectoralis major muscle
17   Pectoralis minor muscle
18   Pulmonary trunk
19   Rhomboid major muscle
20   Right brachiocephalic vein
21   Right main bronchus

22   Serratus anterior muscle
23   Short head of biceps brachii and coracobrachialis muscles
24   Sternal marrow
25   Subscapularis muscle
26   Superior vena cava
27   Trachea
28   Tracheobronchial lymph nodes (subcarinal nodes)
29   Trapezius muscle
30   Triceps muscle
31   Vertebral body

# Abdomen *cross-sections*

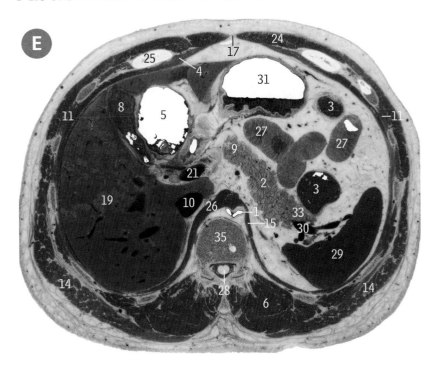

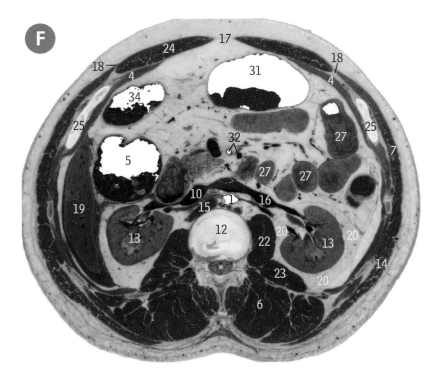

**E** section at L1 vertebral level

**F** section at L2 vertebral level

1 Aorta
2 Body of pancreas
3 Descending colon
4 Diaphragm
5 Duodenum
6 Erector spinae muscle
7 External oblique muscle
8 Gall bladder
9 Head of pancreas
10 Inferior vena cava
11 Intercostal muscle
12 Intervertebral disc
13 Kidney
14 Latissimus dorsi muscle
15 Left crus of diaphragm
16 Left renal vein
17 Linea alba
18 Linea semilunaris
19 Liver
20 Perirenal fat
21 Portal vein
22 Psoas major muscle
23 Quadratus lumborum muscle
24 Rectus abdominis muscle
25 Rib
26 Right crus of diaphragm
27 Small intestine
28 Spinal cord
29 Spleen
30 Splenic artery and vein
31 Stomach
32 Superior mesenteric vessels
33 Tail of pancreas
34 Transverse colon
35 Vertebral body

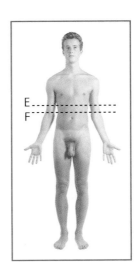

# Pelvic region *cross-sections*

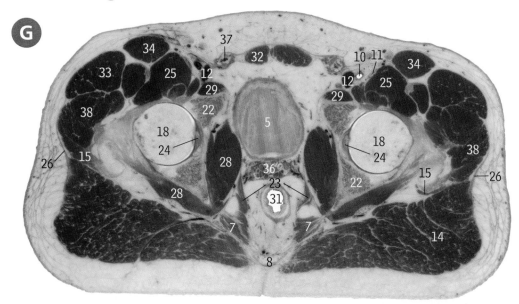

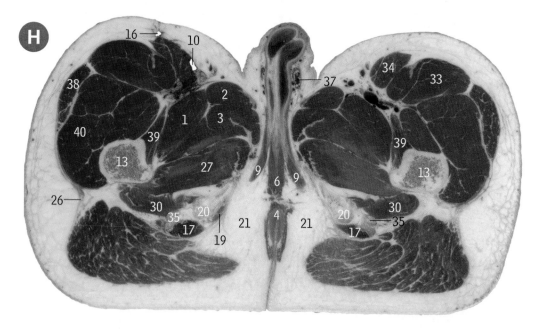

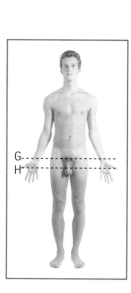

**G** section at level of the hip joint in a male pelvis

**H** section at level of the upper thigh in a male pelvis

| | |
|---|---|
| **1** | Adductor brevis muscle |
| **2** | Adductor longus muscle |
| **3** | Adductor magnus muscle |
| **4** | Anal canal |
| **5** | Bladder |
| **6** | Bulb of penis |
| **7** | Coccygeus part of levator ani muscle |
| **8** | Coccyx |
| **9** | Crus of penis |
| **10** | Femoral artery |
| **11** | Femoral nerve |
| **12** | Femoral vein |
| **13** | Femur |
| **14** | Gluteus maximus muscle |
| **15** | Gluteus minimus muscle |
| **16** | Great saphenous vein |
| **17** | Hamstring origin |
| **18** | Head of femur |
| **19** | Ischiocavernosus muscle |
| **20** | Ischial tuberosity |
| **21** | Ischioanal fossa |
| **22** | Ischium |
| **23** | Levator ani muscle |
| **24** | Ligament of head of femur |
| **25** | Iliopsoas muscle |
| **26** | Iliotibial tract |
| **27** | Obturator externus muscle |
| **28** | Obturator internus muscle |
| **29** | Pectineus muscle |
| **30** | Quadratus femoris muscle |
| **31** | Rectum |
| **32** | Rectus abdominis muscle |
| **33** | Rectus femoris muscle |
| **34** | Sartorius muscle |
| **35** | Sciatic nerve |
| **36** | Seminal vesicles |
| **37** | Spermatic cord |
| **38** | Tensor fasciae latae muscle |
| **39** | Vastus intermedius muscle |
| **40** | Vastus lateralis muscle |

## Skull *from the front*

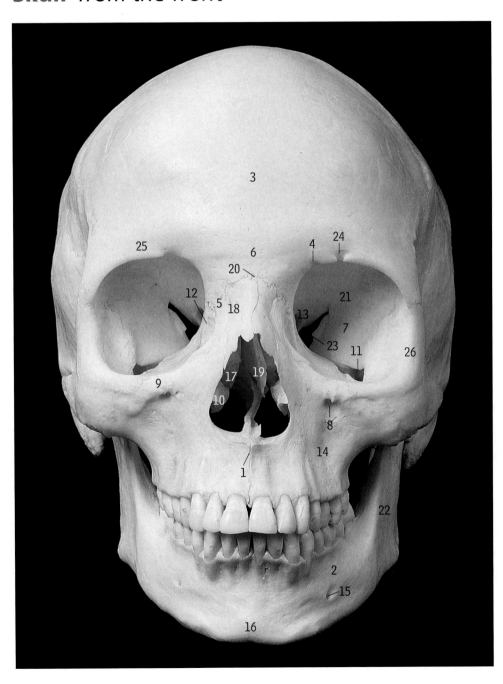

1 Anterior nasal spine
2 Body of mandible
3 Frontal bone
4 Frontal notch
5 Frontal process of maxilla
6 Glabella
7 Greater wing of sphenoid bone
8 Infra-orbital foramen
9 Infra-orbital margin
10 Inferior nasal concha
11 Inferior orbital fissure
12 Lacrimal bone
13 Lesser wing of sphenoid bone
14 Maxilla
15 Mental foramen
16 Mental protuberance
17 Middle nasal concha
18 Nasal bone
19 Nasal septum
20 Nasion
21 Orbit (orbital cavity)
22 Ramus of mandible
23 Superior orbital fissure
24 Supra-orbital foramen
25 Supra-orbital margin
26 Zygomatic bone

The term 'skull' includes the mandible, and 'cranium' refers to the skull without the mandible.

The calvarium is the vault of the skull (cranial vault or skull-cap) and is the upper part of the cranium that encloses the brain.

The front part of the skull forms the facial skeleton.

The supra-orbital, infra-orbital and mental foramina (24, 8 and 15) lie in approximately the same vertical plane.

Details of individual skull bones are given on pages 30–37, of the bones of the orbit and nose on page 22, and of the teeth on page 23.

# Skull *muscle attachments, from the front*

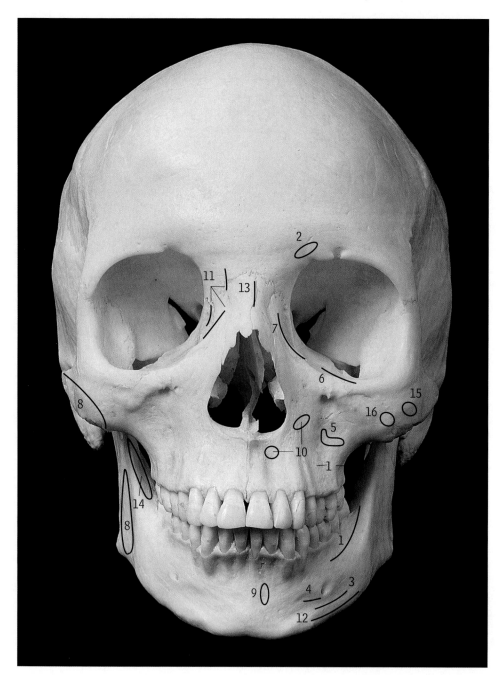

1 Buccinator
2 Corrugator supercilii
3 Depressor anguli oris
4 Depressor labii inferioris
5 Levator anguli oris
6 Levator labii superioris
7 Levator labii superioris alaeque nasi
8 Masseter
9 Mentalis
10 Nasalis
11 Orbicularis oculi
12 Platysma
13 Procerus
14 Temporalis
15 Zygomaticus major
16 Zygomaticus minor

# Skull *radiograph, occipitofrontal 15° projection*

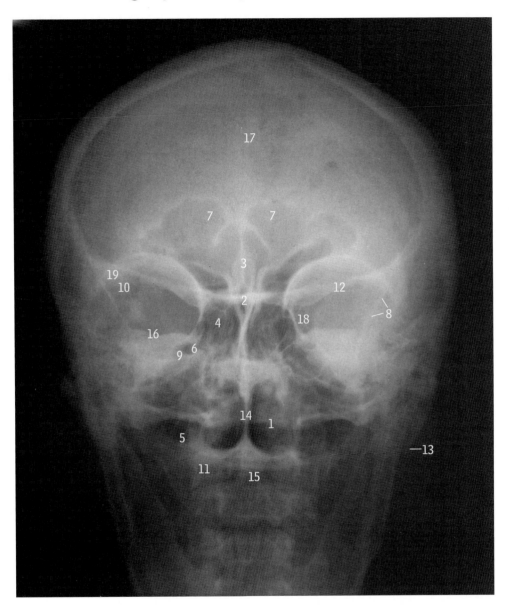

1 Basi-occiput
2 Body of sphenoid
3 Crista galli
4 Ethmoidal air cells
5 Floor of maxillary sinus (antrum)
6 Foramen rotundum
7 Frontal sinus
8 Greater wing of sphenoid
9 Internal acoustic meatus
10 Lambdoid suture
11 Lateral mass of atlas (first cervical vertebra)
12 Lesser wing of sphenoid
13 Mastoid process
14 Nasal septum
15 Odontoid process (dens) of axis (second cervical vertebra)
16 Petrous part of temporal bone
17 Sagittal suture
18 Superior orbital fissure
19 Temporal surface of greater wing of sphenoid

# Skull *from the right*

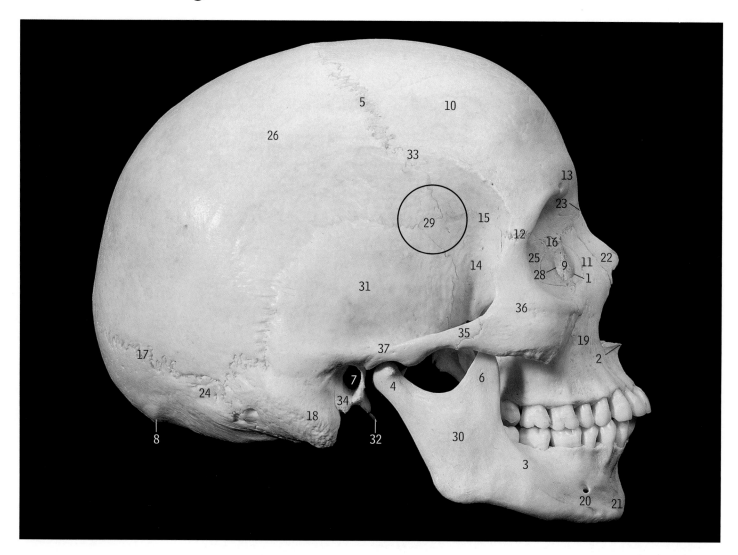

| | | | |
|---|---|---|---|
| **1** Anterior lacrimal crest | **11** Frontal process of maxilla | **21** Mental protuberance | **32** Styloid process of temporal |
| **2** Anterior nasal spine | **12** Frontozygomatic suture | **22** Nasal bone | bone |
| **3** Body of mandible | **13** Glabella | **23** Nasion | **33** Superior temporal line |
| **4** Condyle of mandible | **14** Greater wing of sphenoid | **24** Occipital bone | **34** Tympanic part of temporal |
| **5** Coronal suture | bone | **25** Orbital plate of ethmoid bone | bone |
| **6** Coronoid process of mandible | **15** Inferior temporal line | **26** Parietal bone | **35** Zygomatic arch |
| **7** External acoustic meatus of | **16** Lacrimal bone | **27** Pituitary fossa (sella turcica) | **36** Zygomatic bone |
| temporal bone | **17** Lambdoid suture | **28** Posterior lacrimal crest | **37** Zygomatic process of |
| **8** External occipital | **18** Mastoid process of temporal | **29** Pterion (encircled) | temporal bone |
| protuberance (inion) | bone | **30** Ramus of mandible | |
| **9** Fossa for lacrimal sac | **19** Maxilla | **31** Squamous part of temporal | |
| **10** Frontal bone | **20** Mental foramen | bone | |

Pterion (29) is not a single point but an area where the frontal (10), parietal (26), squamous part of the temporal (31) and greater wing of the sphenoid bone (14) adjoin one another.

It is an important landmark for the anterior branch of the middle meningeal artery, which underlies this area on the inside of the skull (page 27).

*Extradural haemorrhage, see page 90.*

# Skull

## A radiograph, lateral projection

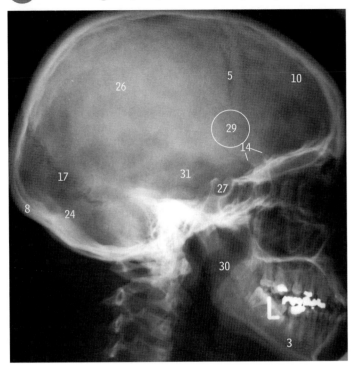

## C coloured bones

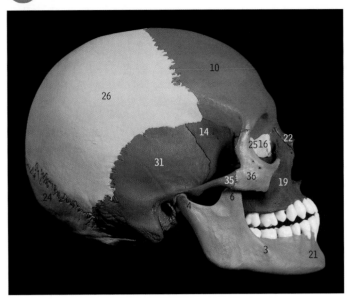

Scalp layers (**S**, skin; **C**, connective tissue; **A**, aponeurosis of occipitofrontalis; **L**, loose areolar tissue; **P**, periosteum). Deep in the pterion Burr hole the middle meningeal artery (MMA) has been revealed.

## B scalp dissection

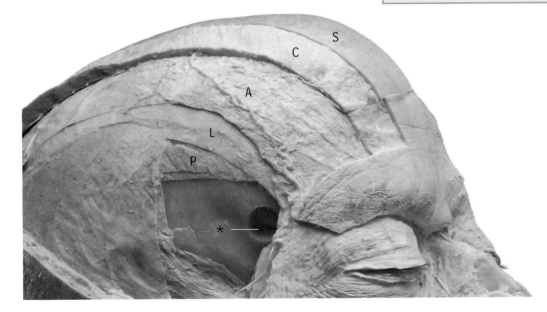

*  Burr hole at pterion.

*Burr holes, see page 90.*

## Skull *muscle attachments, from the right*

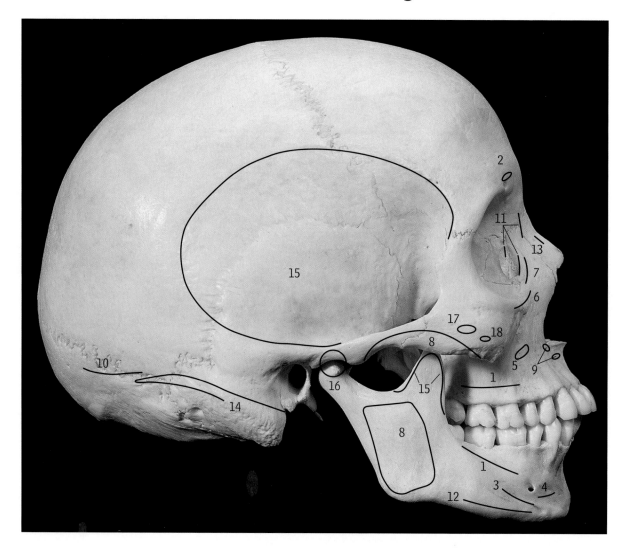

**1** Buccinator
**2** Corrugator supercilii
**3** Depressor anguli oris
**4** Depressor labii inferioris
**5** Levator anguli oris
**6** Levator labii superioris
**7** Levator labii superioris alaeque nasi
**8** Masseter
**9** Nasalis
**10** Occipital part of occipitofrontalis
**11** Orbicularis oculi
**12** Platysma
**13** Procerus
**14** Sternocleidomastoid
**15** Temporalis
**16** Temporomandibular joint
**17** Zygomaticus major
**18** Zygomaticus minor

The bony attachments of the buccinator muscle (1) are to the upper and lower jaws (maxilla and mandible) opposite the three molar teeth. (The teeth are identified on page 23, D.)

The upper attachment of temporalis (upper 15) occupies the temporal fossa (the narrow space above the zygomatic arch at the side of the skull). The lower attachment of temporalis (lower 15) extends from the lowest part of the mandibular notch of the mandible, over the coronoid process and down the front of the ramus almost as far as the last molar tooth.

Masseter (8) extends from the zygomatic arch to the lateral side of the ramus of the mandible.

*Temporomandibular joint (TMJ) reduction, see page 92.*
*Temporomandibular joint (TMJ) reduction, see page 92.*

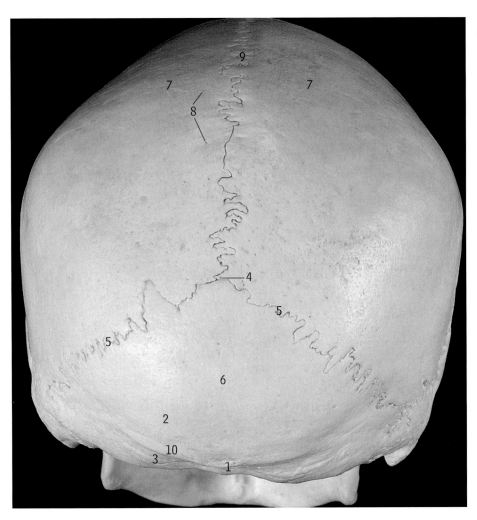

## A Skull *from behind*

1 External occipital protuberance (inion)
2 Highest nuchal line
3 Inferior nuchal line
4 Lambda
5 Lambdoid suture
6 Occipital bone
7 Parietal bone
8 Parietal foramina
9 Sagittal suture
10 Superior nuchal line

## B Skull *right infratemporal region, obliquely from below*

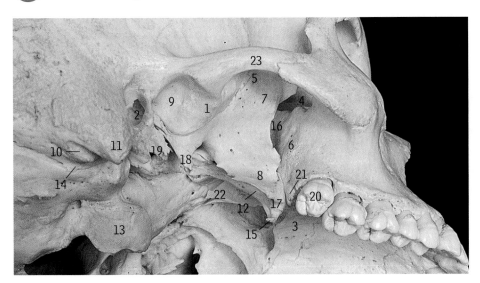

1 Articular tubercle
2 External acoustic meatus
3 Horizontal plate of palatine bone
4 Inferior orbital fissure
5 Infratemporal crest
6 Infratemporal (posterior) surface of maxilla
7 Infratemporal surface of greater wing of
  sphenoid bone
8 Lateral pterygoid plate
9 Mandibular fossa
10 Mastoid notch
11 Mastoid process
12 Medial pterygoid plate
13 Occipital condyle
14 Occipital groove
15 Pterygoid hamulus
16 Pterygomaxillary fissure and
  pterygopalatine fossa
17 Pyramidal process of palatine bone
18 Spine of sphenoid bone
19 Styloid process and sheath
20 Third molar tooth
21 Tuberosity of maxilla
22 Vomer
23 Zygomatic arch

## Ⓐ **Skull** *from above*

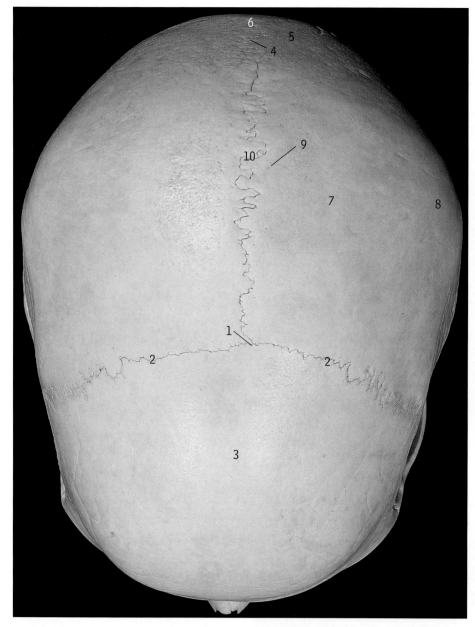

## Ⓑ **Skull** *internal surface of the cranial vault, central part*

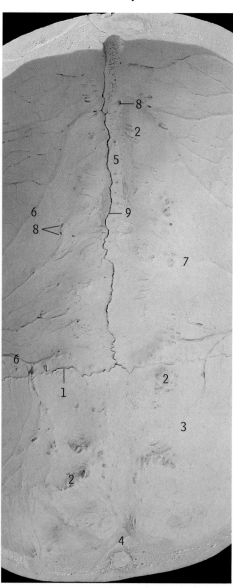

| | |
|---|---|
| **1** | Bregma |
| **2** | Coronal suture |
| **3** | Frontal bone |
| **4** | Lambda |
| **5** | Lambdoid suture |
| **6** | Occipital bone |
| **7** | Parietal bone |
| **8** | Parietal eminence |
| **9** | Parietal foramen |
| **10** | Sagittal suture |

In this skull, the parietal eminences are prominent (A8).

The point where the sagittal suture (A10) meets the coronal suture (A2) is the bregma (A1). At birth, the unossified parts of the frontal and parietal bones in this region form the membranous anterior fontanelle (page 24, D1).

The point where the sagittal suture (A10) meets the lambdoid suture (A5) is the lambda (A4). At birth, the unossified parts of the parietal and occipital bones in this region form the membranous posterior fontanelle (page 24, C13).

The label 3 in the centre of the frontal bone indicates the line of the frontal suture in the fetal skull (page 24, A5). The suture may persist in the adult skull and is sometimes known as the metopic suture.

The arachnoid granulations (page 72, B1), through which cerebrospinal fluid drains into the superior sagittal sinus, cause the irregular depressions (B2) on the parts of the frontal and parietal bones (B3 and 7) that overlie the sinus.

| | |
|---|---|
| **1** | Coronal suture |
| **2** | Depressions for arachnoid granulations |
| **3** | Frontal bone |
| **4** | Frontal crest |
| **5** | Groove for superior sagittal sinus |
| **6** | Grooves for middle meningeal vessels |
| **7** | Parietal bone |
| **8** | Parietal foramina |
| **9** | Sagittal suture |

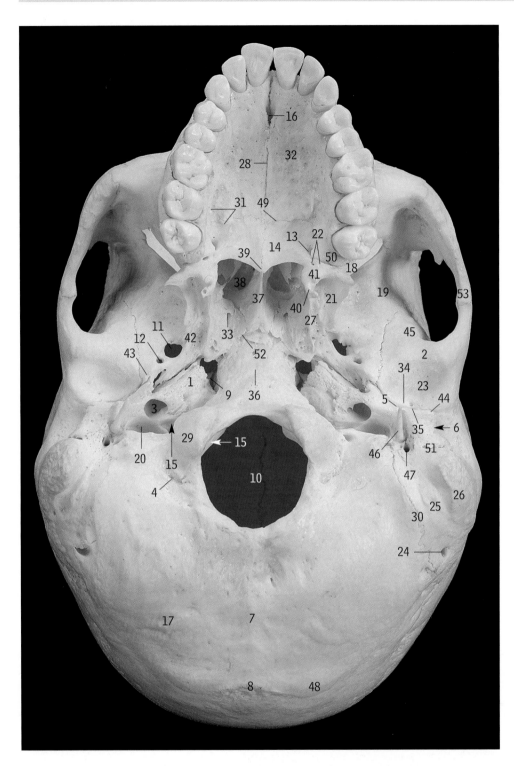

# Skull
## external surface of the base

1 Apex of petrous part of temporal bone
2 Articular tubercle
3 Carotid canal
4 Condylar canal (posterior)
5 Edge of tegmen tympani
6 External acoustic meatus
7 External occipital crest
8 External occipital protuberance
9 Foramen lacerum
10 Foramen magnum
11 Foramen ovale
12 Foramen spinosum
13 Greater palatine foramen
14 Horizontal plate of palatine bone
15 Hypoglossal canal
16 Incisive fossa
17 Inferior nuchal line
18 Inferior orbital fissure
19 Infratemporal crest of greater wing of sphenoid bone
20 Jugular foramen
21 Lateral pterygoid plate
22 Lesser palatine foramina
23 Mandibular fossa
24 Mastoid foramen
25 Mastoid notch
26 Mastoid process
27 Medial pterygoid plate
28 Median palatine (intermaxillary) suture
29 Occipital condyle
30 Occipital groove
31 Palatine grooves and spines
32 Palatine process of maxilla
33 Palatinovaginal canal
34 Petrosquamous fissure
35 Petrotympanic fissure
36 Pharyngeal tubercle
37 Posterior border of vomer
38 Posterior nasal aperture (choana)
39 Posterior nasal spine
40 Pterygoid hamulus
41 Pyramidal process of palatine bone
42 Scaphoid fossa
43 Spine of sphenoid bone
44 Squamotympanic fissure
45 Squamous part of temporal bone
46 Styloid process
47 Stylomastoid foramen
48 Superior nuchal line
49 Transverse palatine (palatomaxillary) suture
50 Tuberosity of maxilla
51 Tympanic part of temporal bone
52 Vomerovaginal canal
53 Zygomatic arch

The palatine process of the maxilla (32) and the horizontal plate of the palatine bone (14) form the hard palate (roof of the mouth and floor of the nose).

The carotid canal (3), recognized by its round shape on the inferior surface of the petrous part of the temporal bone, does not pass straight upwards to open into the inside of the skull but takes a right-angled turn forwards and medially within the petrous temporal to open into the back of the foramen lacerum (9).

*Intracranial spread of infection, see page 91.*

# Skull *muscle attachments, external surface of the base*

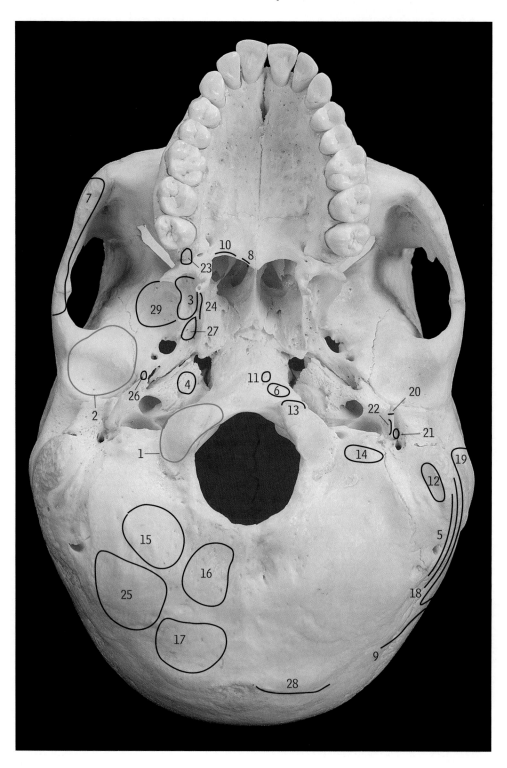

**Green line = capsule attachments of atlanto-occipital and temporomandibular joints**

 1  Capsule attachment of atlanto-occipital joint
 2  Capsule attachment of temporomandibular joint
 3  Deep head of medial pterygoid
 4  Levator veli palatini
 5  Longissimus capitis
 6  Longus capitis
 7  Masseter
 8  Musculus uvulae
 9  Occipital part of occipitofrontalis
10  Palatopharyngeus
11  Pharyngeal raphe
12  Posterior belly of digastric
13  Rectus capitis anterior
14  Rectus capitis lateralis
15  Rectus capitis posterior major
16  Rectus capitis posterior minor
17  Semispinalis capitis
18  Splenius capitis
19  Sternocleidomastoid
20  Styloglossus
21  Stylohyoid
22  Stylopharyngeus
23  Superficial head of medial pterygoid
24  Superior constrictor
25  Superior oblique
26  Tensor tympani
27  Tensor veli palatini
28  Trapezius
29  Upper head of lateral pterygoid

The medial pterygoid plate has no pterygoid muscles attached to it. It passes straight backwards, giving origin at its lower end to part of the superior constrictor of the pharynx (24).

The lateral pterygoid plate has both pterygoid muscles attached to it: medial and lateral muscles from the medial and lateral surfaces, respectively (3 and 29). The plate becomes twisted slightly laterally because of the constant pull of these muscles which pass backwards and laterally to their attachments to the mandible (page 29).

# **Skull** *internal surface of the base (cranial fossae)*

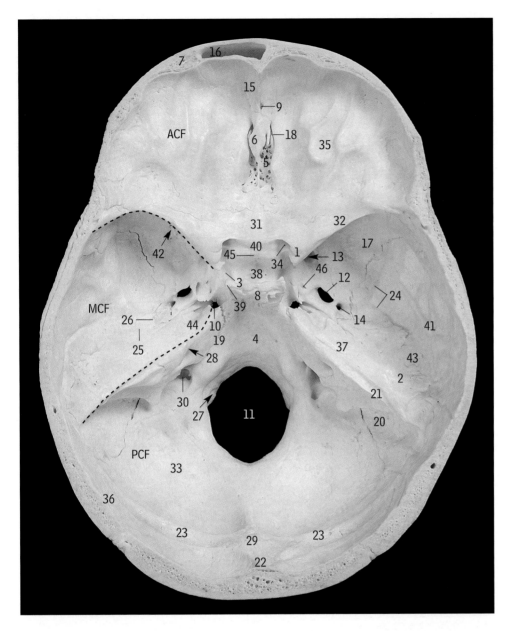

1 Anterior clinoid process
2 Arcuate eminence
3 Carotid groove
4 Clivus
5 Cribriform plate of ethmoid bone
6 Crista galli
7 Diploë
8 Dorsum sellae
9 Foramen caecum
10 Foramen lacerum
11 Foramen magnum
12 Foramen ovale
13 Foramen rotundum
14 Foramen spinosum
15 Frontal crest
16 Frontal sinus
17 Greater wing of sphenoid bone
18 Groove for anterior ethmoidal nerve and vessels
19 Groove for inferior petrosal sinus
20 Groove for sigmoid sinus
21 Groove for superior petrosal sinus
22 Groove for superior sagittal sinus
23 Groove for transverse sinus
24 Grooves for middle meningeal vessels
25 Hiatus and groove for greater petrosal nerve
26 Hiatus and groove for lesser petrosal nerve
27 Hypoglossal canal
28 Internal acoustic meatus
29 Internal occipital protuberance
30 Jugular foramen
31 Jugum of sphenoid bone
32 Lesser wing of sphenoid bone
33 Occipital bone (cerebellar fossa)
34 Optic canal
35 Orbital part of frontal bone
36 Parietal bone (postero-inferior angle only)
37 Petrous part of temporal bone
38 Pituitary fossa (sella turcica)
39 Posterior clinoid process
40 Prechiasmatic groove
41 Squamous part of temporal bone
42 Superior orbital fissure
43 Tegmen tympani
44 Trigeminal impression
45 Tuberculum sellae
46 Venous (emissary) foramen

The anterior cranial fossa (ACF) is limited posteriorly on each side by the free margin of the lesser wing of the sphenoid (32) with its anterior clinoid process (1), and centrally by the anterior margin of the prechiasmatic groove (40).

The middle cranial fossa (MCF) is butterfly-shaped and consists of a central or median part and right and left lateral parts. The central part includes the pituitary fossa (38) on the upper surface of the body of the sphenoid, with the prechiasmatic groove (40) in front and the dorsum sellae (8) with its posterior clinoid processes (39) behind. Each lateral part extends from the posterior border of the lesser wing of the sphenoid (32) to the groove for the superior petrosal sinus (21) on the upper edge of the petrous part of the temporal bone.

The posterior cranial fossa (PCF), whose most obvious feature is the foramen magnum (11), is behind the dorsum sellae (8) and the grooves for the superior petrosal sinuses (21).

For cranial dural attachments and reflections, see pages 61 and 63.

*Anosmia, see page 90.*

## A Skull *bones of the left orbit*

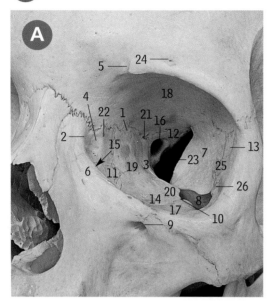

## C Nasal cavity *lateral wall*

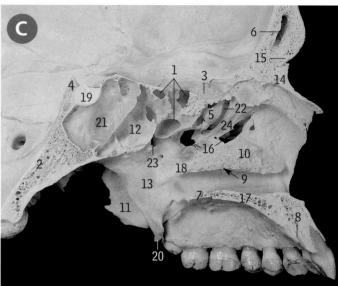

| | |
|---|---|
| **1** Anterior ethmoidal foramen | **14** Maxilla, forming floor |
| **2** Anterior lacrimal crest | **15** Nasolacrimal canal |
| **3** Body of sphenoid bone, forming medial wall | **16** Optic canal |
| **4** Fossa for lacrimal sac | **17** Orbital border of zygomatic bone, forming floor |
| **5** Frontal notch | **18** Orbital part of frontal bone, forming roof |
| **6** Frontal process of maxilla, forming medial wall | **19** Orbital plate of ethmoid bone, forming medial wall |
| **7** Greater wing of sphenoid bone, forming lateral wall | **20** Orbital process of palatine bone, forming floor |
| **8** Inferior orbital fissure | **21** Posterior ethmoidal foramen |
| **9** Infra-orbital foramen | **22** Posterior lacrimal crest |
| **10** Infra-orbital groove | **23** Superior orbital fissure |
| **11** Lacrimal bone, forming medial wall | **24** Supra-orbital foramen |
| **12** Lesser wing of sphenoid bone, forming roof | **25** Zygomatic bone forming lateral wall |
| **13** Marginal tubercle | **26** Zygomatico-orbital foramen |

**In this midline sagittal section of the skull, with the nasal septum removed, the superior and middle nasal conchae have been dissected away to reveal the air cells of the ethmoidal sinus, in particular the ethmoidal bulla (5).**

| | |
|---|---|
| **1** Air cells of ethmoidal sinus | **13** Medial pterygoid plate |
| **2** Clivus | **14** Nasal bone |
| **3** Cribriform plate of ethmoid bone | **15** Nasal spine of frontal bone |
| **4** Dorsum sellae | **16** Opening of maxillary sinus |
| **5** Ethmoidal bulla | **17** Palatine process of maxilla |
| **6** Frontal sinus | **18** Perpendicular plate of palatine bone |
| **7** Horizontal plate of palatine bone | **19** Pituitary fossa (sella turcica) |
| **8** Incisive canal | **20** Pterygoid hamulus |
| **9** Inferior meatus | **21** Right sphenoidal sinus |
| **10** Inferior nasal concha | **22** Semilunar hiatus |
| **11** Lateral pterygoid plate | **23** Sphenopalatine foramen |
| **12** Left sphenoidal sinus | **24** Uncinate process of ethmoid bone |

The roof of the nasal cavity consists mainly of the cribriform plate of the ethmoid bone (C3) with the body of the sphenoid containing the sphenoidal sinuses (C21 and 12) behind, and the nasal bone (C14) and the nasal spine of the frontal bone (C15) at the front.

The floor of the cavity consists of the palatine process of the maxilla (C17) and the horizontal plate of the palatine bone (C7).

The medial wall is the nasal septum which is formed mainly by two bones – the perpendicular plate of the ethmoid and the vomer – and the septal cartilage.

The lateral wall consists of the medial surface of the maxilla with its large opening (C16), overlapped from above by parts of the ethmoid (C1, 5 and 24) and lacrimal bones, from behind by the perpendicular plate of the palatine (C18), and below by the inferior concha (C10).

## B Skull *Left orbit, individual bones*

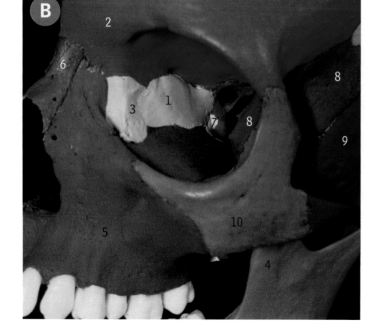

| | |
|---|---|
| **1** Ethmoid | **6** Nasal |
| **2** Frontal | **7** Palatine |
| **3** Lacrimal | **8** Sphenoid |
| **4** Mandible | **9** Temporal |
| **5** Maxilla | **10** Zygomatic |

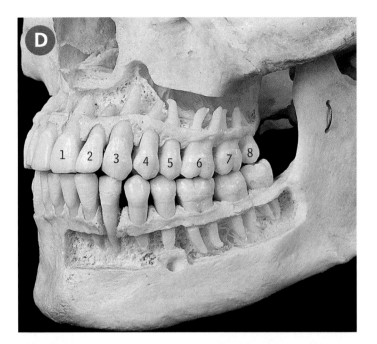

**D** **Permanent teeth**
*from the left and in front*

| | |
|---|---|
| **1** First (central) incisor | **5** Second premolar |
| **2** Second (lateral) incisor | **6** First molar |
| **3** Canine | **7** Second molar |
| **4** First premolar | **8** Third molar |

The corresponding teeth of the upper and lower jaws have similar names. In clinical dentistry, the teeth are usually identified by the numbers 1–8 (as listed here) rather than by name.

The third molar is sometimes called the wisdom tooth.

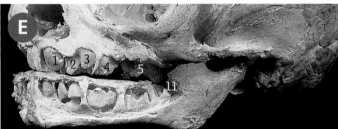

**Upper and lower jaws**
*from the left and in front*

**E** in the newborn with
unerupted deciduous teeth

**F** in a 4-year-old child with erupted deciduous
teeth and unerupted permanent teeth

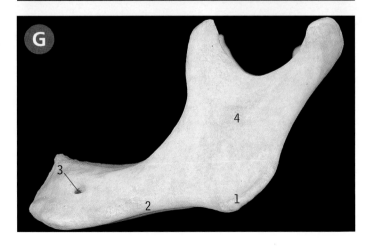

| | |
|---|---|
| **1** First (central) incisor of deciduous dentition | **7** Second (lateral) incisor of permanent dentition |
| **2** Second (lateral) incisor of deciduous dentition | **8** Canine of permanent dentition |
| **3** Canine of deciduous dentition | **9** First premolar of permanent dentition |
| **4** First molar of deciduous dentition | **10** Second premolar of permanent dentition |
| **5** Second molar of deciduous dentition | **11** First molar of permanent dentition |
| **6** First (central) incisor of permanent dentition | **12** Second molar of permanent dentition |

The deciduous molars occupy the positions of the premolars of the permanent dentition.

**G** **Edentulous mandible**
*in old age, from the left*

| | |
|---|---|
| **1** Angle | **3** Mental foramen |
| **2** Body | **4** Ramus |

With the loss of teeth, the alveolar bone becomes resorbed, so that the mental foramen (3) and mandibular canal lie near the upper margin of the bone.

The angle (1) between the ramus (4) and body (2) becomes more obtuse, resembling the infantile angle (as in E and F, above).

# Skull of a full-term fetus

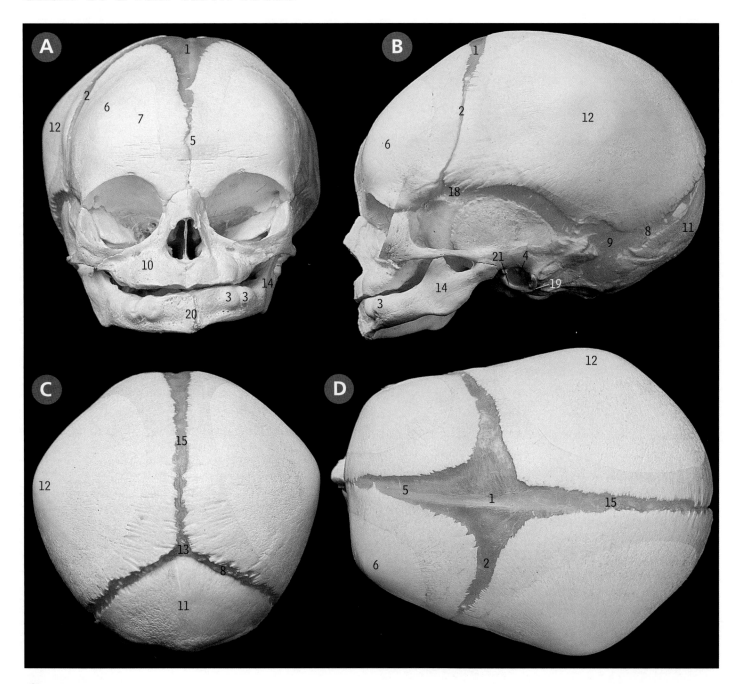

**A**  from the front

**B**  from the left and slightly below

**C**  from behind

**D**  from above

| | | | |
|---|---|---|---|
| **1** | Anterior fontanelle | **11** | Occipital bone |
| **2** | Coronal suture | **12** | Parietal tuberosity |
| **3** | Elevations over deciduous teeth in body of mandible | **13** | Posterior fontanelle |
| **4** | External acoustic meatus | **14** | Ramus of mandible |
| **5** | Frontal suture | **15** | Sagittal suture |
| **6** | Frontal tuberosity | **16** | Sella turcica |
| **7** | Half of frontal bone | **17** | Semicircular canals, superior |
| **8** | Lambdoid suture | **18** | Sphenoidal fontanelle |
| **9** | Mastoid fontanelle | **19** | Stylomastoid foramen |
| **10** | Maxilla | **20** | Symphysis menti |
| | | **21** | Tympanic ring |

# Fetal skull radiographs  **E** *frontal projection*  **F** *lateral projection*

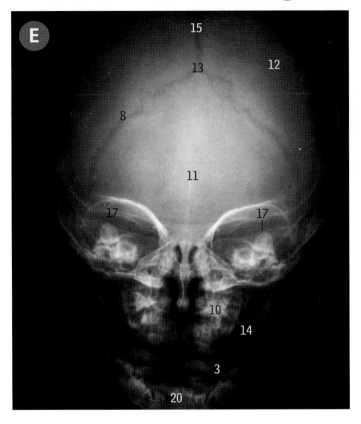

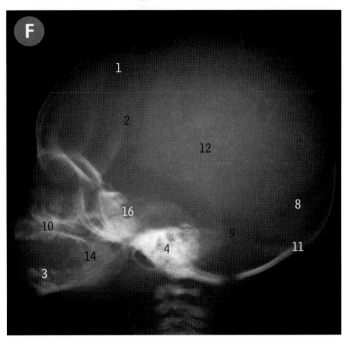

The face at birth forms a relatively smaller proportion of the cranium than in the adult (about one-eighth compared with one-half) because of the small size of the nasal cavity and maxillary sinuses and the lack of erupted teeth.

The posterior fontanelle (C13, E13) closes about 2 months after birth, the anterior fontanelle (A1, D1, F1) in the second year.

Owing to the lack of the mastoid process (which does not develop until the second year), the stylomastoid foramen (B19) and the emerging facial nerve are relatively near the surface and unprotected.

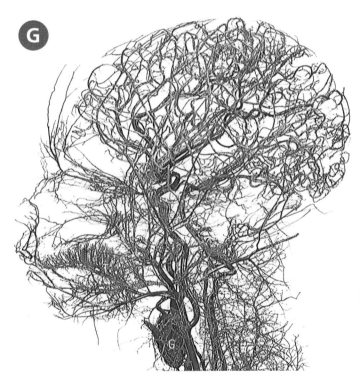

## **G** Resin cast of head and neck arteries *full-term fetus, from the left*

In this cast of fetal arteries, note in the front of the neck the dense arterial pattern indicating the thyroid gland (G), and above and in front of it the fine vessels outlining the tongue (T).

*Hydrocephalus, scalp wounds, see pages 91–92.*

# Skull Ⓐ *coloured left half of the skull in sagittal section*

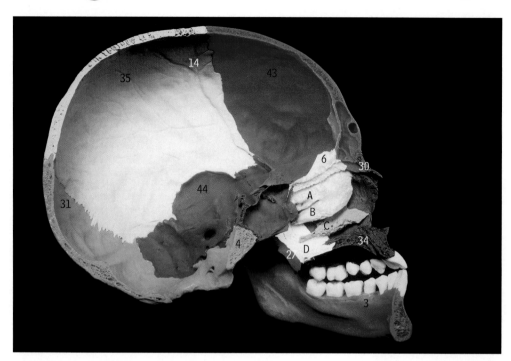

**A**   Superior nasal concha
**B**   Middle nasal concha
**C**   Inferior nasal concha
**D**   Palatine bone
     See page 27 for additional label numbers.

NB: The perpendicular plate of the ethmoid has been removed to expose the conchae.

## Ⓑ *cleared specimen from the front, illuminated from behind*

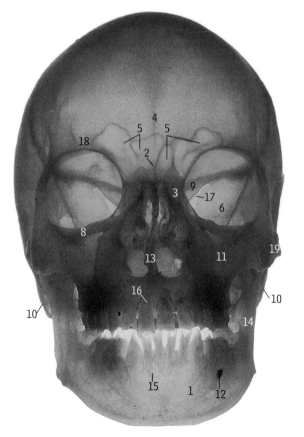

## Ⓒ *radiograph of facial bones, occipitofrontal view*

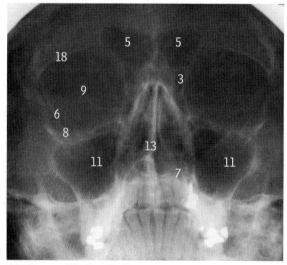

**Compare with the skull on page 11.**

| | |
|---|---|
| **1** Body of mandible | **10** Mastoid process |
| **2** Crista galli | **11** Maxillary sinus |
| **3** Ethmoidal air cells | **12** Mental foramen |
| **4** Frontal crest | **13** Nasal septum |
| **5** Frontal sinus | **14** Ramus of mandible |
| **6** Greater wing of sphenoid bone | **15** Root of lower lateral incisor |
| **7** Inferior nasal concha | **16** Root of upper central incisor |
| **8** Infra-orbital margin | **17** Superior orbital fissure |
| **9** Lesser wing of sphenoid bone | **18** Supra-orbital margin |
| | **19** Zygomatic arch |

*Blow-out fractures, mastoiditis, see pages 90, 91.*

# Skull *left half of the skull in sagittal section*

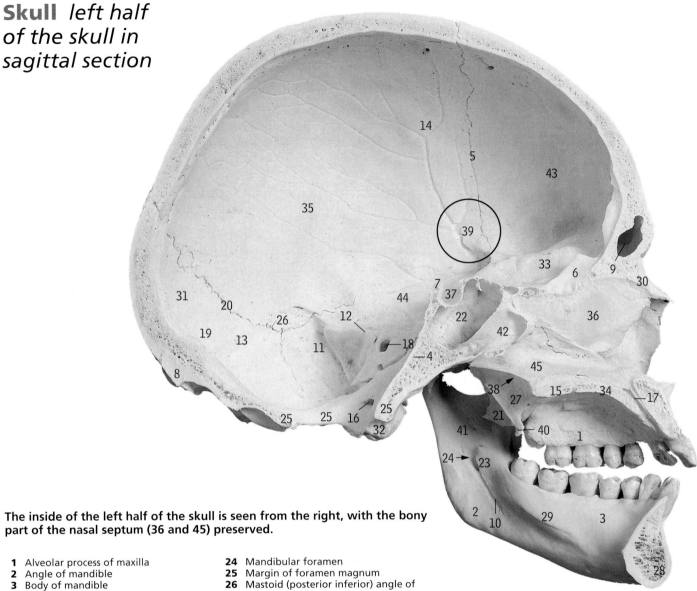

The inside of the left half of the skull is seen from the right, with the bony part of the nasal septum (36 and 45) preserved.

| | |
|---|---|
| **1** Alveolar process of maxilla | **24** Mandibular foramen |
| **2** Angle of mandible | **25** Margin of foramen magnum |
| **3** Body of mandible | **26** Mastoid (posterior inferior) angle of parietal bone |
| **4** Clivus | **27** Medial pterygoid plate |
| **5** Coronal suture | **28** Mental protuberance |
| **6** Crista galli of ethmoid bone | **29** Mylohyoid line |
| **7** Dorsum sellae | **30** Nasal bone |
| **8** External occipital protuberance | **31** Occipital bone |
| **9** Frontal sinus | **32** Occipital condyle |
| **10** Groove for mylohyoid nerve | **33** Orbital part of frontal bone |
| **11** Groove for sigmoid sinus | **34** Palatine process of maxilla |
| **12** Groove for superior petrosal sinus | **35** Parietal bone |
| **13** Groove for transverse sinus | **36** Perpendicular plate of ethmoid bone |
| **14** Grooves for middle meningeal vessels (anterior division) | **37** Pituitary fossa (sella turcica) |
| **15** Horizontal plate of palatine bone | **38** Posterior nasal aperture (choana) |
| **16** Hypoglossal canal | **39** Pterion (encircled) |
| **17** Incisive canal | **40** Pterygoid hamulus of medial pterygoid plate |
| **18** Internal acoustic meatus in petrous part of temporal bone | **41** Ramus of mandible |
| **19** Internal occipital protuberance | **42** Right sphenoidal sinus |
| **20** Lambdoid suture | **43** Squamous part of frontal bone |
| **21** Lateral pterygoid plate | **44** Squamous part of temporal bone |
| **22** Left sphenoidal sinus | **45** Vomer |
| **23** Lingula | |

The bony part of the nasal septum consists of the vomer (45) and the perpendicular plate of the ethmoid bone (36). The anterior part of the septum consists of the septal cartilage (page 83a).

In this skull, the sphenoidal sinuses (42 and 22) are large, and the right one (42) has extended to the left of the midline. The pituitary fossa (37) projects down into the left sinus (22).

The grooves for the middle meningeal vessels (14) pass upwards and backwards. The circle (39) marks the region of the pterion, and corresponds to the position shown on the outside of the skull on page 14, 29.

 *Extradural haemorrhage, pituitary tumour, see pages 90, 92.*

# Mandible

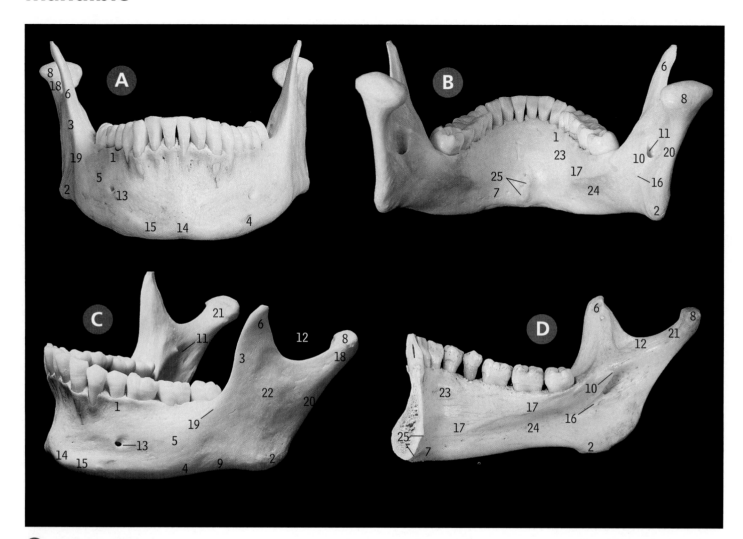

**A** from the front

**B** from behind

**C** from the left and front

**D** internal view from the left

| 1 | Alveolar part | 14 | Mental protuberance |
|---|---|---|---|
| 2 | Angle | 15 | Mental tubercle |
| 3 | Anterior border of ramus | 16 | Mylohyoid groove |
| 4 | Base | 17 | Mylohyoid line |
| 5 | Body | 18 | Neck |
| 6 | Coronoid process | 19 | Oblique line |
| 7 | Digastric fossa | 20 | Posterior border of ramus |
| 8 | Head | 21 | Pterygoid fovea |
| 9 | Inferior border of ramus | 22 | Ramus |
| 10 | Lingula | 23 | Sublingual fossa |
| 11 | Mandibular foramen | 24 | Submandibular fossa |
| 12 | Mandibular notch | 25 | Superior and inferior mental |
| 13 | Mental foramen | | spines (genial tubercles) |

The head (8) and the neck (18, including the pterygoid fovea, 21) constitute the condyle.

The alveolar part (1) contains the sockets for the roots of the teeth.

The base (4) is the inferior border of the body (5), and becomes continuous with the inferior border (9) of the ramus (22).

# Mandible *muscle attachments*

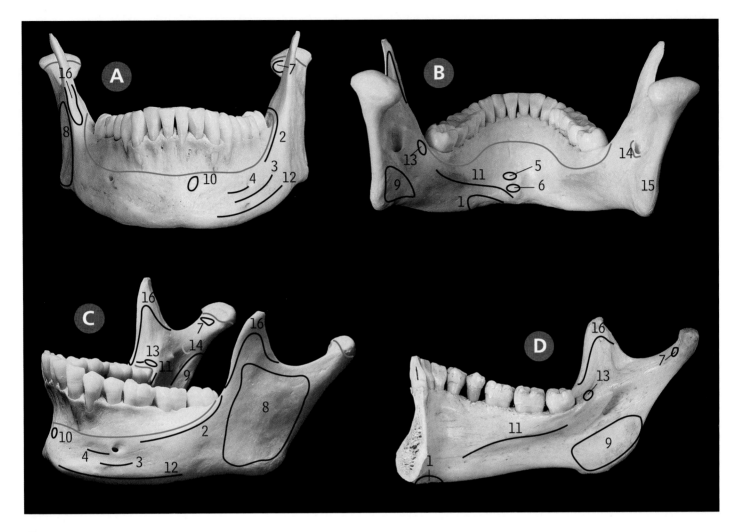

**A** from the front

**B** from behind

**C** from the left and front

**D** internal view from the left

**Green line = capsular attachment of temporomandibular joint; blue line = limit of attachment of the oral mucous membrane; pale green line = ligament attachment**

| | | | |
|---|---|---|---|
| **1** | Anterior belly of digastric | **10** | Mentalis |
| **2** | Buccinator | **11** | Mylohyoid |
| **3** | Depressor anguli oris | **12** | Platysma |
| **4** | Depressor labii inferioris | **13** | Pterygomandibular raphe |
| **5** | Genioglossus | | and superior constrictor |
| **6** | Geniohyoid | **14** | Sphenomandibular ligament |
| **7** | Lateral pterygoid | **15** | Stylomandibular ligament |
| **8** | Masseter | **16** | Temporalis |
| **9** | Medial pterygoid | | |

The lateral pterygoid (A7) is attached to the pterygoid fovea on the neck of the mandible (and also to the capsule of the temporomandibular joint and the articular disc – see page 52, A27, A28).

The medial pterygoid (B9, C9) is attached to the medial surface of the angle of the mandible, below the groove for the mylohyoid nerve.

Masseter (C8) is attached to the lateral surface of the ramus.

Temporalis (C16) is attached over the coronoid process, extending back as far as the deepest part of the mandibular notch and downwards over the front of the ramus almost as far as the last molar tooth.

Buccinator (C2) is attached opposite the three molar teeth, at the back reaching the pterygomandibular raphe (C13).

Genioglossus (B5) is attached to the upper mental spine and geniohyoid (B6) to the lower.

Mylohyoid (11) is attached to the mylohyoid line.

The attachment of the lateral temporomandibular ligament to the lateral aspect of the neck of the condyle is not shown.

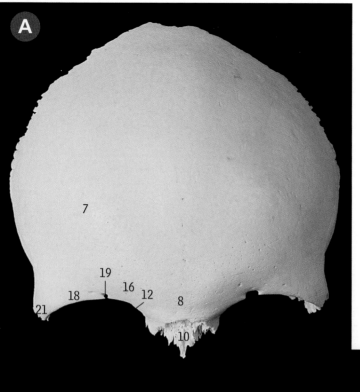

# Frontal bone

**A** external surface from the front

**B** external surface from the left

**C** from below

**D** internal surface from above and behind (right half removed; ethmoidal notch is inferior)

1 Anterior ethmoidal canal (position of groove)
2 Ethmoidal notch
3 Foramen caecum
4 Fossa for lacrimal gland
5 Frontal crest
6 Frontal sinus
7 Frontal tuberosity
8 Glabella
9 Inferior temporal line
10 Nasal spine
11 Orbital part
12 Position of frontal notch or foramen
13 Posterior ethmoidal canal (position of groove)
14 Roof of ethmoidal air cells
15 Sagittal crest
16 Superciliary arch
17 Superior temporal line
18 Supra-orbital margin
19 Supra-orbital notch or foramen
20 Trochlear fovea (or tubercle)
21 Zygomatic process

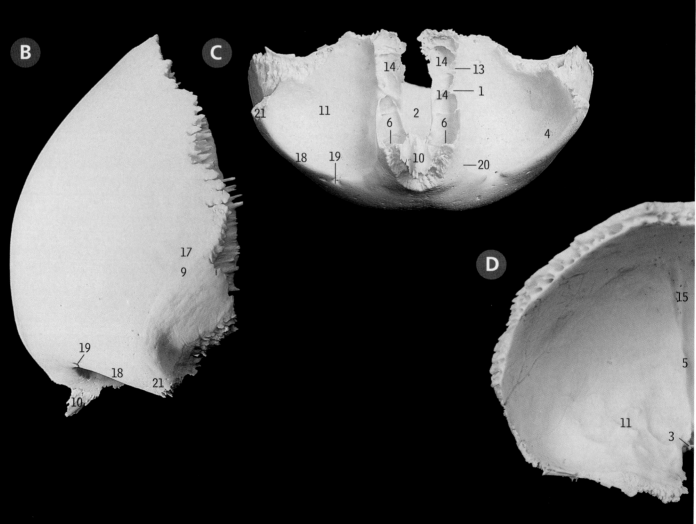

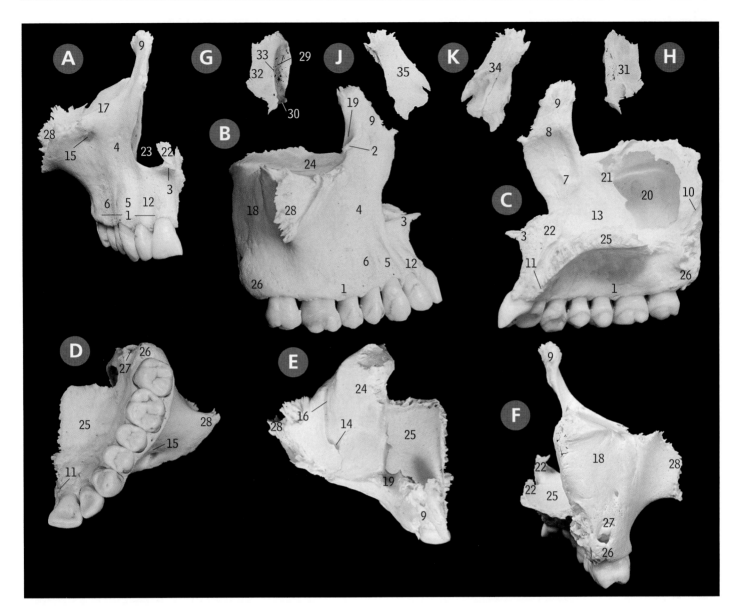

# Right maxilla

**A** from the front

**B** from the lateral side

**C** from the medial side

**D** from below

**E** from above

**F** from behind

| | |
|---|---|
| 1 Alveolar process | 15 Infra-orbital foramen |
| 2 Anterior lacrimal crest | 16 Infra-orbital groove |
| 3 Anterior nasal spine | 17 Infra-orbital margin |
| 4 Anterior surface | 18 Infratemporal surface |
| 5 Canine eminence | 19 Lacrimal groove |
| 6 Canine fossa | 20 Maxillary hiatus and sinus |
| 7 Conchal crest | 21 Middle meatus |
| 8 Ethmoidal crest | 22 Nasal crest |
| 9 Frontal process | 23 Nasal notch |
| 10 Greater palatine canal | 24 Orbital surface |
|     (position of groove) | 25 Palatine process |
| 11 Incisive canal | 26 Tuberosity |
| 12 Incisive fossa | 27 Unerupted third molar |
| 13 Inferior meatus |     tooth |
| 14 Infra-orbital canal | 28 Zygomatic process |

# Right lacrimal bone

**G** from the lateral (orbital) side

**H** from the medial (nasal) side

29 Lacrimal groove
30 Lacrimal hamulus
31 Nasal surface
32 Orbital surface
33 Posterior lacrimal crest

# Right nasal bone

**J** from the lateral side

**K** from the medial side

34 Internal surface and groove for anterior
    ethmoidal nerve
35 Lateral surface

# Right palatine bone

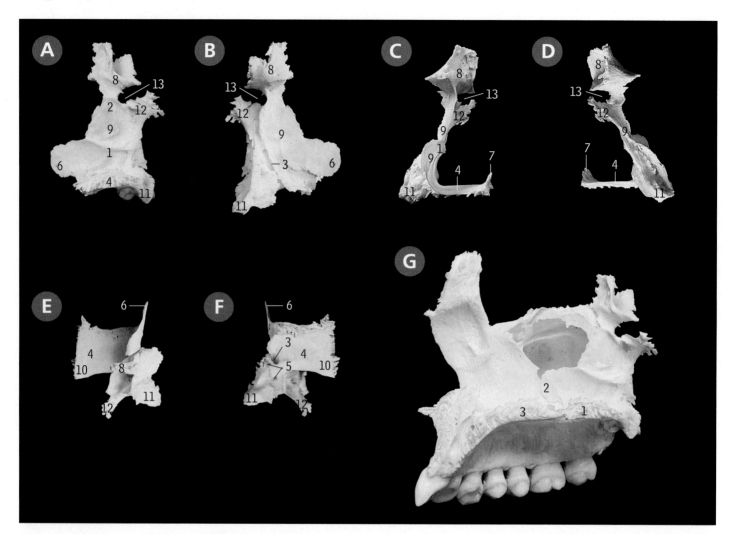

<table>
<tr><td>**A**</td><td>**from the medial side**</td><td>**D**</td><td>**from behind**</td></tr>
<tr><td>**B**</td><td>**from the lateral side**</td><td>**E**</td><td>**from above**</td></tr>
<tr><td>**C**</td><td>**from the front**</td><td>**F**</td><td>**from below**</td></tr>
</table>

**G** **Articulation of the right maxilla and the palatine bone, from the medial side**

1 Conchal crest
2 Ethmoidal crest
3 Greater palatine groove
4 Horizontal plate
5 Lesser palatine canals
6 Maxillary process
7 Nasal crest
8 Orbital process
9 Perpendicular plate
10 Posterior nasal spine
11 Pyramidal process
12 Sphenoidal process
13 Sphenopalatine notch

1 Horizontal plate of palatine
2 Maxillary process of palatine
3 Palatine process of maxilla

# Right temporal bone

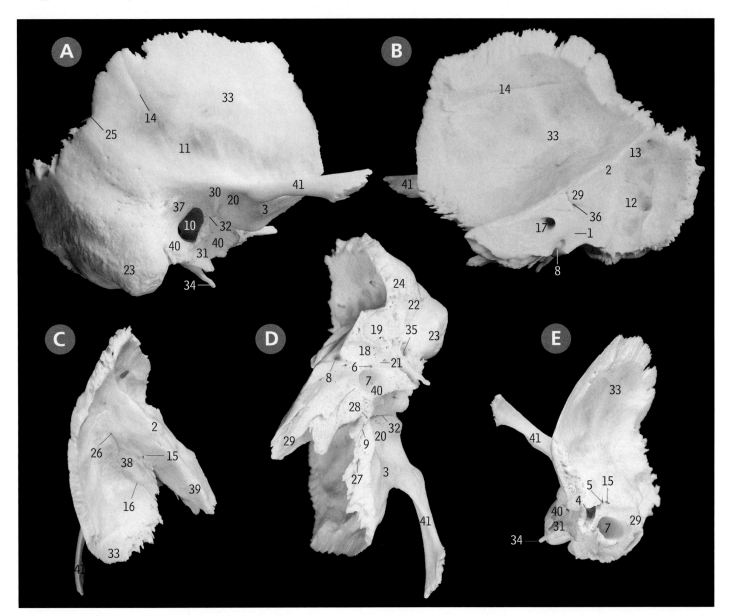

| | |
|---|---|
| **A** | **external aspect** |
| **B** | **internal aspect** |
| **C** | **from above** |
| **D** | **from below** |
| **E** | **from the front** |

**1** Aqueduct of vestibule
**2** Arcuate eminence
**3** Articular tubercle
**4** Auditory (eustachian) tube
**5** Canal for tensor tympani
**6** Canaliculus for tympanic branch of glossopharyngeal nerve
**7** Carotid canal
**8** Cochlear canaliculus
**9** Edge of tegmen tympani
**10** External acoustic meatus
**11** Groove for middle temporal artery
**12** Groove for sigmoid sinus
**13** Groove for superior petrosal sinus
**14** Grooves for branches of middle meningeal vessels

**15** Hiatus and groove for greater petrosal nerve
**16** Hiatus and groove for lesser petrosal nerve
**17** Internal acoustic meatus
**18** Jugular fossa
**19** Jugular surface
**20** Mandibular fossa
**21** Mastoid canaliculus for auricular branch of vagus nerve
**22** Mastoid notch
**23** Mastoid process
**24** Occipital groove
**25** Parietal notch
**26** Petrosquamous fissure (from above)
**27** Petrosquamous fissure (from below)

**28** Petrotympanic fissure
**29** Petrous part
**30** Postglenoid tubercle
**31** Sheath of styloid process
**32** Squamotympanic fissure
**33** Squamous part
**34** Styloid process
**35** Stylomastoid foramen
**36** Subarcuate fossa
**37** Suprameatal triangle
**38** Tegmen tympani
**39** Trigeminal impression on apex of petrous part
**40** Tympanic part
**41** Zygomatic process

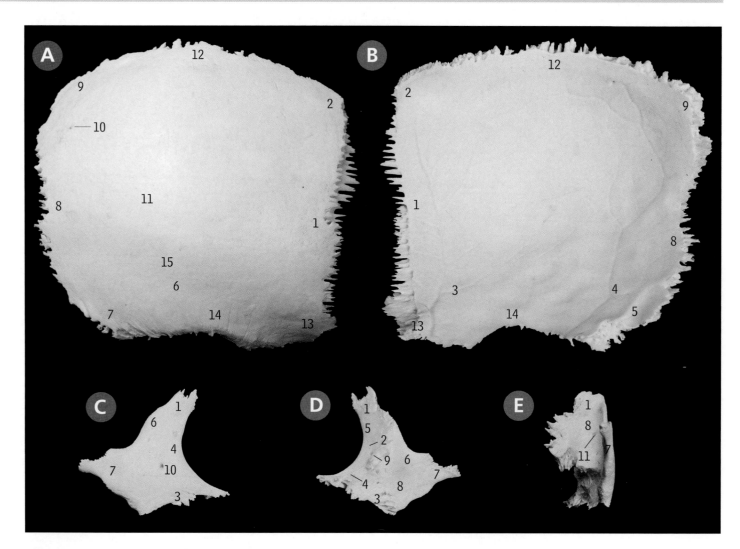

# Right parietal bone

**A** external surface

**B** internal surface

1 Frontal (anterior) border
2 Frontal (antero-superior) angle
3 Furrows for frontal branch of middle meningeal vessels (anterior division)
4 Furrows for parietal branch of middle meningeal vessels (posterior division)
5 Groove for sigmoid sinus at mastoid angle
6 Inferior temporal line
7 Mastoid (postero-inferior) angle
8 Occipital (posterior) border
9 Occipital (postero-superior) angle
10 Parietal foramen
11 Parietal tuberosity
12 Sagittal (superior) border
13 Sphenoidal (antero-inferior) angle
14 Squamosal (inferior) border
15 Superior temporal line

# Right zygomatic bone

**C** lateral surface

**D** from the medial side

**E** from behind

1 Frontal process
2 Marginal tubercle
3 Maxillary border
4 Orbital border
5 Orbital surface
6 Temporal border
7 Temporal process
8 Temporal surface
9 Zygomatico-orbital foramen
10 Zygomaticofacial foramen
11 Zygomaticotemporal foramen

The zygomatic process of the temporal bone (page 33, 41) and the temporal process of the zygomatic bone (C7, D7) form the zygomatic arch (page 14, 35).

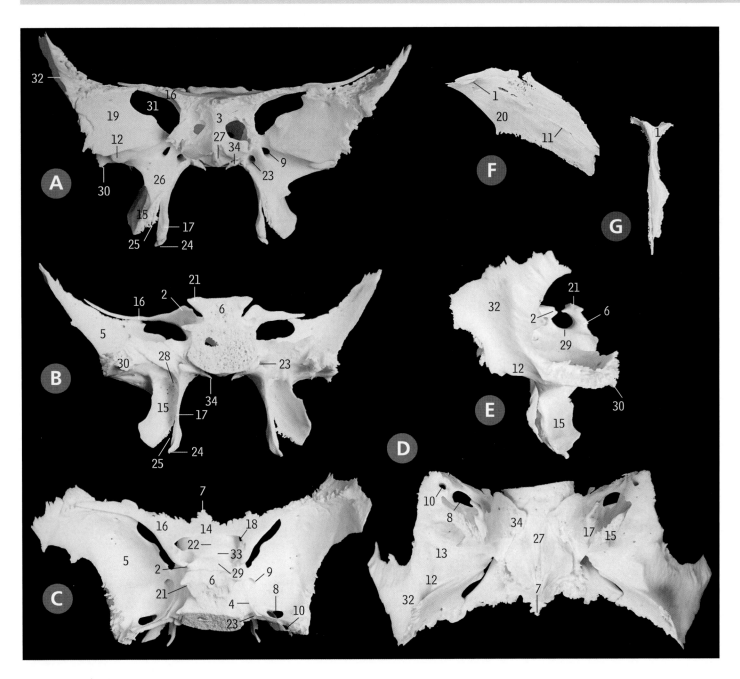

# Sphenoid bone

**A** from the front
**D** from below
**B** from behind
**E** from the left
**C** from above and behind

# Vomer

**F** from the right
**G** from behind

| | | | |
|---|---|---|---|
| **1** Ala | **9** Foramen rotundum | **16** Lesser wing | **26** Pterygoid process |
| **2** Anterior clinoid process | **10** Foramen spinosum | **17** Medial pterygoid plate | **27** Rostrum |
| **3** Body with openings of | **11** Groove for nasopalatine | **18** Optic canal | **28** Scaphoid fossa |
| sphenoidal sinuses | nerve and vessels | **19** Orbital surface of greater wing | **29** Sella turcica (pituitary fossa) |
| **4** Carotid groove | **12** Infratemporal crest of greater | **20** Posterior border | **30** Spine |
| **5** Cerebral surface of greater | wing | **21** Posterior clinoid process | **31** Superior orbital fissure |
| wing | **13** Infratemporal surface of | **22** Prechiasmatic groove | **32** Temporal surface of greater |
| **6** Dorsum sellae | greater wing | **23** Pterygoid canal | wing |
| **7** Ethmoidal spine | **14** Jugum | **24** Pterygoid hamulus | **33** Tuberculum sellae |
| **8** Foramen ovale | **15** Lateral pterygoid plate | **25** Pterygoid notch | **34** Vaginal process |

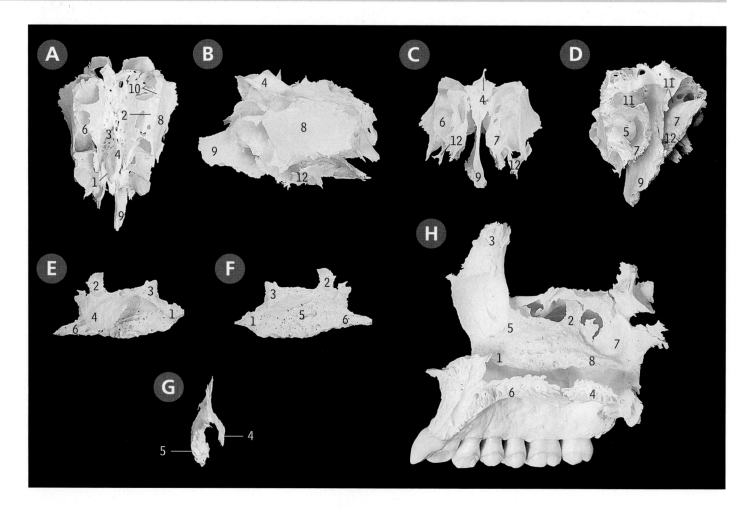

# Ethmoid bone

**A** from above

**B** from the left

**C** from the front

**D** from the left, below and behind

1 Ala of crista galli
2 Anterior ethmoidal groove
3 Cribriform plate
4 Crista galli
5 Ethmoidal bulla
6 Ethmoidal labyrinth (containing ethmoidal air cells)
7 Middle nasal concha
8 Orbital plate
9 Perpendicular plate
10 Posterior ethmoidal groove
11 Superior nasal concha (meatus)
12 Uncinate process

# Right inferior nasal concha

**E** from the lateral side

**F** from the medial side

**G** from behind

1 Anterior end
2 Ethmoidal process
3 Lacrimal process
4 Maxillary process
5 Medial surface
6 Posterior end

# Maxilla

**H** Articulation of right maxilla, palatine bone and inferior nasal concha, from the medial side

1 Anterior end of inferior nasal concha
2 Ethmoidal process of inferior nasal concha
3 Frontal process of maxilla
4 Horizontal plate of palatine
5 Lacrimal process of inferior nasal concha
6 Palatine process of maxilla
7 Perpendicular plate of palatine
8 Posterior end of inferior nasal concha

# Occipital bone

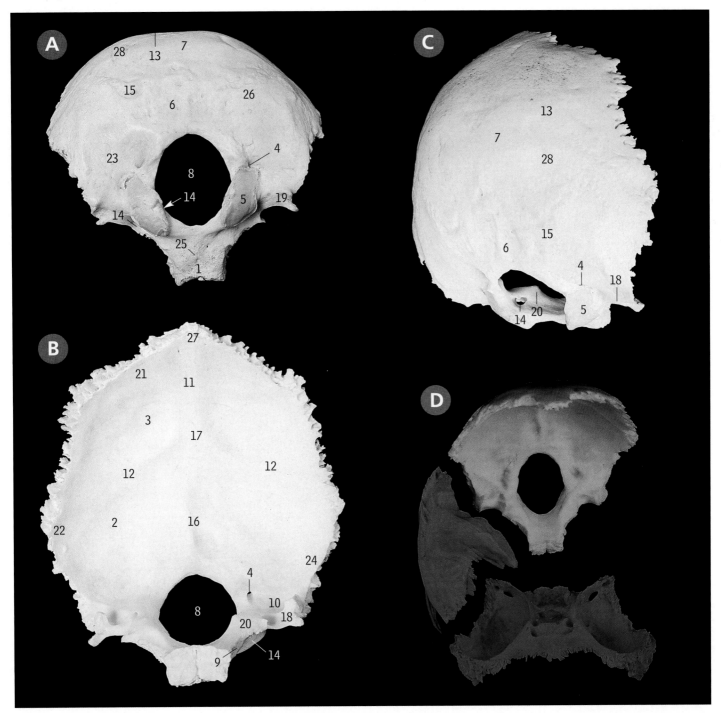

**A**  external surface from below

**B**  internal surface

**C**  external surface from the right and below

**D**  bones of the base of the skull

orange, occipital; red, temporal; blue, sphenoid

1  Basilar part
2  Cerebellar fossa
3  Cerebral fossa
4  Condylar fossa (and condylar canal in B and C)
5  Condyle
6  External occipital crest
7  External occipital protuberance
8  Foramen magnum
9  Groove for inferior petrosal sinus

10  Groove for sigmoid sinus
11  Groove for superior sagittal sinus
12  Groove for transverse sinus
13  Highest nuchal line
14  Hypoglossal canal
15  Inferior nuchal line
16  Internal occipital crest
17  Internal occipital protuberance
18  Jugular notch

19  Jugular process
20  Jugular tubercle
21  Lambdoid margin
22  Lateral angle
23  Lateral part
24  Mastoid margin
25  Pharyngeal tubercle
26  Squamous part
27  Superior angle
28  Superior nuchal line

# Neck *surface markings of the front and right side*

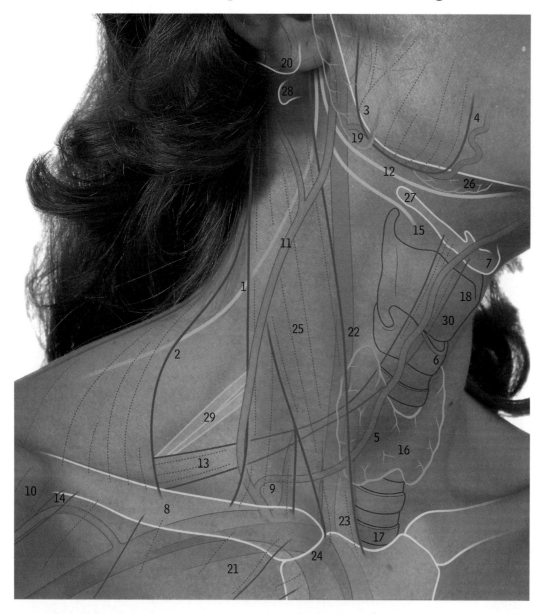

The pulsation of the common carotid artery (22, opposite page, 8) can be felt by backward pressure in the angle between the lower anterior border of sternocleidomastoid and the side of the larynx and trachea.

The cricoid cartilage (6) is about 5 cm (2 in) above the jugular notch of the manubrium of the sternum (17).

The lower end of the internal jugular vein lies behind the interval between the sternal (23) and clavicular (9) heads of sternocleidomastoid (when viewed from the front), just above the point where it joins the subclavian vein to form the brachiocephalic vein (24).

The trunks of the brachial plexus (29) can be felt as a cord-like structure in the lower part of the posterior triangle.

| | | |
|---|---|---|
| **1** Accessory nerve emerging from sternocleidomastoid | **10** Deltoid | **22** Site for palpation of common carotid artery |
| **2** Accessory nerve passing under anterior border of trapezius | **11** External jugular vein | **23** Sternal head of sternocleidomastoid |
| **3** Angle of mandible | **12** Hypoglossal nerve | **24** Sternoclavicular joint and union of internal jugular and subclavian veins to form brachiocephalic vein |
| **4** Anterior border of masseter and facial artery | **13** Inferior belly of omohyoid | |
| **5** Anterior jugular vein | **14** Infraclavicular fossa and cephalic vein | **25** Sternocleidomastoid |
| **6** Arch of cricoid cartilage | **15** Internal laryngeal nerve | **26** Submandibular gland |
| **7** Body of hyoid bone | **16** Isthmus of thyroid gland | **27** Tip of greater horn of hyoid bone |
| **8** Clavicle | **17** Jugular notch and trachea | **28** Tip of transverse process of atlas |
| **9** Clavicular head of sternocleidomastoid | **18** Laryngeal prominence (Adam's apple) | **29** Upper trunk of brachial plexus |
| | **19** Lowest part of parotid gland | **30** Vocal cord position |
| | **20** Mastoid process | |
| | **21** Pectoralis major | |

*Torticollis, see page 92.*

# Side of the neck *right side, deep dissection*

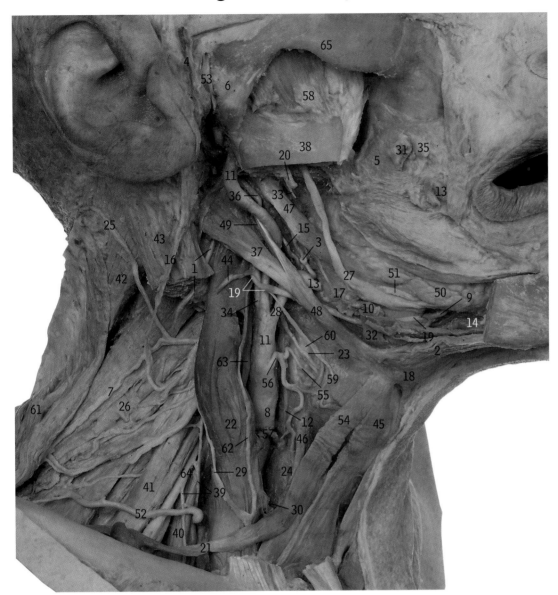

The lingual nerve (27) lies superficial to hyoglossus (17) and at this level is a flattened band rather than a typical round nerve, with the deep part of the submandibular gland (10) below it. The nerve crosses underneath the submandibular duct (51), lying first lateral to the duct and then medial to it.

The thyrohyoid membrane (60) is pierced by the internal laryngeal nerve (23) and the superior laryngeal artery (55).

Apart from supplying muscles of the tongue, the hypoglossal nerve (19) gives branches to geniohyoid (14) and thyrohyoid (59) and forms the upper root of the ansa cervicalis (62). These three branches consist of the fibres from the first cervical nerve that have joined the hypoglossal nerve higher in the neck; they are not derived from the hypoglossal nucleus. The C1 fibres in the upper root of the ansa contribute to the supply of sternohyoid (45) and omohyoid (21, 54).

| | |
|---|---|
| **1** | Accessory nerve |
| **2** | Anterior belly of digastric and nerve |
| **3** | Ascending palatine artery |
| **4** | Auriculotemporal nerve |
| **5** | Buccinator |
| **6** | Capsule of temporomandibular joint |
| **7** | Cervical nerves to trapezius |
| **8** | Common carotid artery |
| **9** | Deep lingual artery |
| **10** | Deep part of submandibular gland |
| **11** | External carotid artery |
| **12** | External laryngeal nerve |
| **13** | Facial artery |
| **14** | Geniohyoid |
| **15** | Glossopharyngeal nerve |
| **16** | Great auricular nerve |
| **17** | Hyoglossus |
| **18** | Hyoid bone |
| **19** | Hypoglossal nerve |
| **20** | Inferior alveolar nerve |
| **21** | Inferior belly of omohyoid |
| **22** | Internal jugular vein |
| **23** | Internal laryngeal nerve |
| **24** | Lateral lobe of thyroid gland |
| **25** | Lesser occipital nerve |
| **26** | Levator scapulae |
| **27** | Lingual nerve |
| **28** | Linguofacial trunk |
| **29** | Lower root of ansa cervicalis |
| **30** | Middle thyroid vein |
| **31** | Molar salivary glands |
| **32** | Mylohyoid and nerve |
| **33** | Nerve to mylohyoid |
| **34** | Occipital artery |
| **35** | Parotid duct |
| **36** | Posterior auricular artery |
| **37** | Posterior belly of digastric |
| **38** | Ramus of mandible |
| **39** | Roots of phrenic nerve |
| **40** | Scalenus anterior |
| **41** | Scalenus medius |
| **42** | Splenius capitis |
| **43** | Sternocleidomastoid |
| **44** | Sternocleidomastoid branch of occipital artery |
| **45** | Sternohyoid |
| **46** | Sternothyroid |
| **47** | Styloglossus |
| **48** | Stylohyoid |
| **49** | Stylohyoid ligament |
| **50** | Sublingual gland |
| **51** | Submandibular duct |
| **52** | Superficial cervical artery |
| **53** | Superficial temporal artery |
| **54** | Superior belly of omohyoid |
| **55** | Superior laryngeal artery |
| **56** | Superior thyroid artery |
| **57** | Superior thyroid vein |
| **58** | Temporalis |
| **59** | Thyrohyoid and nerve |
| **60** | Thyrohyoid membrane |
| **61** | Trapezius |
| **62** | Upper root of ansa cervicalis |
| **63** | Vagus nerve |
| **64** | Ventral ramus of fifth cervical nerve |
| **65** | Zygomatic arch |

# Front of the neck *superficial dissection*

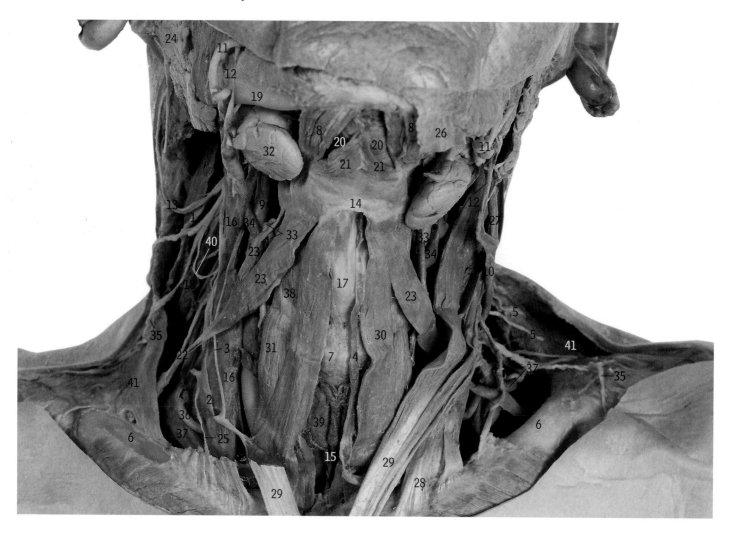

| | | | |
|---|---|---|---|
| **1** | Accessory nerve | **16** | Internal jugular vein |
| **2** | Ansa cervicalis, lower root | **17** | Laryngeal prominence |
| **3** | Ansa cervicalis, upper root | **18** | Levator scapulae |
| **4** | Anterior jugular vein | **19** | Mandible |
| **5** | Cervical nerves to trapezius | **20** | Mylohyoid |
| **6** | Clavicle | **21** | Mylohyoid, anomalous fibres |
| **7** | Cricoid cartilage | **22** | Omohyoid, intermediate |
| **8** | Digastric, anterior belly | | tendon |
| **9** | External carotid artery | **23** | Omohyoid, superior belly |
| **10** | External jugular vein | **24** | Parotid gland |
| **11** | Facial artery | **25** | Phrenic nerve |
| **12** | Facial vein | **26** | Platysma |
| **13** | Great auricular nerve | **27** | Retromandibular vein |
| **14** | Hyoid bone, body | **28** | Sternocleidomastoid, |
| **15** | Inferior thyroid vein | | clavicular head |

| | | | |
|---|---|---|---|
| **29** | Sternocleidomastoid, sternal head | **37** | Suprascapular vein |
| **30** | Sternohyoid | **38** | Thyrohyoid |
| **31** | Sternothyroid | **39** | Thyroid gland, isthmus |
| **32** | Submandibular gland | **40** | Transverse cervical nerve |
| **33** | Superior thyroid artery | **41** | Trapezius |
| **34** | Superior thyroid vein | | |
| **35** | Supraclavicular nerve | | |
| **36** | Suprascapular artery | | |

Midline landmarks in the neck include the body of the hyoid bone (14), the laryngeal prominence (Adam's apple, 17) and the arch of the cricoid cartilage (7).

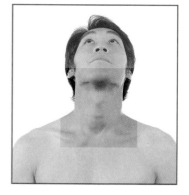

*Tracheostomy, see page 92.*

# Front of the neck *deeper dissection*

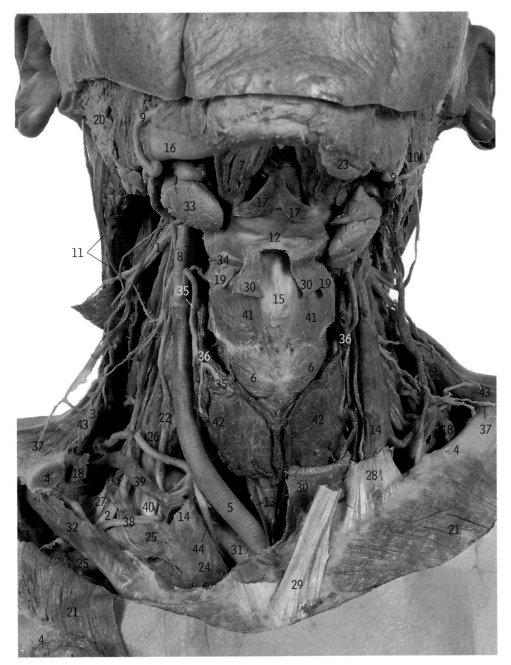

1. Accessory nerve
2. Brachial plexus (roots)
3. Cervical nerves to trapezius
4. Clavicle
5. Common carotid artery
6. Cricothyroid
7. Digastric, anterior belly
8. External carotid artery
9. Facial artery
10. Facial vein
11. Great auricular nerve
12. Hyoid bone, body
13. Inferior thyroid vein
14. Internal jugular vein
15. Laryngeal prominence
16. Mandible
17. Mylohyoid, anomalous fibres
18. Omohyoid, inferior belly
19. Omohyoid, superior belly
20. Parotid gland
21. Pectoralis major
22. Phrenic nerve
23. Platysma
24. Right brachiocephalic vein
25. Right subclavian vein
26. Scalenus anterior
27. Scalenus medius
28. Sternocleidomastoid, clavicular head
29. Sternocleidomastoid, sternal head
30. Sternohyoid
31. Subclavian artery
32. Subclavius
33. Submandibular gland
34. Superior laryngeal artery
35. Superior thyroid artery
36. Superior thyroid vein
37. Supraclavicular nerve
38. Suprascapular artery
39. Suprascapular vein
40. Tendon of scalenus anterior
41. Thyrohyoid
42. Thyroid gland, lateral lobe
43. Trapezius
44. Vagus nerve

On the right hand side, the clavicle (4) has been cut and retracted forwards to reveal the underlying subclavius (32).

*Accessory nerve paralysis, goitre, sialectasis, see pages 90–92.*

# Right side of the neck

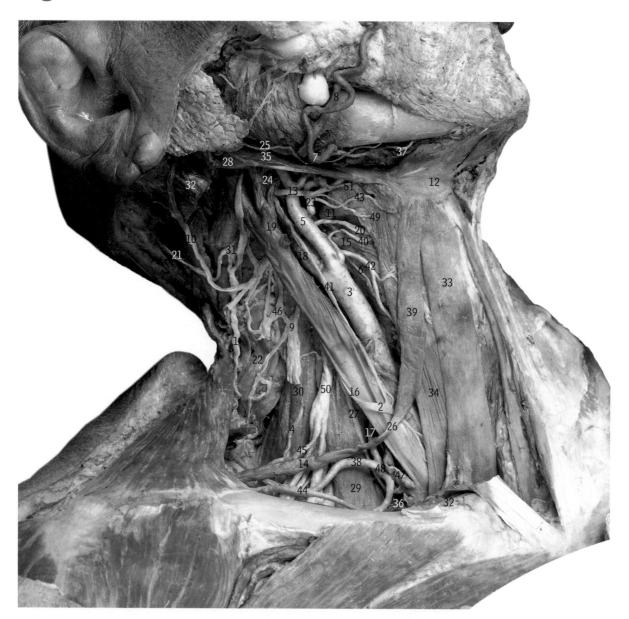

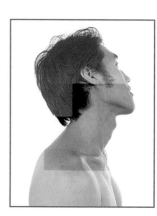

| | | |
|---|---|---|
| **1** Accessory nerve | **19** Internal jugular vein (double at upper end) | **35** Stylohyoid |
| **2** Ansa cervicalis | **20** Internal laryngeal nerve and thyrohyoid membrane | **36** Subclavian vein |
| **3** Common carotid artery | **21** Lesser occipital nerve | **37** Submental artery |
| **4** Dorsal scapular nerve | **22** Levator scapulae | **38** Transverse cervical artery (superficial) |
| **5** External carotid artery | **23** Lingual artery | **39** Superior belly of omohyoid |
| **6** External laryngeal nerve | **24** Lingual vein | **40** Superior laryngeal artery |
| **7** Facial artery | **25** Marginal mandibular branch of facial nerve | **41** Superior root of ansa cervicalis |
| **8** Facial vein | **26** Omohyoid tendon | **42** Superior thyroid artery |
| **9** Fourth cervical nerve ventral rami | **27** Phrenic nerve | **43** Suprahyoid artery on hyoglossus |
| **10** Great auricular nerve | **28** Posterior belly of digastric | **44** Suprascapular artery |
| **11** Greater horn of hyoid bone | **29** Scalenus anterior | **45** Suprascapular nerve |
| **12** Hyoid bone | **30** Scalenus medius | **46** Third cervical nerve ventral rami |
| **13** Hypoglossal nerve | **31** Second cervical nerve ventral rami | **47** The right lymphatic duct termination |
| **14** Inferior belly of omohyoid | **32** Sternocleidomastoid | **48** Thyrocervical trunk |
| **15** Inferior constrictor of pharynx | **33** Sternohyoid | **49** Thyrohyoid and nerve |
| **16** Inferior root of ansa cervicalis | **34** Sternothyroid | **50** Upper trunk of brachial plexus |
| **17** Inferior thyroid artery | | **51** Vena comitans of hypoglossal nerve |
| **18** Internal carotid artery | | |

# Left side of the neck *from the left and front*

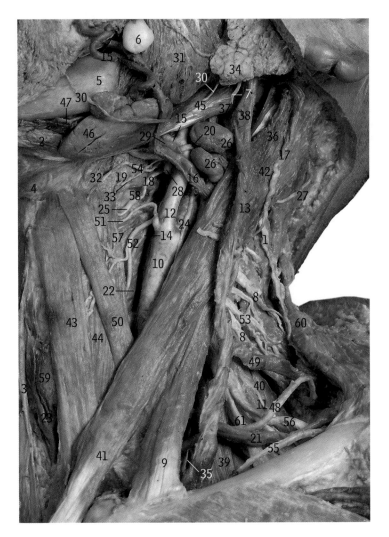

**Platysma and the deep cervical fascia have been removed.**

In 20% of faces, as in this specimen, the marginal mandibular branch of the facial nerve (30) arches downwards off the face for part of its course and overlies the submandibular gland (46).

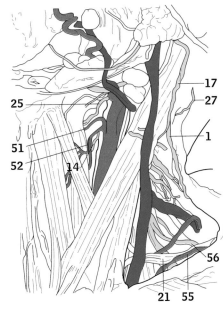

| | |
|---|---|
| **1** Accessory nerve | **20** Hypoglossal nerve |
| **2** Anterior belly of digastric | **21** Inferior belly of omohyoid |
| **3** Anterior jugular vein | **22** Inferior constrictor of |
| **4** Body of hyoid bone | pharynx |
| **5** Body of mandible | **23** Inferior thyroid vein |
| **6** Buccal fat pad | **24** Internal carotid artery and |
| **7** Cervical branch of facial | superior root of ansa |
| nerve | cervicalis |
| **8** Cervical nerves to trapezius | **25** Internal laryngeal nerve |
| **9** Clavicular head of | **26** Jugulodigastric lymph nodes |
| sternocleidomastoid | **27** Lesser occipital nerve |
| **10** Common carotid artery | **28** Lingual artery |
| **11** Dorsal scapular nerve | **29** Lingual vein |
| **12** External carotid artery | **30** Marginal mandibular branch |
| **13** External jugular vein | of facial nerve |
| **14** External laryngeal nerve | **31** Masseter |
| **15** Facial artery | **32** Mylohyoid |
| **16** Facial vein | **33** Nerve to thyrohyoid |
| **17** Great auricular nerve | **34** Parotid gland |
| **18** Greater horn of hyoid bone | **35** Phrenic nerve (on scalenus |
| (underlying 25) | anterior) |
| **19** Hyoglossus | **36** Posterior auricular vein |

| | |
|---|---|
| **37** Posterior belly of digastric | **55** Suprascapular artery |
| **38** Posterior branch of | **56** Suprascapular nerve |
| retromandibular vein | **57** Thyrohyoid |
| **39** Scalenus anterior | **58** Thyrohyoid membrane |
| **40** Scalenus medius | **59** Thyroid gland (left lobe) |
| **41** Sternal head of | **60** Trapezius |
| sternocleidomastoid | **61** Upper trunk of brachial |
| **42** Sternocleidomastoid | plexus |
| **43** Sternohyoid | |
| **44** Sternothyroid | |
| **45** Stylohyoid | |
| **46** Submandibular gland | |
| **47** Submental artery and vein | |
| **48** Superficial cervical artery | |
| **49** Superficial cervical vein | |
| **50** Superior belly of | |
| omohyoid | |
| **51** Superior laryngeal artery | |
| **52** Superior thyroid artery | |
| **53** Supraclavicular nerve | |
| (cut upper edge) | |
| **54** Suprahyoid artery | |

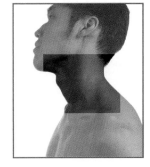

*Carotid artery bruits, cervical lymph node enlargement, see page 90.*

# Right lower face and upper neck

**A** *parotid and upper cervical regions*  **B** *submandibular region*

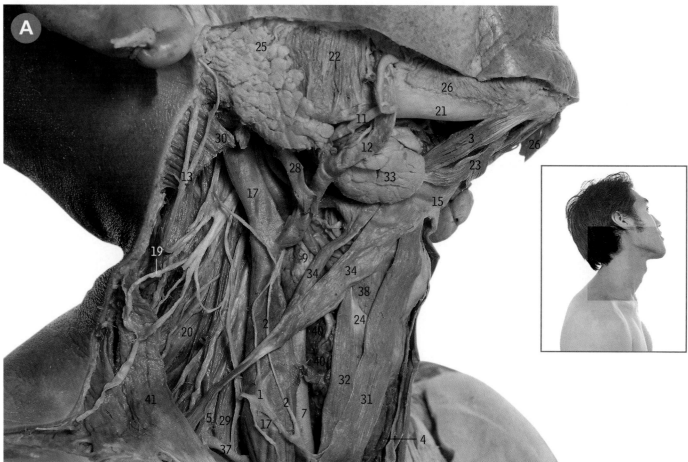

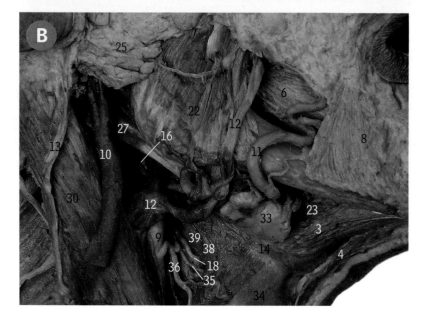

| | |
|---|---|
| **1** Ansa cervicalis, inferior branch | **22** Masseter |
| **2** Ansa cervicalis, superior branch | **23** Mylohyoid |
| **3** Anterior belly of digastric | **24** Oblique line of the thyroid cartilage |
| **4** Anterior jugular vein | **25** Parotid gland and facial nerve branches at anterior border |
| **5** Brachial plexus (roots) | **26** Platysma |
| **6** Buccinator | **27** Posterior belly of digastric |
| **7** Common carotid artery | **28** Retromandibular vein |
| **8** Depressor anguli oris | **29** Scalenus anterior |
| **9** External carotid artery | **30** Sternocleidomastoid |
| **10** External jugular vein | **31** Sternohyoid |
| **11** Facial artery | **32** Sternothyroid |
| **12** Facial vein | **33** Submandibular gland |
| **13** Great auricular nerve | **34** Superior belly of omohyoid (bifid) |
| **14** Greater horn of hyoid bone | **35** Superior laryngeal artery |
| **15** Hyoid bone | **36** Superior thyroid artery |
| **16** Hypoglossal nerve | **37** Suprascapular artery |
| **17** Internal jugular vein | **38** Thyrohyoid |
| **18** Internal laryngeal nerve | **39** Thyrohyoid membrane |
| **19** Lesser occipital nerve | **40** Thyroid gland (right lobe) |
| **20** Levator scapulae | **41** Trapezius |
| **21** Mandible | |

*Mumps, parotidectomy (removal of parotid gland), parotid tumours, see pages 91, 92.*

# Right side of the neck *deep dissection*

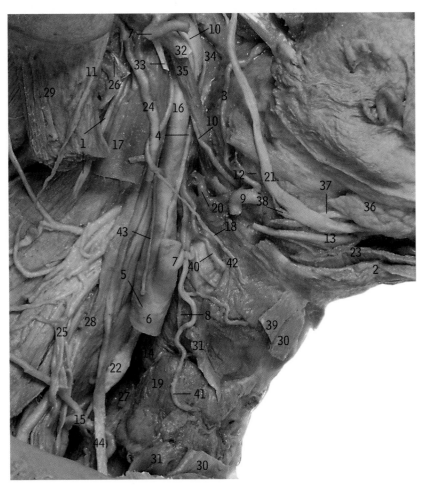

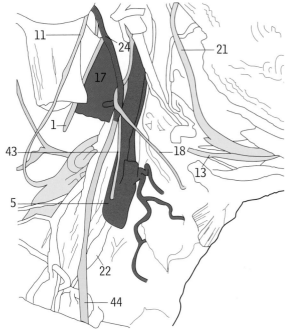

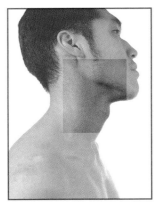

| | |
|---|---|
| **1** Accessory nerve | **23** Mylohyoid |
| **2** Anterior belly of digastric | **24** Occipital artery |
| **3** Ascending palatine artery | **25** Phrenic nerve |
| **4** Ascending pharyngeal artery | **26** Posterior belly of digastric |
| **5** Carotid sinus | **27** Recurrent laryngeal nerve |
| **6** Common carotid artery | **28** Scalenus anterior |
| **7** External carotid artery | **29** Sternocleidomastoid |
| **8** External laryngeal nerve | **30** Sternohyoid |
| **9** Facial artery | **31** Sternothyroid |
| **10** Glossopharyngeal nerve | **32** Styloglossus |
| **11** Great auricular nerve | **33** Stylohyoid (cut end displaced medially) |
| **12** Hyoglossus | **34** Stylohyoid ligament |
| **13** Hypoglossal nerve | **35** Stylopharyngeus |
| **14** Inferior constrictor | **36** Sublingual gland |
| **15** Inferior thyroid artery | **37** Submandibular duct |
| **16** Internal carotid artery | **38** Submandibular ganglion |
| **17** Internal jugular vein | **39** Superior belly of omohyoid |
| **18** Internal laryngeal nerve | **40** Superior laryngeal artery |
| **19** Lateral lobe of thyroid gland | **41** Superior thyroid artery |
| **20** Lingual artery | **42** Thyrohyoid and nerve |
| **21** Lingual nerve | **43** Upper root of ansa cervicalis |
| **22** Middle cervical sympathetic ganglion | **44** Vagus nerve |

The hypoglossal nerve (13) passes downwards, curling around the occipital artery (24) and lying superficial to the external carotid (7) and lingual (20) arteries.

The glossopharyngeal nerve (10) passes downwards and forwards, curling round the lateral side of stylopharyngeus (35).

The removal of parts of the sternohyoid (30), omohyoid (39) and sternothyroid (31) displays the lateral lobe of the thyroid gland (19). Note the inferior thyroid artery (15) behind the lower part of the lobe, with the recurrent laryngeal nerve (27) passing deep to this looping vessel to enter the pharynx beneath the inferior constrictor (14).

*Carotid endarterectomy, see page 90.*

# Prevertebral region

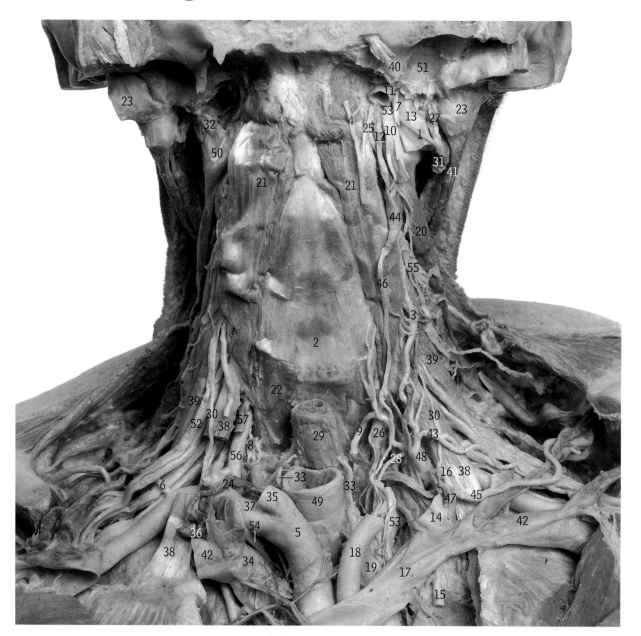

| | | |
|---|---|---|
| **1** Accessory nerve (spinal root) | **21** Longus capitis | **39** Scalenus medius |
| **2** Anterior longitudinal ligament | **22** Longus colli | **40** Spine of sphenoid bone |
| **3** Ascending cervical artery and vein | **23** Mastoid process | **41** Sternocleidomastoid |
| **4** Ascending pharyngeal artery | **24** Mediastinal lymphatic trunk | **42** Subclavian vein |
| **5** Brachiocephalic artery | **25** Meningeal branch of ascending | **43** Superficial cervical artery |
| **6** Dorsal scapular artery | pharyngeal artery | **44** Superior cervical ganglion |
| **7** Glossopharyngeal nerve | **26** Middle cervical ganglion | **45** Suprascapular artery |
| **8** Inferior cervical ganglion | **27** Occipital artery | **46** Sympathetic trunk |
| **9** Inferior thyroid artery | **28** Oesophageal branch of inferior thyroid | **47** Thoracic duct |
| **10** Inferior vagal ganglion | artery | **48** Thyrocervical trunk |
| **11** Internal carotid artery | **29** Oesophagus | **49** Trachea |
| **12** Internal carotid nerve | **30** Phrenic nerve | **50** Transverse process of atlas |
| **13** Internal jugular vein, upper end | **31** Posterior belly of digastric | **51** Tympanic part of temporal bone |
| **14** Internal jugular vein, lower end | **32** Rectus capitis lateralis | **52** Upper trunk of brachial plexus |
| **15** Internal thoracic artery | **33** Recurrent laryngeal nerve | **53** Vagus nerve, on left |
| **16** Jugular lymphatic trunk | **34** Right brachiocephalic vein | **54** Vagus nerve, on right |
| **17** Left brachiocephalic vein | **35** Right common carotid artery | **55** Ventral ramus of third cervical nerve |
| **18** Left common carotid artery | **36** Right lymphatic duct | **56** Vertebral artery |
| **19** Left subclavian artery | **37** Right subclavian artery | **57** Vertebral vein |
| **20** Levator scapulae | **38** Scalenus anterior | |

# Root of the neck

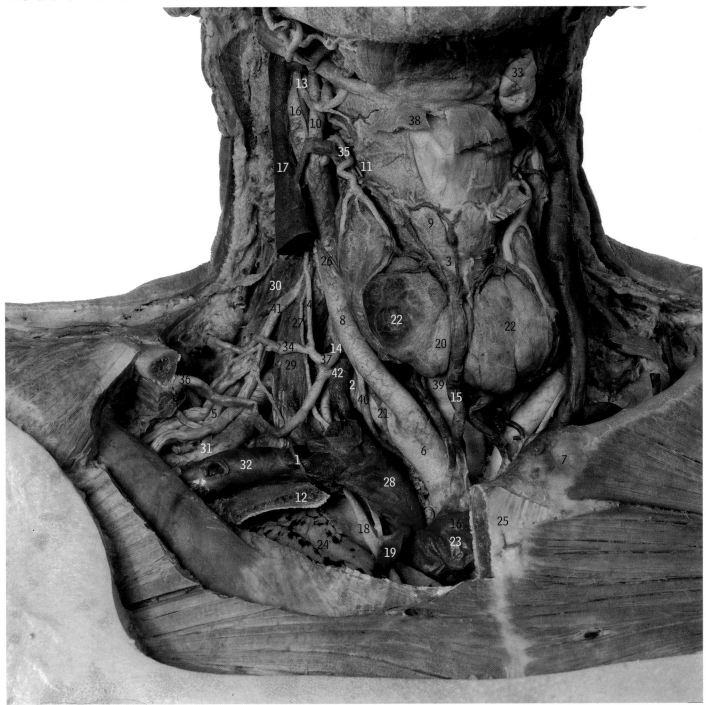

| | | |
|---|---|---|
| **1** Accessory phrenic nerve | **15** Inferior thyroid veins | **29** Scalenus anterior |
| **2** Ansa subclavia | **16** Internal carotid artery | **30** Scalenus medius |
| **3** Arch of cricoid cartilage | **17** Internal jugular vein | **31** Subclavian artery |
| **4** Ascending cervical artery | **18** Internal thoracic artery | **32** Subclavian vein |
| **5** Brachial plexus | **19** Internal thoracic vein | **33** Submandibular gland |
| **6** Brachiocephalic artery | **20** Isthmus of thyroid gland | **34** Superficial cervical artery |
| **7** Capsule of sternoclavicular joint | **21** Jugular lymphatic trunk | **35** Superior thyroid artery and vein |
| **8** Common carotid artery | **22** Lateral lobe of thyroid gland | **36** Suprascapular artery |
| **9** Cricothyroid muscle | **23** Left brachiocephalic vein | **37** Thyrocervical trunk |
| **10** External carotid artery | **24** Lung apex | **38** Thyrohyoid |
| **11** External laryngeal nerve | **25** Manubrium of sternum | **39** Trachea |
| **12** First rib (sectioned) | **26** Middle thyroid vein | **40** Vagus nerve |
| **13** Hypoglossal nerve | **27** Phrenic nerve | **41** Ventral ramus of fifth cervical nerve |
| **14** Inferior thyroid artery | **28** Right brachiocephalic vein | **42** Vertebral vein |

*Internal jugular vein catheterisation, subclavian vein catheterisation, see pages 91, 92.*

# Face *surface markings on the front and right side*

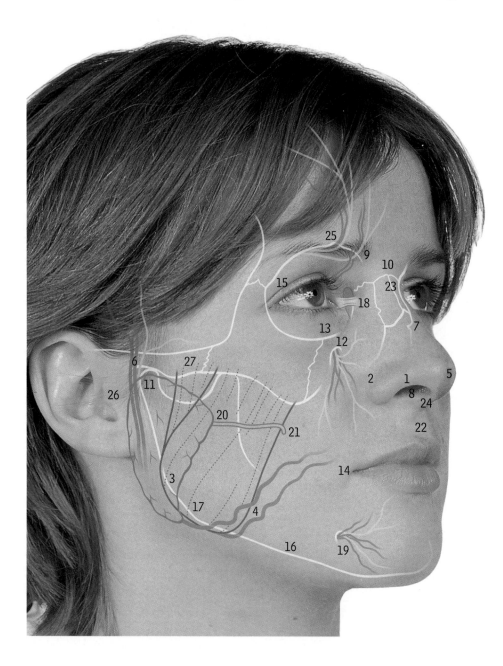

1 Ala
2 Alar groove (nasolabial groove)
3 Angle of mandible
4 Anterior border of masseter and facial vessels
5 Apex of external nose
6 Auriculotemporal nerve and superficial temporal vessels
7 Dorsum of nose
8 External aperture (anterior naris)
9 Frontal notch and supratrochlear nerve and vessels
10 Glabella of nose
11 Head of mandible
12 Infra-orbital foramen, nerve and vessels
13 Infra-orbital margin
14 Lateral angle of mouth
15 Lateral part of supra-orbital margin
16 Lower border of body of mandible
17 Lower border of ramus of mandible
18 Medial palpebral ligament anterior to lacrimal sac
19 Mental foramen, nerve and vessels
20 Parotid duct emerging from gland
21 Parotid duct turning medially at anterior border of masseter
22 Philtrum
23 Root of nose
24 Septum of nose (nasal columella)
25 Supra-orbital notch (or foramen), nerve and vessels
26 Tragus
27 Zygomatic arch

The pulsation of the superficial temporal artery (6) is palpable in front of the tragus of the ear (26).

The parotid duct (20 and 21) lies under the middle-third of a line drawn from the tragus of the ear (26) to the midpoint of the philtrum (22).

The pulsation of the facial artery (4) is palpable where the vessel crosses the lower border of the mandible at the anterior margin of the masseter muscle, about 2.5 cm (1 in) in front of the angle of the mandible (3).

*Ophthalmic herpes zoster, see page 91.*

# Face *superficial dissection from the front and the right*

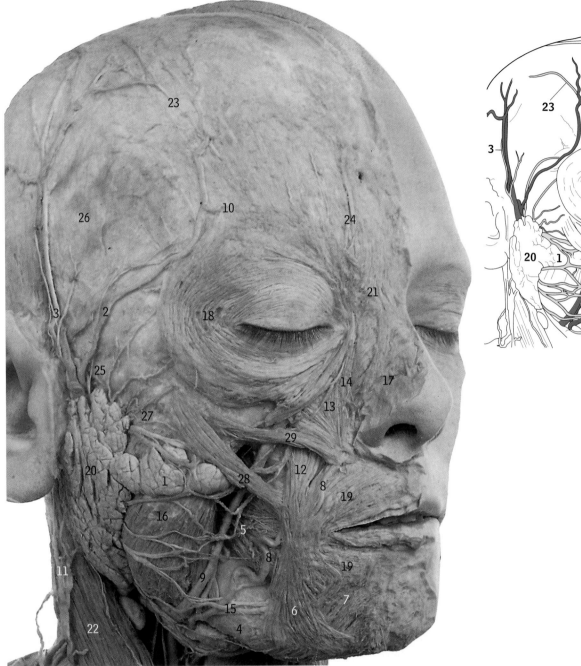

1 Accessory parotid gland overlying parotid duct
2 Anterior branch of superficial temporal artery
3 Auriculotemporal nerve and superficial temporal vessels
4 Body of mandible
5 Buccinator and buccal branches of facial nerve
6 Depressor anguli oris
7 Depressor labii inferioris
8 Facial artery
9 Facial vein
10 Frontalis part of occipitofrontalis
11 Great auricular nerve
12 Levator anguli oris
13 Levator labii superioris
14 Levator labii superioris alaeque nasi
15 Marginal mandibular branch of facial nerve
16 Masseter
17 Nasalis
18 Orbicularis oculi
19 Orbicularis oris
20 Parotid gland
21 Procerus
22 Sternocleidomastoid
23 Supra-orbital nerve
24 Supratrochlear nerve
25 Temporal branch of facial nerve
26 Temporalis underlying temporal fascia
27 Zygomatic branch of facial nerve
28 Zygomaticus major
29 Zygomaticus minor

*Facial nerve palsy, intracranial spread of infection, surgical flaps of the scalp, see pages 90–92.*

# Face *superficial dissection from the right*

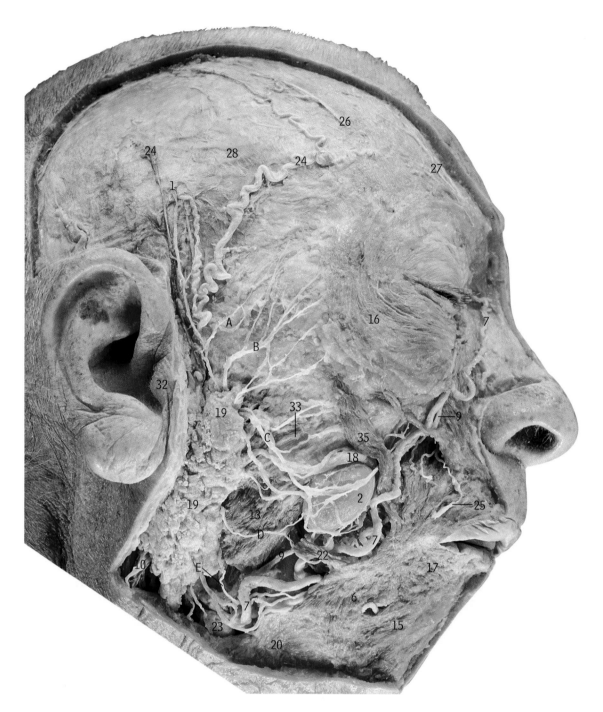

After removal of skin and some fat (A, B, C, D, E = temporal, zygomatic, buccal, mandibular and cervical branches of facial nerve, respectively).

| | | | |
|---|---|---|---|
| **1** Auriculotemporal nerve | **9** Facial vein | **19** Parotid gland | **28** Temporal fascia |
| **2** Buccal fat pad | **10** Great auricular nerve | **20** Platysma | **29** Temporal line, inferior |
| **3** Buccal nerve (V3) | **11** Infra-orbital nerve | **21** Retromandibular vein | **30** Temporal line, superior |
| **4** Buccinator | **12** Mandible, body | **22** Risorius, overlying facial | **31** Temporalis |
| **5** Capsule of | **13** Masseter | artery and vein | **32** Tragus |
| temporomandibular joint | **14** Mental nerve | **23** Submandibular gland | **33** Transverse facial artery |
| **6** Depressor anguli oris | **15** Mentalis | **24** Superficial temporal vessels | **34** Zygomatic arch |
| **7** Facial artery | **16** Orbicularis oculi | **25** Superior labial artery | **35** Zygomaticus major |
| **8** Facial nerve (A, B, C, D, E | **17** Orbicularis oris | **26** Supraorbital nerve | |
| branches) | **18** Parotid duct | **27** Supratrochlear nerve | |

# Right temporal fossa

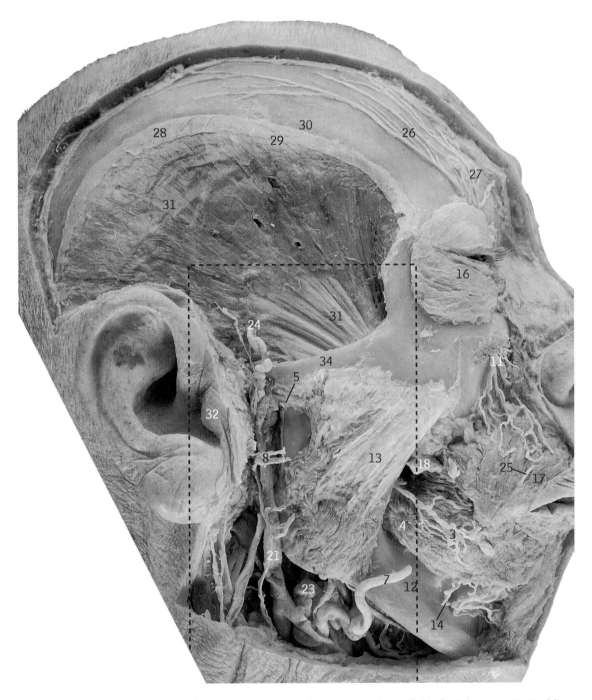

After removal of temporal fascia, parotid gland and most branches of the facial nerve. Dotted line indicates field of deeper dissections shown on next page.

# Infratemporal fossa *progressively deeper dissections*

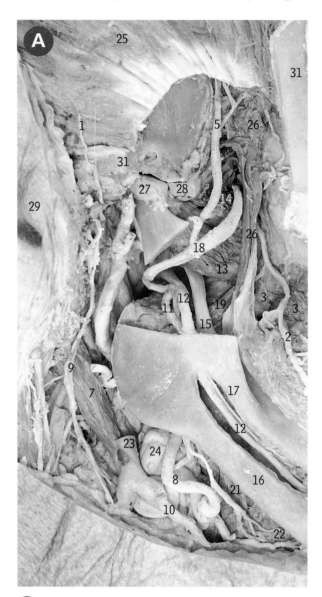

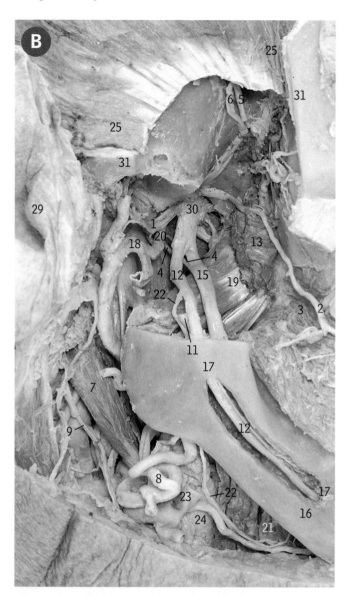

**A** Removal of the masseter, part of the zygomatic arch, most of the superficial and inferior parts of temporalis, the superior half of the mandibular ramus (except the neck and condyle) and the pterygoid venous plexus reveals the superficial contents of the infratemporal fossa.

**B** Removal of the deep head of temporalis, the lateral pterygoid and the neck and condyle of the mandible exposes the deepest structures.

| | | | |
|---|---|---|---|
| **1** | Auriculotemporal nerve | **13** | Lateral pterygoid, inferior head |
| **2** | Buccal nerve (V3) | **14** | Lateral pterygoid, superior head |
| **3** | Buccinator | **15** | Lingual nerve |
| **4** | Chorda tympani | **16** | Mandible, body |
| **5** | Deep temporal artery | **17** | Mandibular canal (opened) |
| **6** | Deep temporal nerve | **18** | Maxillary artery |
| **7** | Digastric, posterior belly | **19** | Medial pterygoid |
| **8** | Facial artery | **20** | Middle meningeal artery |
| **9** | Facial nerve, cervical branch | **21** | Mylohyoid |
| **10** | Facial vein | **22** | Nerve to mylohyoid |
| **11** | Inferior alveolar artery | | |
| **12** | Inferior alveolar nerve | | |

| | |
|---|---|
| **23** | Retromandibular vein |
| **24** | Submandibular gland |
| **25** | Temporalis |
| **26** | Temporalis, deep head (sphenomandibularis) |
| **27** | Temporomandibular joint, capsule |
| **28** | Temporomandibular joint, disc |
| **29** | Tragus |
| **30** | Trigeminal nerve, mandibular division (V3) |
| **31** | Zygomatic arch |

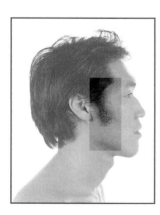

## A Coronal section of cadaveric face *temporalis heads*

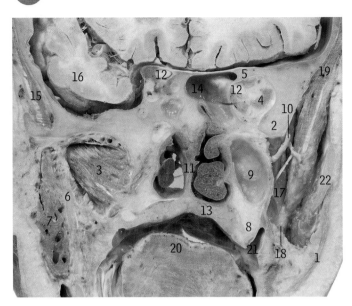

1 Buccinator
2 Greater wing of sphenoid
3 Lateral pterygoid
4 Lateral rectus
5 Lesser wing of sphenoid
6 Mandible
7 Masseter
8 Maxilla
9 Maxillary air (paranasal) sinus
10 Maxillary artery, muscular branches
11 Nasal septum
12 Optic nerve
13 Palate
14 Sphenoidal sinus
15 Temporal bone
16 Temporal lobe, brain
17 Temporalis, deep head (sphenomandibularis – Zenker 1955)
18 Temporalis, insertion
19 Temporalis, superficial head
20 Tongue
21 Vestibule of oral cavity
22 Zygoma

## C Endoscopic view of nasal septum (choanae)

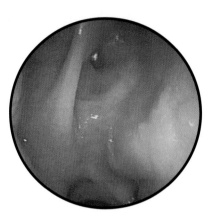

## B Coronal MRI of face *muscles of mastication*

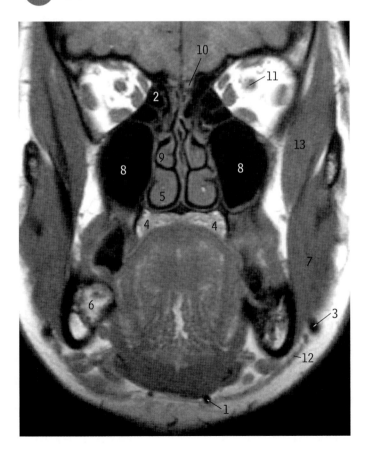

1 Anterior jugular vein
2 Ethmoid air cells
3 Facial artery
4 Hard palate
5 Inferior concha
6 Mandible
7 Masseter
8 Maxillary sinus
9 Middle concha
10 Olfactory tract
11 Optic nerve
12 Platysma
13 Temporalis

*Inferior alveolar nerve block, see page 91.*

# Right trigeminal, facial and petrosal nerves *with associated ganglia*

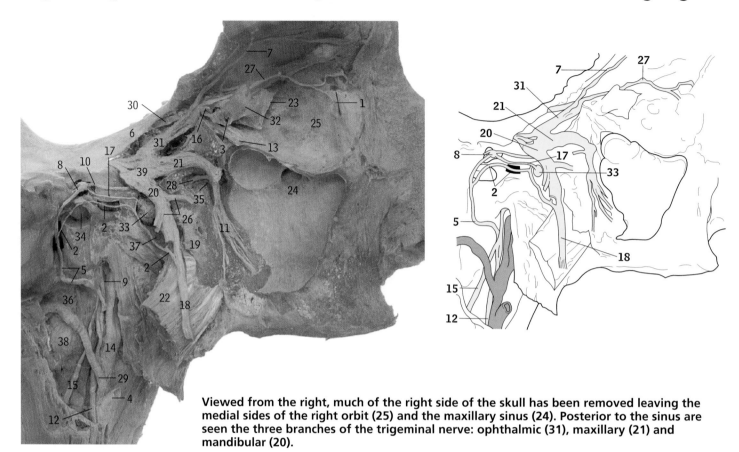

Viewed from the right, much of the right side of the skull has been removed leaving the medial sides of the right orbit (25) and the maxillary sinus (24). Posterior to the sinus are seen the three branches of the trigeminal nerve: ophthalmic (31), maxillary (21) and mandibular (20).

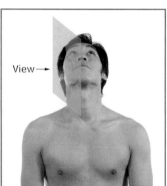

View→

| | | |
|---|---|---|
| **1** Bristle in lacrimal canaliculus | **14** Internal carotid artery | **26** Muscular branches of |
| **2** Chorda tympani | **15** Internal jugular vein and | mandibular nerve |
| **3** Ciliary ganglion | accessory nerve | **27** Nasociliary nerve |
| **4** External carotid artery | **16** Lacrimal nerve | **28** Nerve of pterygoid canal |
| **5** Facial nerve | **17** Lesser petrosal nerve | **29** Occipital artery |
| **6** Free margin of tentorium | **18** Lingual nerve | **30** Oculomotor nerve |
| cerebelli | **19** Lower head of lateral | **31** Ophthalmic nerve |
| **7** Frontal nerve | pterygoid and lateral | **32** Optic nerve |
| **8** Geniculate ganglion of facial | pterygoid plate | **33** Otic ganglion |
| nerve | **20** Mandibular nerve | **34** Position of tympanic |
| **9** Glossopharyngeal nerve | **21** Maxillary nerve | membrane |
| **10** Greater petrosal nerve | **22** Medial pterygoid | **35** Pterygopalatine ganglion |
| **11** Greater and lesser palatine | **23** Medial rectus | **36** Rectus capitis lateralis |
| nerves | **24** Medial wall of maxillary sinus | **37** Tensor veli palatini |
| **12** Hypoglossal nerve | and ostium | **38** Transverse process of atlas |
| **13** Inferior rectus | **25** Medial wall of orbit | **39** Trigeminal ganglion |

The greater petrosal nerve (10) is a branch of the geniculate ganglion of the facial nerve (8) and can be remembered as the nerve of tear secretion (though it also supplies nasal glands). It carries preganglionic fibres from the superior salivary nucleus in the pons, and runs in the groove on the floor of the middle cranial fossa (page 21, 25) to enter the foramen lacerum and become the nerve of the pterygoid canal (28) which joins the pterygopalatine ganglion (35). Postganglionic fibres leave the ganglion to join the maxillary nerve and enter the orbit by the zygomatic branch which communicates with the lacrimal nerve, supplying the gland.

The lesser petrosal nerve (17), although having a communication with the facial nerve, is a branch of the glossopharyngeal nerve, being de-rived from the tympanic branch which supplies the mucous membrane of the middle ear by the tympanic plexus (page 70, C19). Its fibres are derived from the inferior salivary nucleus in the pons, and after leaving the middle ear and running in its groove on the floor of the middle

cranial fossa (17, and page 21, 26), the nerve reaches the otic ganglion (33) via the foramen ovale. From the ganglion secretomotor fibres join the mandibular nerve (20) to be distributed to the parotid gland by filaments from the auriculotemporal nerve.

The chorda tympani (2) arises from the facial nerve before the latter leaves the stylomastoid foramen (5, upper leader line). It crosses the upper part of the tympanic membrane (34) underneath its mucosal covering and runs through the temporal bone, emerging from the petrotympanic fissure (page 19, 35) to join the lingual nerve (18). It carries preganglionic fibres to the submandibular ganglion (page 69, C35) for the submandibular and sublingual salivary glands, and also taste fibres for the anterior two-thirds of the tongue.

The otic ganglion (33), which normally adheres to the deep surface of the mandibular nerve (20), has been teased off from the nerve and a black marker has been placed behind it.

# Pharynx *posterior surface, from behind*

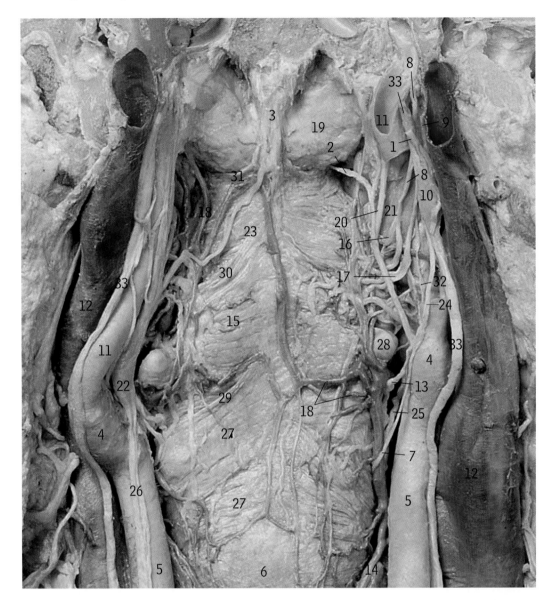

1 Accessory nerve
2 Ascending pharyngeal artery
3 Attachment of pharyngeal raphe to pharyngeal tubercle of base of skull
4 Carotid sinus
5 Common carotid artery
6 Cricopharyngeal part of inferior constrictor
7 External laryngeal nerve
8 Glossopharyngeal nerve
9 Hypoglossal nerve
10 Inferior ganglion of vagus nerve
11 Internal carotid artery
12 Internal jugular vein
13 Internal laryngeal nerve
14 Lateral lobe of thyroid gland
15 Middle constrictor
16 Pharyngeal branch of glossopharyngeal nerve
17 Pharyngeal branch of vagus nerve

18 Pharyngeal veins
19 Pharyngobasilar fascia
20 Posterior meningeal artery
21 Stylopharyngeus
22 Superior cervical sympathetic ganglion
23 Superior constrictor
24 Superior laryngeal branch of vagus nerve
25 Superior thyroid artery
26 Sympathetic trunk
27 Thyropharyngeal part of inferior constrictor
28 Tip of greater horn of hyoid bone
29 Upper border of inferior constrictor
30 Upper border of middle constrictor
31 Upper border of superior constrictor
32 Vagal branch to carotid body
33 Vagus nerve

**The vertebral column has been removed to reveal the carotid sheath and constrictor muscles of the pharynx.**

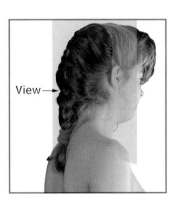

View→

*Gag reflex, see page 90.*

# Posterior pharyngeal wall *from behind*

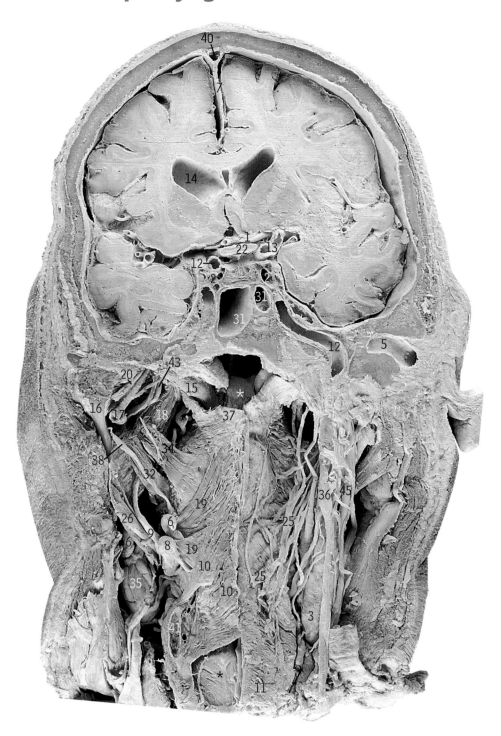

Slightly oblique coronal section of the head and neck in the plane of the posterior pharyngeal wall, with the right side slightly posterior to the left.

Sections of the posterior pharyngeal wall have been removed (asterisks – superiorly the pharyngobasilar fascia and inferiorly the lower border of the inferior constrictor) to reveal parts of the nasopharynx and the laryngopharynx, respectively.

Refer to the key on page 57 for the numbers on this figure.

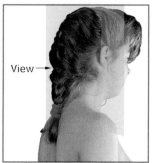

View →

# A  'Opened' pharynx *from behind*

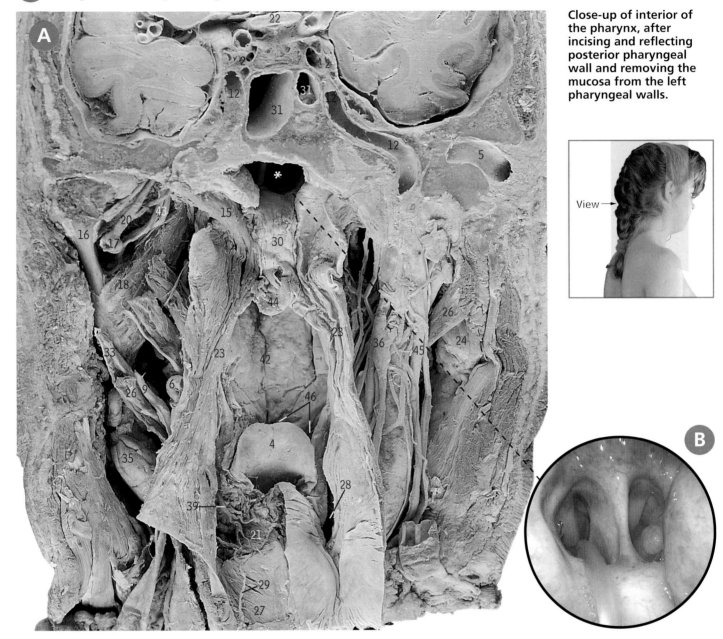

Close-up of interior of the pharynx, after incising and reflecting posterior pharyngeal wall and removing the mucosa from the left pharyngeal walls.

View→

| | | |
|---|---|---|
| **1** | Anterior cerebral artery | |
| **2** | Cavernous sinus | |
| **3** | Common carotid | |
| **4** | Epiglottis | |
| **5** | External auditory canal | |
| **6** | Facial artery | |
| **7** | Falx cerebri | |
| **8** | Hyoid-tip of greater horn | |
| **9** | Hypoglossal nerve | |
| **10** | Inferior constrictor | |
| **11** | Inferior constrictor-cricopharyngeus part | |
| **12** | Internal carotid | |
| **13** | Internal carotid giving off middle cerebral | |
| **14** | Lateral ventricle | |
| **15** | Levator veli palatini | |
| **16** | Mandible, neck | |

| | |
|---|---|
| **17** | Maxillary artery |
| **18** | Medial pterygoid |
| **19** | Middle constrictor |
| **20** | Middle meningeal artery |
| **21** | Oblique arytenoid |
| **22** | Optic chiasm |
| **23** | Palatopharyngeus |
| **24** | Parotid gland |
| **25** | Pharyngeal plexus of veins |
| **26** | Posterior belly of digastric |
| **27** | Posterior crico-arytenoid |
| **28** | Piriform fossa (recess) |
| **29** | Recurrent laryngeal nerve |
| **30** | Soft palate, nasal surface |
| **31** | Sphenoidal sinus |
| **32** | Styloglossus muscle |
| **33** | Stylohyoid muscle |

| | |
|---|---|
| **34** | Stylopharyngeus, with glossopharyngeal nerve |
| **35** | Submandibular gland |
| **36** | Superior cervical ganglion |
| **37** | Superior constrictor |
| **38** | Superior pharyngeal branch of vagus |
| **39** | Superior laryngeal nerve, internal branch |
| **40** | Superior sagittal sinus |
| **41** | Thyroid cartilage lamina, cut |
| **42** | Tongue, dorsum, posterior third |
| **43** | Trigeminal nerve, mandibular division |
| **44** | Uvula |
| **45** | Vagus |
| **46** | Vallecula |

# B  Endoscopic view of Choanae and posterior nasal septum

NB: Nasogastric tube in situ.

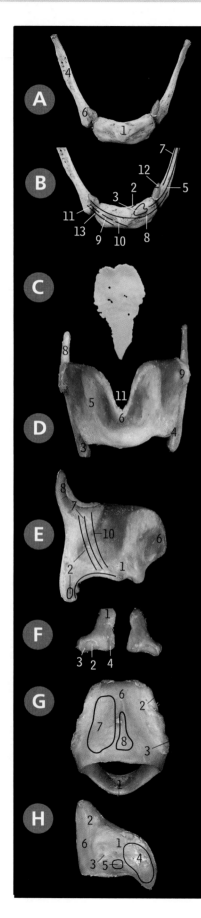

# Hyoid bone

**A**   from above and in front

**B**   with muscle attachments

| | |
|---|---|
| **1** Body | **8** Mylohyoid |
| **2** Genioglossus | **9** Omohyoid |
| **3** Geniohyoid | **10** Sternohyoid |
| **4** Greater horn | **11** Stylohyoid |
| **5** Hyoglossus | **12** Stylohyoid |
| **6** Lesser horn |     ligament |
| **7** Middle | **13** Thyrohyoid |
|     constrictor | |

# Epiglottis

**C**   cartilage, from the front

# Thyroid

**D**   cartilage, from the front

**E**   from the right,
with attachments

**1** Cricothyroid
**2** Inferior constrictor
**3** Inferior horn
**4** Inferior tubercle
**5** Lamina
**6** Laryngeal prominence
(Adam's apple)
**7** Sternothyroid
**8** Superior horn
**9** Superior tubercle
**10** Thyrohyoid
**11** Thyroid notch

# Arytenoid cartilages

**F**   from behind

**1** Apex
**2** Articular surface for cricoid cartilage
**3** Muscular process
**4** Vocal process

# Cricoid cartilage and muscle attachments

**G**   from behind and below

**H**   from the right

**1** Arch
**2** Articular surface for arytenoid
cartilage
**3** Articular surface for inferior horn of
thyroid cartilage
**4** Cricothyroid
**5** Inferior constrictor
**6** Lamina
**7** Posterior crico-arytenoid
**8** Tendon of oesophagus

# Laryngeal *surface anatomy*

**I**   lateral view

**J**   anterior view

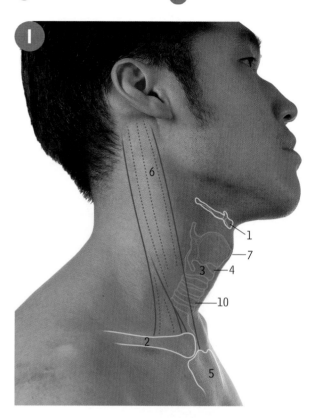

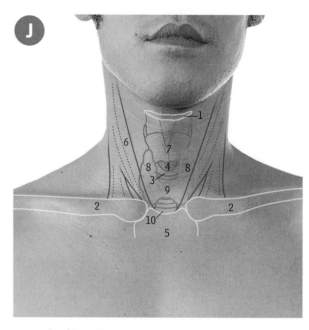

| | |
|---|---|
| **1** Body of hyoid bone | **7** Thyroid cartilage, |
| **2** Clavicle |     laryngeal prominence |
| **3** Cricoid cartilage | **8** Thyroid gland, lateral |
| **4** Cricothyroid |     lobe |
|     ligament/membrane | **9** Thyroid gland, isthmus |
| **5** Manubrium | **10** Tracheal ring |
| **6** Sternomastoid muscle | |

## A Tongue and the inlet of the larynx *from above*

The V-shaped sulcus terminalis (10), behind the row of vallate papillae (11), is not well marked in this tongue.

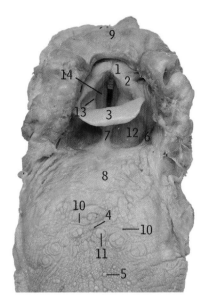

**1** Corniculate cartilage in aryepiglottic fold
**2** Cuneiform cartilage in aryepiglottic fold
**3** Epiglottis
**4** Foramen caecum
**5** Fungiform papilla
**6** Lateral glosso-epiglottic fold
**7** Median glosso-epiglottic fold
**8** Pharyngeal part of dorsum of tongue
**9** Posterior wall of pharynx
**10** Sulcus terminalis
**11** Vallate papilla
**12** Vallecula
**13** Vestibular fold (false vocal cord)
**14** Vocal fold (true vocal cord)

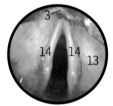

**Endoscopic view of laryngeal inlet**

## B Larynx *from behind*

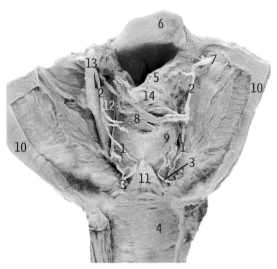

**1** Anastomosis between internal and recurrent laryngeal nerves
**2** Branch of internal laryngeal nerve
**3** Branches of recurrent laryngeal nerve
**4** Circular fibres of oesophagus
**5** Corniculate cartilage in aryepiglottic fold
**6** Epiglottis
**7** Internal branch of superior laryngeal nerve, piercing mucosa and thyrohyoid membrane
**8** Oblique arytenoid muscle
**9** Posterior crico-arytenoid muscle
**10** Posterior pharyngeal wall
**11** Tendon of oesophagus (crico-oesphageal tendon)
**12** Thyroid cartilage, lamina, posterior surface
**13** Thyroid cartilage, superior horn
**14** Transverse arytenoid muscle

# Intrinsic muscles of the larynx

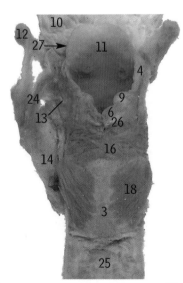

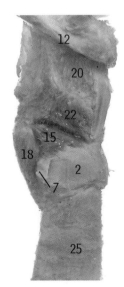

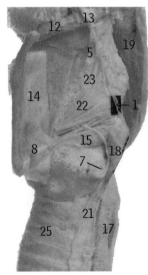

**1** Anastomosis of internal and recurrent laryngeal nerves
**2** Arch of cricoid cartilage
**3** Area on lamina of cricoid cartilage for tendon of oesophagus
**4** Aryepiglottic fold
**5** Aryepiglottic muscle
**6** Corniculate cartilage
**7** Cricothyroid joint
**8** Cricothyroid muscle (reflected from cricoid attachment)
**9** Cuneiform cartilage
**10** Dorsum of tongue
**11** Epiglottis
**12** Greater horn of hyoid bone
**13** Internal laryngeal nerve
**14** Lamina of thyroid cartilage
**15** Lateral crico-arytenoid muscle
**16** Oblique arytenoid muscle
**17** Oesophagus
**18** Posterior crico-arytenoid muscle
**19** Posterior wall of pharynx
**20** Quadrangular membrane
**21** Recurrent laryngeal nerve
**22** Thyro-arytenoid muscle
**23** Thyro-epiglottic muscle
**24** Thyrohyoid membrane
**25** Trachea
**26** Transverse arytenoid muscle
**27** Vallecula

## C *from behind*  D *from the right*  E *from the left*

In D the right lamina of the thyroid cartilage has been removed, and in E part of the thyroid lamina has been turned forwards.

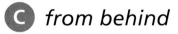

*Recurrent laryngeal nerve damage, see page 92.*

## A Larynx *in sagittal section, from the right*

## B Larynx *internal view, hemisection*

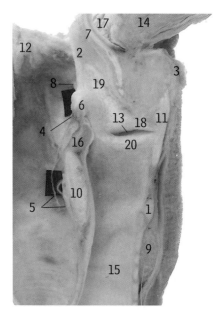

*Endoscopic view of cricoid and tracheal rings*

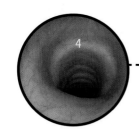

**The vocal fold (vocal cord, 20) lies below the vestibular fold (false vocal cord, 18)**

| | |
|---|---|
| **1** Arch of cricoid cartilage | **9** Isthmus of thyroid gland |
| **2** Aryepiglottic fold and inlet of larynx | **10** Lamina of cricoid cartilage |
| **3** Body of hyoid bone | **11** Lamina of thyroid cartilage |
| **4** Branches of internal laryngeal nerve anastomosing with recurrent laryngeal nerve | **12** Pharyngeal wall |
| | **13** Sinus of larynx (laryngeal ventricle) |
| **5** Branches of recurrent laryngeal nerve | **14** Tongue |
| | **15** Trachea |
| **6** Corniculate cartilage and apex of arytenoid cartilage | **16** Transverse arytenoid muscle |
| | **17** Vallecula |
| **7** Epiglottis | **18** Vestibular fold |
| **8** Internal laryngeal nerve entering piriform recess | **19** Vestibule of larynx |
| | **20** Vocal fold |

**1** Articular facet on cricoid for left arytenoid cartilage
**2** Articulation site of thyroid and cricoid cartilages
**3** Arytenoid cartilage, right, medial surface
**4** Cricoid cartilage, lamina
**5** Epiglottis, hemisected
**6** Hyoid arch, cross-section
**7** Hyoid, greater horn
**8** Quadrangular membrane
**9** Thyrohyoid membrane
**10** Thyroid cartilage, lamina, cross-section
**11** Vestibular fold (false vocal cord)
**12** Vocal fold (true vocal cord)

**Medial view of the membranes and ligaments of the right side of the superior larynx, after removal of the left half above the cricoid cartilage.**

The space between the vestibular and vocal folds is the sinus of the larynx (A13), and this is continuous with the saccule, a small pouch that extends upwards for a few millimetres between the vestibular fold and the inner surface of the thyroarytenoid muscle.

The fissure between the two vestibular folds (A18) is the rima of the vestibule. The fissure between the vocal folds is the rima of the glottis.

The vestibular folds are often called the false vocal cords.

The intrinsic muscles of the larynx are supplied by the recurrent laryngeal nerve, except the cricothyroid (page 41, 6) which is supplied by the external laryngeal nerve (page 43, 14).

The mucous membrane of the larynx above the level of the vocal folds is supplied by the internal laryngeal nerve, and below the vocal folds by the recurrent laryngeal nerve (A4 and 5 above).

The recurrent laryngeal nerve (E21 on page 59) enters the larynx by passing beneath the lower border of the inferior constrictor of the pharynx, and here it lies immediately behind the cricothyroid joint (E7 on page 59).

The anterior part of the vocal fold (A20 and B12 above) is formed by the upper margin of the cricovocal membrane, and the posterior part by the vocal process of the arytenoid cartilage (page 58, F4).

The vestibular fold (false vocal cord, A18 above) is formed by the lower margin of the quadrangular membrane (B8), whose upper margin forms the aryepiglottic fold (A2 above).

The central (anterior) part of the cricothyroid membrane is usually known as the conus elasticus but sometimes this term is used for the cricovocal membrane.

# Cranial fossae Ⓐ *with dura mater intact* Ⓑ *with some dura removed*

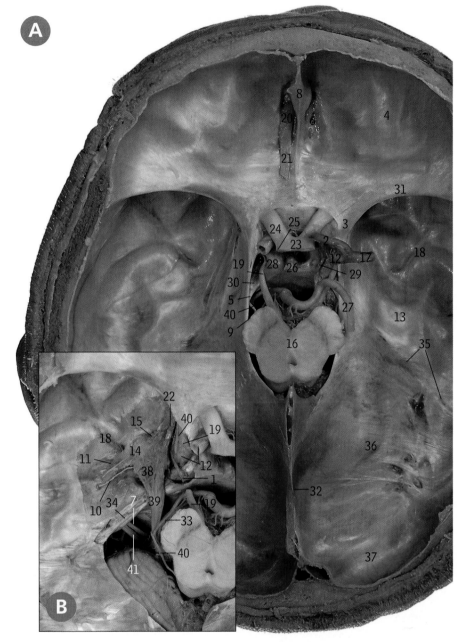

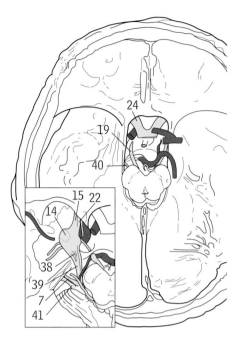

| | | |
|---|---|---|
| **1** Abducent nerve | **16** Midbrain (superior colliculus level) | **31** Sphenoparietal sinus (at posterior border of lesser wing of sphenoid bone) |
| **2** Anterior cerebral artery | **17** Middle cerebral artery | |
| **3** Anterior clinoid process | **18** Middle meningeal vessels | **32** Straight sinus (at junction of falx cerebri and tentorium cerebelli) |
| **4** Anterior cranial fossa | **19** Oculomotor nerve | |
| **5** Attached margin of tentorium cerebelli | **20** Olfactory bulb | **33** Superior cerebellar artery |
| **6** Cribriform plate of ethmoid bone | **21** Olfactory tract | **34** Superior petrosal sinus |
| **7** Facial nerve | **22** Ophthalmic nerve | **35** Superior petrosal sinus (at attached margin of tentorium cerebelli) |
| **8** Falx cerebri attached to crista galli | **23** Optic chiasma | |
| **9** Free margin of tentorium cerebelli | **24** Optic nerve | **36** Tentorium cerebelli |
| **10** Hiatus for greater petrosal nerve | **25** Optic tract | **37** Transverse sinus (at attached margin of tentorium cerebelli) |
| **11** Hiatus for lesser petrosal nerve | **26** Pituitary stalk | |
| **12** Internal carotid artery | **27** Posterior cerebral artery | **38** Trigeminal ganglion |
| **13** Lateral part of middle cranial fossa | **28** Posterior clinoid process | **39** Trigeminal nerve |
| **14** Mandibular nerve | **29** Posterior communicating artery | **40** Trochlear nerve |
| **15** Maxillary nerve | **30** Roof of cavernous sinus | **41** Vestibulocochlear nerve |

*Cavernous sinus thrombosis, see page 90.*

# Sagittal section of the head

**A** *right half, from the left*

**B** *endoscopic view of nasopharynx*

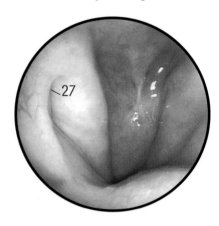

**C** *MRI (magnetic resonance image)*

The falx cerebri (10) separates the two cerebral hemispheres. The tentorium cerebelli (39) separates the posterior parts of the cerebral hemispheres from the cerebellum (5).

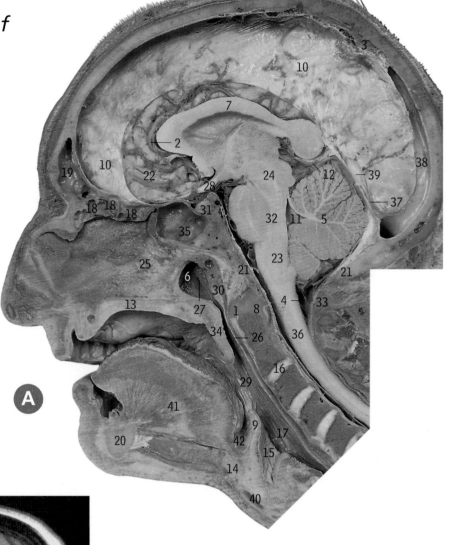

**A**

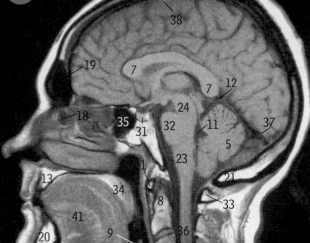

**C**

| | |
|---|---|
| **1** Anterior arch of atlas | **22** Medial surface of right |
| **2** Anterior cerebral artery | cerebral hemisphere |
| **3** Arachnoid granulations | **23** Medulla oblongata |
| **4** Cerebellomedullary cistern | **24** Midbrain |
| (cisterna magna) | **25** Nasal septum (bony part) |
| **5** Cerebellum | **26** Nasopharynx |
| **6** Choana (posterior nasal | **27** Opening of auditory tube |
| aperture) | **28** Optic chiasma |
| **7** Corpus callosum | **29** Oral part of pharynx |
| **8** Dens of axis | (oropharynx) |
| **9** Epiglottis | **30** Pharyngeal (nasopharyngeal) |
| **10** Falx cerebri | tonsil (adenoids) |
| **11** Fourth ventricle | **31** Pituitary gland |
| **12** Great cerebral vein | **32** Pons |
| **13** Hard palate | **33** Posterior arch of atlas |
| **14** Hyoid bone | **34** Soft palate |
| **15** Inlet of larynx | **35** Sphenoidal sinus |
| **16** Intervertebral disc between | **36** Spinal cord |
| axis and third cervical vertebra | **37** Straight sinus |
| **17** Laryngeal part of pharynx | **38** Superior sagittal sinus |
| **18** Left ethmoidal air cells | **39** Tentorium cerebelli |
| **19** Left frontal sinus | **40** Thyroid cartilage |
| **20** Mandible | **41** Tongue |
| **21** Margin of foramen magnum | **42** Vallecula |

*Adenoid (pharyngeal tonsil) enlargement, see page 89.*

## A Cerebral dura mater and cranial nerves

1 Abducent nerve
2 Arachnoid granulations
3 Attached margin of tentorium cerebelli
4 Choana (posterior nasal aperture)
5 Clivus
6 Dens of axis
7 Falx cerebri
8 Free margin of tentorium cerebelli
9 Glossopharyngeal, vagus and accessory nerves
10 Inferior sagittal sinus
11 Internal carotid artery
12 Margin of foramen magnum
13 Medulla oblongata
14 Motor root of facial nerve
15 Nasal septum
16 Oculomotor nerve
17 Olfactory tract
18 Optic nerve
19 Pituitary gland
20 Posterior arch of atlas
21 Rootlets of hypoglossal nerve
22 Sensory root (nervus intermedius) of facial nerve
23 Sphenoidal sinus
24 Sphenoparietal sinus
25 Spinal cord
26 Spinal part of accessory nerve
27 Straight sinus
28 Superior sagittal sinus
29 Tentorium cerebelli
30 Transverse sinus
31 Trigeminal nerve
32 Trochlear nerve
33 Vertebral artery
34 Vestibulocochlear nerve

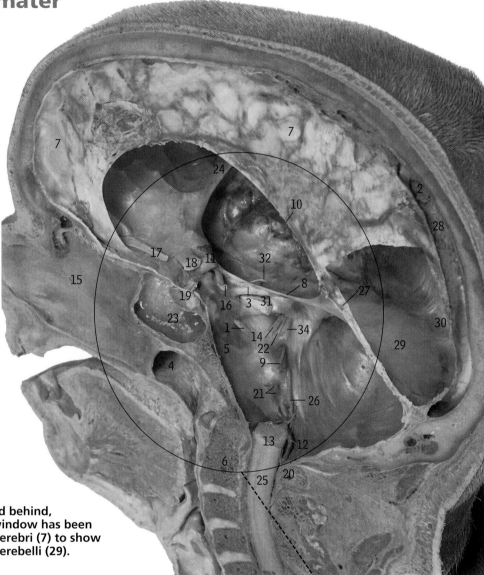

In this oblique view from the left and behind, the brain has been removed and a window has been cut in the posterior part of the falx cerebri (7) to show the upper surface of the tentorium cerebelli (29).

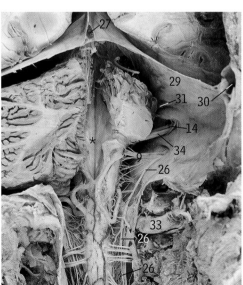

## B Right posterior cranial fossa *viewed from behind*

After removal of posterior skull, dura, upper cervical vertebral laminae, all of right cerebellar hemisphere and much of left to expose the floor of the fourth ventricle (asterisk).

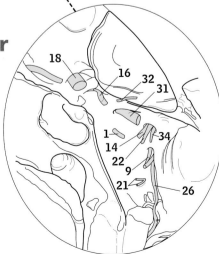

*Subdural haemorrhages, see pages 89–90.*

# Left eye

## A   *surface features*

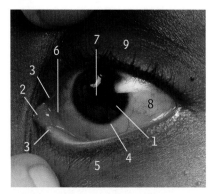

With the eyelids in the normal open position, the lower margin of the upper lid (9) overlaps approximately the upper half of the iris (1); the margin of the lower lid (5) is level with the lower margin of the iris (1).

| | | | |
|---|---|---|---|
| **1** | Iris behind cornea | **5** | Lower lid |
| **2** | Lacrimal caruncle | **6** | Plica semilunaris |
| **3** | Lacrimal papilla | **7** | Pupil behind cornea |
| **4** | Limbus (corneoscleral junction) | **8** | Sclera |
| | | **9** | Upper lid |

The cornea is the transparent anterior part of the outer coat of the eyeball and is continuous with the sclera (8) at the limbus (4).

The pupil (7) is the central aperture of the iris (1), the circular pigmented diaphragm that lies in front of the lens.

Each lacrimal papilla (3) contains the lacrimal punctum, the minute opening of the lacrimal canaliculus (B8) which runs medially to open into the lacrimal sac, lying deep to the medial palpebral ligament (B10) and continuing downwards as the nasolacrimal duct (B12) within the nasolacrimal canal.

## B   Nasolacrimal duct

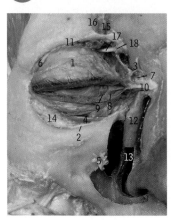

1 Aponeurosis of levator palpebrae superioris
2 Cut edge of orbital septum and periosteum
3 Dorsal nasal artery
4 Inferior oblique
5 Infra-orbital nerve
6 Lacrimal gland
7 Lacrimal sac (upper extremity)
8 Lower lacrimal canaliculus
9 Lower lacrimal papilla and punctum
10 Medial palpebral ligament
11 Muscle fibres of levator palpebrae superioris
12 Nasolacrimal duct
13 Opening of nasolacrimal duct (anterior wall removed) in inferior meatus of nose
14 Orbital fat pad
15 Supra-orbital artery
16 Supra-orbital nerve
17 Tendon of superior oblique
18 Trochlea

In B, the facial muscles and part of the skull have been dissected away to display the nasolacrimal duct (12) opening into the inferior meatus of the nose (13).

1 Anterior cerebral artery
2 Anterior communicating artery
3 Anterior ethmoidal artery and nerve
4 Cribriform plate of ethmoid bone
5 Eyeball
6 Frontal nerve
7 Infratrochlear nerve and ophthalmic artery
8 Internal carotid artery
9 Lacrimal artery
10 Lacrimal gland
11 Lacrimal nerve
12 Lateral rectus
13 Levator palpebrae superioris
14 Medial rectus
15 Middle cerebral artery
16 Nasociliary nerve
17 Ophthalmic artery
18 Optic chiasma
19 Optic nerve (with overlying short ciliary nerves in left orbit)
20 Posterior ciliary artery
21 Superior oblique
22 Superior rectus
23 Supra-orbital artery
24 Supra-orbital nerve
25 Supratrochlear nerve
26 Trochlear nerve

## C   Macrodacryocystogram

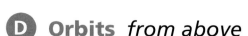

1 Common canaliculus
2 Hard palate
3 Inferior canaliculus
4 Lacrimal catheters
5 Lacrimal sac
6 Nasolacrimal duct
7 Site of lacrimal punctum
8 Superior canaliculus

## D   Orbits *from above*

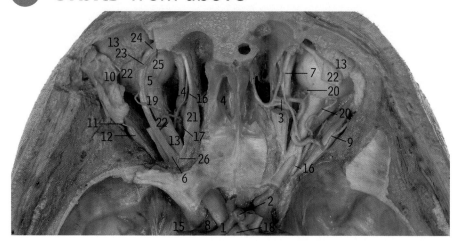

*Central retinal artery occlusion, corneal reflex, meibomian cyst, ophthalmoscopy, pupillary reflex, see pages 90–92.*

# Internal view left orbit

## A *medial*

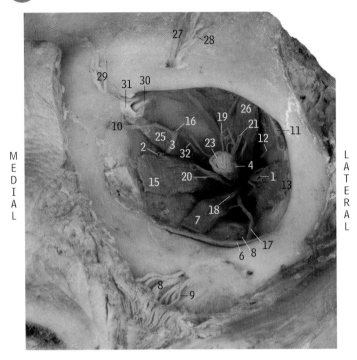

## B *lateral*

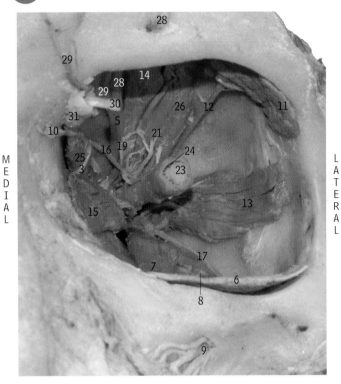

## C *frontal*

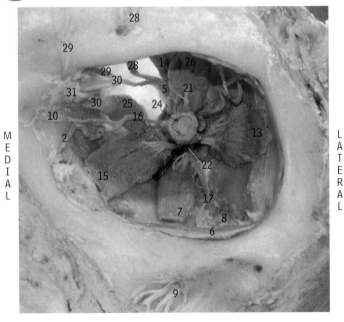

| | | | |
|---|---|---|---|
| **1** | Abducent nerve | **18** | Nerve to inferior rectus |
| **2** | Anterior ethmoidal artery | **19** | Nerve to levator palpebrae superioris |
| **3** | Anterior ethmoidal nerve | **20** | Nerve to medial rectus |
| **4** | Dural sheath of optic nerve | **21** | Nerve to superior rectus |
| **5** | Frontal nerve | **22** | Oculomotor nerve |
| **6** | Inferior oblique | **23** | Optic nerve surrounding central artery of retina |
| **7** | Inferior rectus | **24** | Subarachnoid space |
| **8** | Infra-orbital artery | **25** | Superior oblique |
| **9** | Infra-orbital nerve | **26** | Superior rectus |
| **10** | Infratrochlear nerve | **27** | Supra-orbital artery |
| **11** | Lacrimal gland | **28** | Supra-orbital nerve |
| **12** | Lacrimal nerve | **29** | Supratrochlear nerve |
| **13** | Lateral rectus | **30** | Tendon of superior oblique |
| **14** | Levator palpebrae superioris | **31** | Trochlea |
| **15** | Medial rectus | **32** | Trochlear nerve |
| **16** | Nasociliary nerve | | |
| **17** | Nerve to inferior oblique | | |

# Superior view of right orbit

**A** *superficial*

ANTERIOR

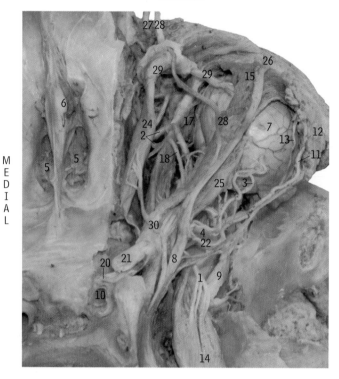

**B** *deep*

ANTERIOR

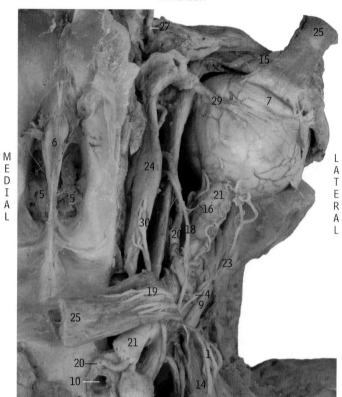

**1** Abducent nerve
**2** Anterior ethmoidal artery and nerve
**3** Ciliary arteries
**4** Ciliary ganglion
**5** Cribriform plate of ethmoid bone
**6** Crista galli
**7** Eyeball
**8** Frontal nerve
**9** Infra-orbital nerve
**10** Internal carotid artery
**11** Lacrimal artery
**12** Lacrimal gland
**13** Lacrimal nerve
**14** Lateral rectus
**15** Levator palpebrae superioris
**16** Long ciliary nerve
**17** Medial rectus
**18** Nasociliary nerve
**19** Nerve to superior rectus
**20** Ophthalmic artery
**21** Optic nerve
**22** Posterior ciliary artery
**23** Short ciliary nerves
**24** Superior oblique
**25** Superior rectus
**26** Supra-orbital nerve
**27** Supratrochlear artery
**28** Supratrochlear nerve
**29** Tendon of superior oblique
**30** Trochlear nerve

*Abducent nerve palsy, oculomotor nerve palsy, trochlear nerve palsy, see pages 90–92.*

# Lateral view of orbit

**A** *superficial* **B** *deep*

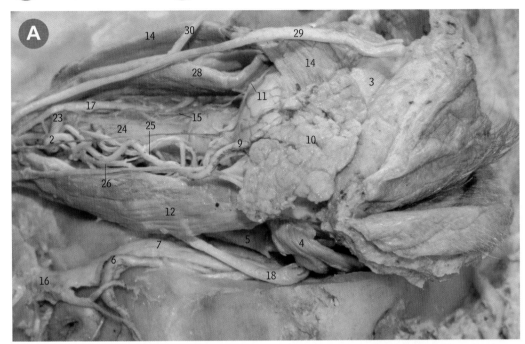

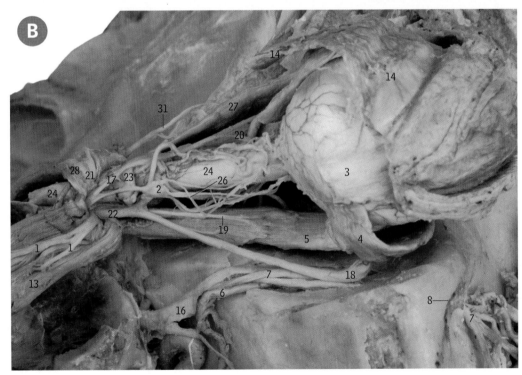

1 Abducent nerve
2 Ciliary ganglion
3 Eyeball
4 Inferior oblique
5 Inferior rectus
6 Infra-orbital artery
7 Infra-orbital nerve
8 Infra-orbital foramen
9 Lacrimal artery
10 Lacrimal gland
11 Lacrimal nerve
12 Lateral rectus
13 Lateral rectus (reflected backwards)
14 Levator palpebrae superioris
15 Long ciliary nerve
16 Maxillary branch of trigeminal nerve
17 Nasociliary nerve
18 Nerve to inferior oblique
19 Nerve to inferior rectus
20 Nerve to medial rectus
21 Nerve to superior rectus
22 Oculomotor nerve, inferior division
23 Ophthalmic artery
24 Optic nerve
25 Short ciliary artery
26 Short ciliary nerves
27 Superior oblique
28 Superior rectus
29 Supra-orbital nerve
30 Supratrochlear nerve
31 Trochlear nerve

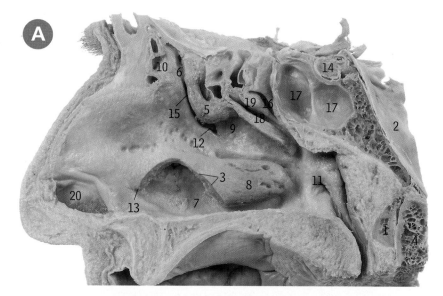

## A Lateral wall of the right nasal cavity

1 Anterior arch of atlas
2 Clivus
3 Cut edge of inferior nasal concha
4 Dens of axis
5 Ethmoidal bulla
6 Ethmoidal infundibulum
7 Inferior meatus
8 Inferior nasal concha
9 Middle meatus
10 Opening of anterior ethmoidal air cells
11 Opening of auditory tube
12 Opening of maxillary sinus
13 Opening of nasolacrimal duct
14 Pituitary gland
15 Semilunar hiatus
16 Sphenoethmoidal recess
17 Sphenoidal sinus
18 Superior meatus
19 Superior nasal concha
20 Vestibule

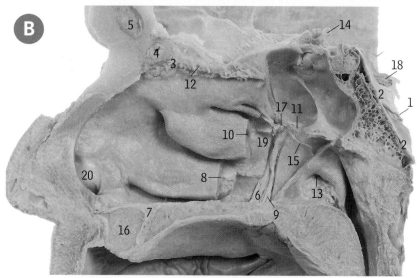

## B Right nasal cavity and pterygopalatine ganglion
*from the left*

1 Abducent nerve
2 Clivus
3 Cribriform plate of ethmoid
4 Ethmoidal air cell (anterior)
5 Frontal sinus
6 Greater palatine nerve
7 Incisive foramen
8 Inferior nasal concha, cut edge of mucoperiosteum
9 Lesser palatine nerves
10 Middle nasal concha, cut
11 Nerve of pterygoid canal
12 Olfactory nerve fibres
13 Opening of auditory tube
14 Optic nerve
15 Pharyngeal branch to ganglion
16 Premaxilla
17 Pterygopalatine ganglion
18 Trigeminal nerve
19 Vertical plate of palatine bone
20 Vestibule

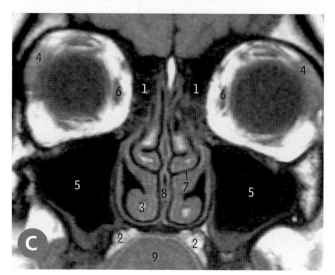

## C Face
*coronal MR image*

1 Ethmoid air cells
2 Hard palate
3 Inferior concha
4 Lacrimal gland
5 Maxillary sinus
6 Medial rectus muscle
7 Middle meatus
8 Nasal septum
9 Tongue

*Middle ear pressure equalisation, nasogastric intubation, see page 91.*

# Right trigeminal nerve branches *from the midline*

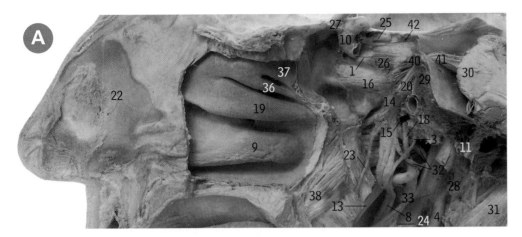

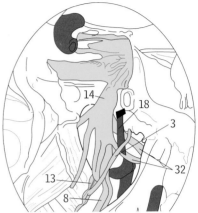

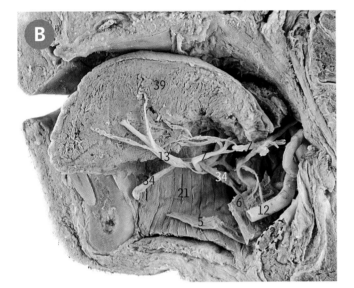

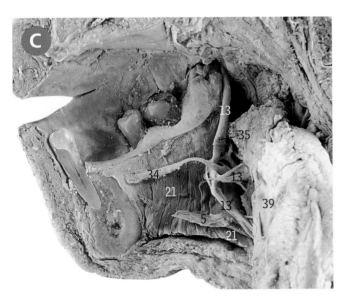

**A** sagittal section just left of midline

**B** **C** sagittal sections just right of the midline after removal of geniohyoid muscle, sublingual gland and oral mucosa. Tongue reflected medially in C.

**1** Abducent nerve
**2** Body of hyoid bone
**3** Chorda tympani
**4** External carotid artery
**5** Geniohyoid
**6** Hyoglossus
**7** Hypoglossal nerve
**8** Inferior alveolar nerve
**9** Inferior nasal concha
**10** Internal carotid artery
**11** Jugular bulb
**12** Lingual artery
**13** Lingual nerve
**14** Mandibular branch of trigeminal nerve
**15** Marker in auditory tube
**16** Maxillary branch of trigeminal nerve
**17** Medial pterygoid
**18** Middle meningeal artery
**19** Middle nasal concha
**20** Motor root of trigeminal nerve
**21** Mylohyoid
**22** Nasal septum (cartilaginous part)
**23** Nerve to medial pterygoid
**24** Nerve to mylohyoid
**25** Oculomotor nerve
**26** Ophthalmic branch of trigeminal nerve
**27** Optic nerve
**28** Parotid gland
**29** Petrous part of temporal bone
**30** Pons
**31** Posterior belly of digastric
**32** Roots of auriculotemporal nerve
**33** Sphenomandibular ligament and maxillary artery
**34** Submandibular duct
**35** Submandibular ganglion
**36** Superior nasal concha
**37** Supreme nasal concha
**38** Tensor veli palatini
**39** Tongue
**40** Trigeminal ganglion
**41** Trigeminal nerve
**42** Trochlear nerve

*Hypoglossal nerve palsy, see page 91.*

## A Right external ear

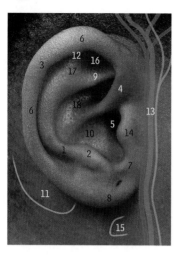

1 Antihelix
2 Antitragus
3 Auricular tubercle
4 Crus of helix
5 External acoustic meatus
6 Helix
7 Intertragic notch
8 Lobule
9 Lower crus of antihelix
10 Lower part of concha
11 Mastoid process
12 Scaphoid fossa
13 Superficial temporal vessels and auriculotemporal nerve
14 Tragus
15 Transverse process of atlas
16 Triangular fossa
17 Upper crus of antihelix
18 Upper part of concha

## B Right tympanic membrane *as seen using auriscope*

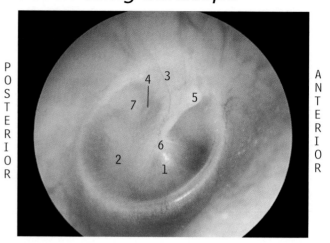

1 Cone of light (light reflex)
2 Pars tensa
3 Pars flaccida
4 Chorda tympani
5 Malleus, lateral process
6 Umbo
7 Incus, long process

## C Right temporal bone and ear

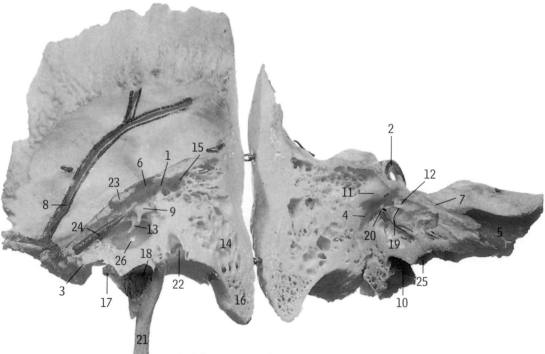

The bone has been bisected and opened out like a book, with some removal of the upper part of the petrous part. The section has opened up the tympanic (middle ear) cavity. On the left side of the figure the lateral wall of the middle ear, which includes the tympanic membrane (26), is seen from the medial side, while on the right the main features of the medial wall are in view.

1 Aditus to mastoid antrum
2 Anterior (superior) semicircular canal
3 Bony part of auditory tube
4 Canal for facial nerve (yellow)
5 Carotid canal (red)
6 Epitympanic recess
7 Groove for greater petrosal nerve (yellow)
8 Groove for middle meningeal vessels
9 Incus
10 Jugular bulb (blue)
11 Lateral semicircular canal
12 Lesser petrosal nerve
13 Malleus
14 Mastoid air cells
15 Mastoid antrum
16 Mastoid process
17 Part of carotid canal (red)
18 Part of jugular bulb (blue)
19 Promontory with overlying tympanic plexus
20 Stapes in oval window and stapedius muscle
21 Styloid process
22 Stylomastoid foramen
23 Tegmen tympani
24 Tensor tympani muscle in its canal
25 Tympanic branch of glossopharyngeal nerve entering its canaliculus
26 Tympanic membrane

*Hyperacuisis, otalgia (referred pain), see page 91.*

# Ear *right temporal bone*

**A** middle ear and the facial nerve and branches

**B** enlarged view of A

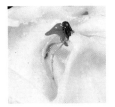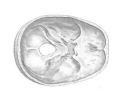

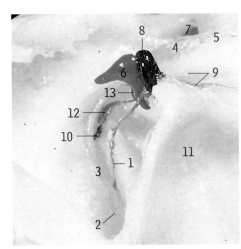

This dissection is seen from the right and above, looking forwards and medially. Bone has been removed to show the upper parts of the malleus (8) and incus (6), which normally project up into the epitympanic recess. The upper part of the facial canal (2) has been opened to show the facial nerve (3) giving off the chorda tympani (1) and the nerve to stapedius (10). The geniculate ganglion of the facial nerve (4) is seen giving off the greater petrosal nerve (5).

1 Chorda tympani
2 Facial canal leading to stylomastoid foramen
3 Facial nerve
4 Geniculate ganglion of facial nerve
5 Greater petrosal nerve
6 Incus
7 Internal acoustic meatus
8 Malleus
9 Margin of auditory tube
10 Nerve to stapedius
11 Paraffin wax (for support) overlying tympanic membrane
12 Stapedius
13 Stapes

> The stapedius (12) tendon emerges from a small conical projection on the posterior wall of the tympanic cavity, the pyramid (here dissected away).

# Ear

**C** right temporal bone; middle ear and inner ear, enlarged

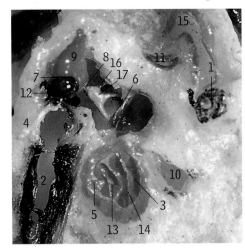

This dissection is viewed from above, looking slightly backwards and laterally. Within the cavity of the middle ear are the three auditory ossicles – malleus (12), incus (9) and stapes (17). The tympanic membrane and external acoustic meatus are not seen but lie below the label 7. The cochlea has been opened up to show its internal bony structure (3, 5, 13 and 14).

1 Anterior (superior) semicircular canal
2 Auditory tube
3 Bony canal of cochlea
4 Chorda tympani
5 Cupola of cochlea
6 Footplate of stapes in oval window of vestibule
7 Incudomalleolar joint
8 Incudostapedial joint
9 Incus
10 Internal acoustic meatus
11 Lateral semicircular canal
12 Malleus
13 Modiolus of cochlea
14 Osseous spiral lamina of cochlea
15 Posterior semicircular canal
16 Stapedius tendon
17 Stapes

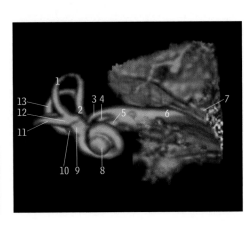

# Right ear

**D** from above, diagram of parts

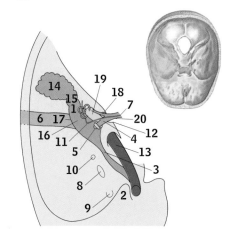

1 Aditus to mastoid antrum
2 Anterior clinoid process
3 Auditory tube
4 Cochlear nerve
5 Cochlear part of inner ear
6 External acoustic meatus
7 Facial nerve
8 Foramen ovale
9 Foramen rotundum
10 Foramen spinosum
11 Geniculate ganglion of facial nerve
12 Internal acoustic meatus
13 Internal carotid artery emerging from foramen lacerum
14 Mastoid air cells
15 Mastoid antrum
16 Middle ear
17 Tympanic membrane
18 Vestibular nerve
19 Vestibular part of inner ear
20 Vestibulocochlear nerve

**E** Inner ear CT (3D reconstruction)

1 Anterior (superior) semicircular canals (SSC)
2 Common crus
3 Labyrinthine segment of facial nerve
4 Superior vestibular nerve
5 Cochlear nerve
6 Vestibulocochlear nerve
7 Abducent nerve CN VI
8 Cochlea
9 Vestibule
10 Oval window
11 Lateral SCC
12 Lateral SCC, ampulla
13 Posterior SCC

## A Cranial vault and falx *from below*

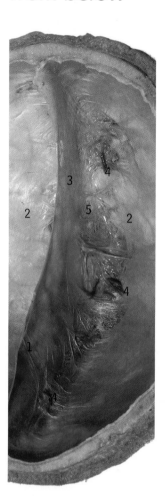

Looking up into the cranial vault from below, the falx cerebri (3) is seen to be continuous with the dura over the vault (2), and has been cut off at the back (1) from the tentorium cerebelli.

1 Cut edge of falx cerebri
2 Dura mater over cranial vault
3 Falx cerebri
4 Superior cerebral veins
5 Superior sagittal sinus

## B Brain *from above*

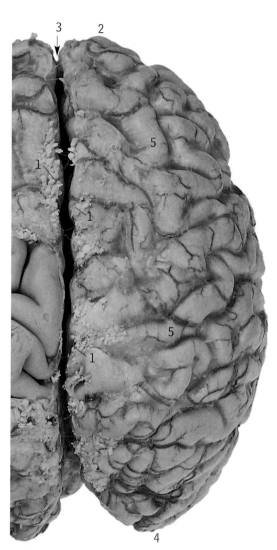

The right cerebral hemisphere is seen with the overlying arachnoid mater and arachnoid granulations (1) adjacent to the longitudinal fissure (3). Over the small part of the left hemisphere shown, a window has been cut in the arachnoid revealing the subarachnoid space.

1 Arachnoid granulations
2 Frontal pole
3 Longitudinal fissure
4 Occipital pole
5 Superolateral surface

## C Brain *right cerebral hemisphere, from above*

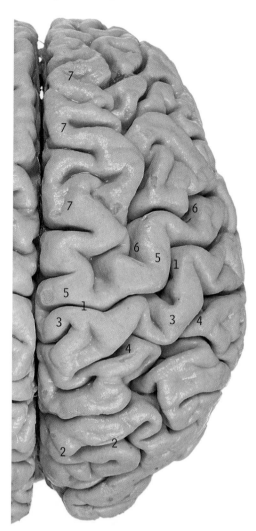

Removal of the arachnoid and the underlying vessels displays the gyri and sulci. Only a small number are named here; the most important are the central sulcus (1) and the precentral and postcentral gyri (5 and 3).

1 Central sulcus
2 Parieto-occipital sulcus
3 Postcentral gyrus
4 Postcentral sulcus
5 Precentral gyrus
6 Precentral sulcus
7 Superior frontal gyrus

*Subarachnoid haemorrhage, see page 92.*

# Brain Ⓐ *from the right* Ⓑ *right cerebral hemisphere, from the right*

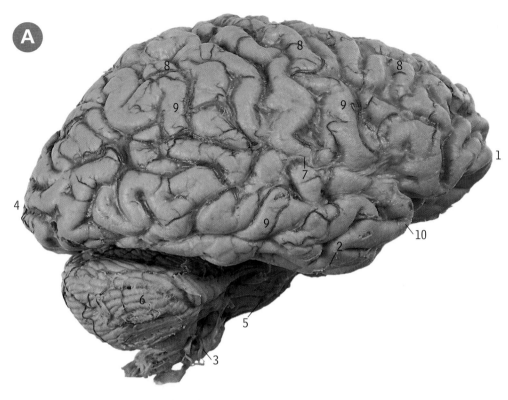

**Ⓐ**

As in B (page 72), the arachnoid mater has been left intact and vessels are seen beneath it; the larger ones are veins (as at 7).

1 Frontal pole
2 Inferior cerebral veins
3 Medulla oblongata and vertebral artery
4 Occipital pole
5 Pons and basilar artery
6 Right cerebellar hemisphere
7 Superficial middle cerebral vein overlying lateral sulcus
8 Superior cerebral veins
9 Superolateral surface of right cerebral hemisphere
10 Temporal pole

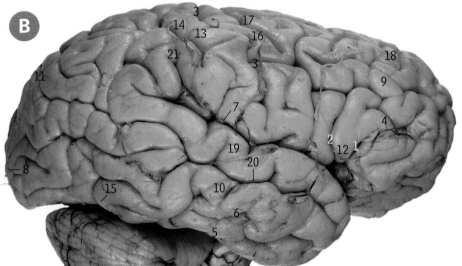

**Ⓑ**

The arachnoid mater has been removed, leaving some of the larger branches of the middle cerebral artery (unlabelled) after they have emerged from the lateral sulcus (7). Only the main gyri and sulci are named here: the most important are the precentral and postcentral gyri (16 and 13) and the central and lateral sulci (3 and 7).

1 Anterior ramus of lateral sulcus
2 Ascending ramus of lateral sulcus
3 Central sulcus
4 Inferior frontal gyrus
5 Inferior temporal gyrus
6 Inferior temporal sulcus
7 Lateral sulcus (posterior ramus)
8 Lunate sulcus
9 Middle frontal gyrus
10 Middle temporal gyrus
11 Parieto-occipital sulcus
12 Pars triangularis
13 Postcentral gyrus
14 Postcentral sulcus
15 Pre-occipital notch
16 Precentral gyrus
17 Precentral sulcus
18 Superior frontal gyrus
19 Superior temporal gyrus
20 Superior temporal sulcus
21 Supramarginal gyrus

The central sulcus (C1 (page 72) and B3, above) marks the boundary between the frontal and parietal lobes.

An arbitrary line from the pre-occipital notch (B15) to the parieto-occipital sulcus (B11) marks the boundary between the parietal and occipital lobes, and the part of the hemisphere in front of this line and below the lateral sulcus (strictly, the posterior ramus of the lateral sulcus, B7) forms the temporal lobe.

The precentral and postcentral gyri (B16 and 13) contain the classically described 'motor' and 'sensory' areas of the cortex.

The motor speech areas (usually in the left cerebral hemisphere) are in the region of the ascending and anterior rami of the lateral sulcus and the pars triangularis (B2, 1 and 12).

The auditory areas of the cortex probably comprise parts of the superior temporal gyrus (B19), especially the upper surface of it within the lateral sulcus (B7).

## A Brain *from below*

This is the view of the under-surface of the brain as typically seen when first removed from the skull, without any dissection. Arachnoid mater, torn in places and with blood vessels beneath it, remains on the outer surface.

1 Abducent nerve
2 Anterior perforated substance
3 Arachnoid mater overlying mamillary bodies
4 Basilar artery
5 Cerebellar hemisphere
6 Crus of cerebral peduncle (midbrain)
7 Facial nerve
8 Frontal pole
9 Gyrus rectus
10 Inferior surface of frontal lobe
11 Inferior surface of temporal lobe
12 Internal carotid artery
13 Longitudinal fissure
14 Medulla oblongata
15 Oculomotor nerve
16 Olfactory bulb
17 Olfactory tract
18 Optic chiasma
19 Optic nerve
20 Pituitary stalk (infundibulum)
21 Pons
22 Posterior communicating artery
23 Spinal part of accessory nerve
24 Temporal pole
25 Trigeminal nerve
26 Uncus
27 Vertebral artery
28 Vestibulocochlear nerve

## B Optic tract and geniculate bodies *from below*

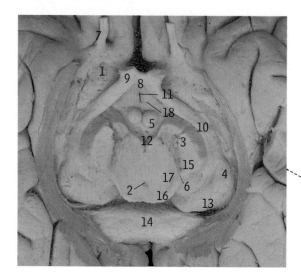

The brainstem has been mostly removed, leaving only the upper part of the midbrain. The most medial parts of each cerebral hemisphere have also been dissected away. To find the geniculate bodies (4 and 6), which are on the under-surface of the posterior part (pulvinar, 13) of the thalamus, identify the optic chiasma (8) and then follow the optic tract (10) backwards round the side of the midbrain (3).

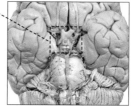

1 Anterior perforated substance
2 Aqueduct of midbrain
3 Crus of midbrain
4 Lateral geniculate body
5 Mamillary body
6 Medial geniculate body
7 Olfactory tract
8 Optic chiasma
9 Optic nerve
10 Optic tract
11 Pituitary stalk (infundibulum)
12 Posterior perforated substance
13 Pulvinar of thalamus
14 Splenium of corpus callosum
15 Substantia nigra of midbrain
16 Tectum of midbrain
17 Tegmentum of midbrain
18 Tuber cinereum

## A  **Brain** *from below*

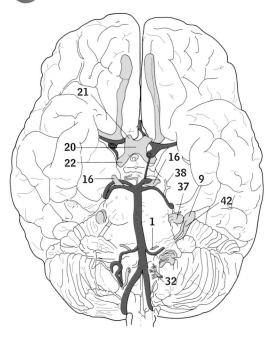

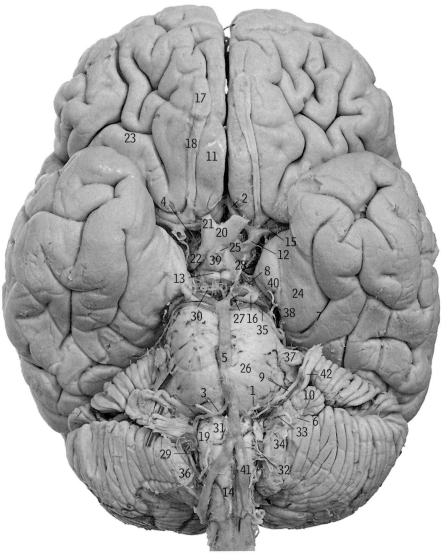

1  Abducent nerve
2  Anterior cerebral artery
3  Anterior inferior cerebellar artery
4  Anterior perforated substance
5  Basilar artery
6  Choroid plexus from lateral recess of
   fourth ventricle
7  Collateral sulcus
8  Crus of cerebral peduncle
9  Facial nerve
10  Flocculus of cerebellum
11  Gyrus rectus
12  Internal carotid artery
13  Mamillary body
14  Medulla oblongata
15  Middle cerebral artery
16  Oculomotor nerve
17  Olfactory bulb
18  Olfactory tract
19  Olive of medulla oblongata
20  Optic chiasma
21  Optic nerve
22  Optic tract
23  Orbital sulcus
24  Parahippocampal gyrus
25  Pituitary stalk (infundibulum)
26  Pons
27  Posterior cerebral artery
28  Posterior communicating artery
29  Posterior inferior cerebellar artery
30  Posterior perforated substance
31  Pyramid of medulla oblongata
32  Rootlets of hypoglossal nerve
   (superficial to marker)
33  Roots of glossopharyngeal,
   vagus and accessory nerves
34  Spinal part of accessory nerve
35  Superior cerebellar artery
36  Tonsil of cerebellum
37  Trigeminal nerve
38  Trochlear nerve
39  Tuber cinereum and median eminence
40  Uncus
41  Vertebral artery
42  Vestibulocochlear nerve

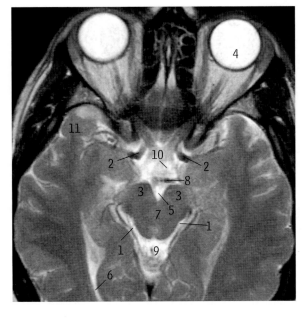

## B  **Brain**
*axial MR image
showing cisterns*

1  Ambient cistern
2  Carotid artery, internal
3  Cerebral peduncle
4  Globe
5  Interpeduncular cistern
6  Lateral ventricle, posterior horn
7  Midbrain
8  Posterior cerebral artery
9  Quadrigeminal cistern
10  Suprachiasmatic cistern
11  Temporal lobe

## A  **Right half of the brain** *in a midline sagittal section, from the left*

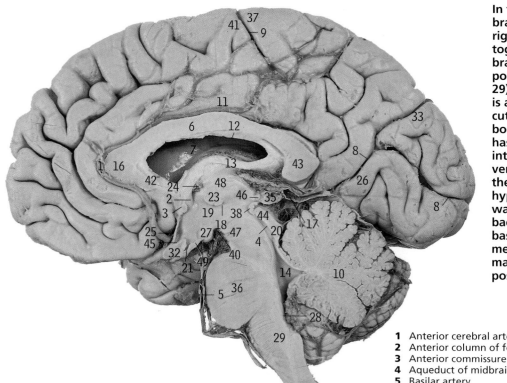

In this typical half-section of the brain, the medial surface of the right cerebral hemisphere is seen, together with the sectioned brainstem (midbrain, 4, 20, 44, 47; pons, 36; and medulla oblongata, 29). The septum pellucidum, which is a midline structure and whose cut edge (12) is seen below the body of the corpus callosum (6), has been removed to show the interior of the body of the lateral ventricle (7). The third ventricle has the thalamus (48) and hypothalamus (19) in its lateral wall, while in its floor from front to back are the optic chiasma (32), the base of the pituitary stalk (21), the median eminence (49), the mamillary bodies (27), and the posterior perforated substance (40).

## B  **Carotid arteriogram**
*digitally subtracted arterial phase of carotid arteriogram, lateral projection*

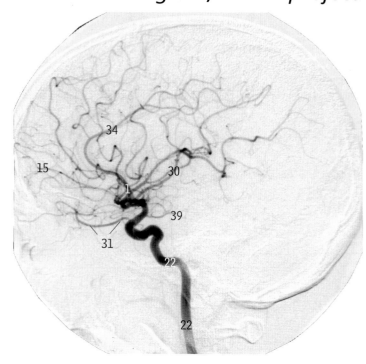

| | | | |
|---|---|---|---|
| **1** | Anterior cerebral artery | **27** | Mamillary body |
| **2** | Anterior column of fornix | **28** | Median aperture of |
| **3** | Anterior commissure | | fourth ventricle |
| **4** | Aqueduct of midbrain | **29** | Medulla oblongata |
| **5** | Basilar artery | **30** | Middle cerebral artery |
| **6** | Body of corpus callosum | **31** | Ophthalmic artery |
| **7** | Body of lateral ventricle | **32** | Optic chiasma |
| **8** | Calcarine sulcus | **33** | Parieto-occipital sulcus |
| **9** | Central sulcus | **34** | Pericallosal artery |
| **10** | Cerebellum | **35** | Pineal body |
| **11** | Cingulate gyrus | **36** | Pons |
| **12** | Cut edge of septum | **37** | Postcentral gyrus |
| | pellucidum | **38** | Posterior commissure |
| **13** | Fornix | **39** | Posterior communicating |
| **14** | Fourth ventricle | | artery |
| **15** | Frontopolar artery | **40** | Posterior perforated |
| **16** | Genu of corpus callosum | | substance |
| **17** | Great cerebral vein | **41** | Precentral gyrus |
| **18** | Hypothalamic sulcus | **42** | Rostrum of corpus |
| **19** | Hypothalamus | | callosum |
| **20** | Inferior colliculus of | **43** | Splenium of corpus |
| | midbrain | | callosum |
| **21** | Infundibular recess (base | **44** | Superior colliculus of |
| | of pituitary stalk) | | midbrain |
| **22** | Internal carotid artery | **45** | Supra-optic recess |
| **23** | Interthalamic connexion | **46** | Suprapineal recess |
| **24** | Interventricular foramen | **47** | Tegmentum of midbrain |
| | and choroid plexus | **48** | Thalamus |
| **25** | Lamina terminalis | **49** | Tuber cinereum and |
| **26** | Lingual gyrus | | median eminence |

The third ventricle is the cavity which has in its lateral wall the thalamus (A48) and hypothalamus (A19).

The fourth ventricle (A14) is largely between the pons (A36) and cerebellum (A10), although its lower end is behind the upper part of the medulla oblongata (A29) (see page 78, D).

The aqueduct of the midbrain (A4) connects the third and fourth ventricles; cerebrospinal fluid normally flows through it from the third to the fourth ventricle.

The interventricular foramen (A24) connects the third to the lateral ventricle, and is bounded in front by the anterior column of the fornix (A2) and behind by the thalamus (A48).

## C Brain *medial surface of the right cerebral hemisphere*

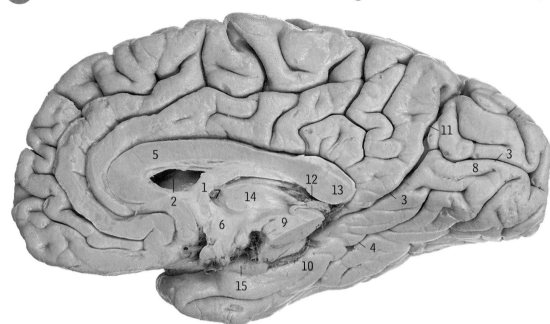

The brainstem has been removed through the midbrain (9) so that the lower part of the hemisphere can be seen; in A, on page 76, the brainstem hides this part.

1 Anterior column of fornix
2 Anterior horn of lateral ventricle
3 Calcarine sulcus
4 Collateral sulcus
5 Corpus callosum
6 Hypothalamus in lateral wall of third ventricle
7 Interventricular foramen
8 Lingual gyrus
9 Midbrain
10 Parahippocampal gyrus
11 Parieto-occipital sulcus
12 Pineal body
13 Splenium of corpus callosum
14 Thalamus in lateral wall of third ventricle
15 Uncus

## D Cranial nerves

## E Endoscopy – base of brain

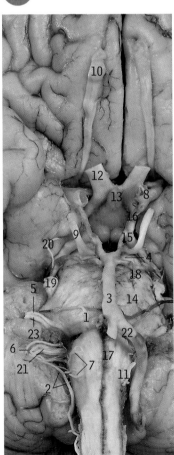

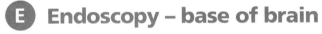

In this ventral view of the central part of the brain, the right vertebral artery (on the left of the picture) has been removed almost at the junction with its fellow (22). The filaments of the first nerve (olfactory) are not seen entering the olfactory bulb (10) as they are torn off when removing the brain. The roots forming the glossopharyngeal, vagus and accessory nerves (6, 21 and 2) cannot be clearly identified from one another, but the spinal part of the accessory nerve (2) is seen running up beside the medulla to join the cranial part.

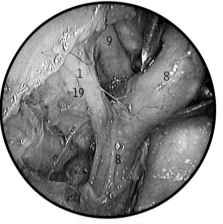

1 Abducent nerve
2 Accessory nerve, spinal root
3 Basilar artery
4 Crus of cerebral peduncle
5 Facial nerve
6 Glossopharyngeal nerve
7 Hypoglossal nerve
8 Internal carotid artery
9 Oculomotor nerve
10 Olfactory bulb
11 Olive of medulla oblongata
12 Optic nerve
13 Pituitary stalk
14 Pons
15 Posterior cerebral artery
16 Posterior communicating artery
17 Pyramid of medulla oblongata
18 Superior cerebellar artery
19 Trigeminal nerve
20 Trochlear nerve
21 Vagus nerve
22 Vertebral artery
23 Vestibulocochlear nerve

The oculomotor nerve (D9) emerges on the medial side of the crus of the cerebral peduncle (D4), and the trochlear nerve (D20) winds round the lateral side of the peduncle. Both nerves pass between the posterior cerebral and superior cerebellar arteries (D15 and 18).

The trochlear nerve (D20) is the only cranial nerve to emerge from the dorsal surface of the brainstem.

The trigeminal nerve (D19) emerges from the lateral side of the pons (D14).

The abducent nerve (D1) emerges between the pons and the pyramid (D14 and 17).

The facial and vestibulocochlear nerves (D5 and 23) emerge from the lateral pontomedullary angle.

The glossopharyngeal and vagus nerves (D6, 21) and the cranial root of the accessory nerve emerge from the medulla oblongata lateral to the olive (D11).

The hypoglossal nerve (D7) emerges as two series of rootlets from the medulla oblongata between the pyramid (D17) and the olive (D11).

The spinal part of the accessory nerve emerges from the lateral surface of the upper five or six cervical segments of the spinal cord, dorsal to the denticulate ligament (page 79, G5).

# Arteries of the base of the brain Ⓐ *injected arteries*
Ⓑ *arterial circle (Willis) and basilar artery*

Ⓒ *MR angiogram of arterial circle (Willis)*

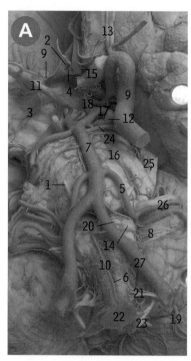

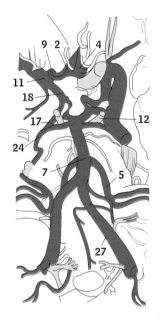

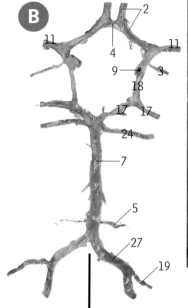

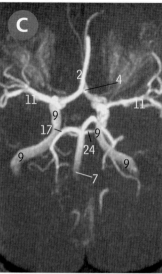

Part of the right cerebral hemisphere (on the left of the picture) has been removed to show the right middle cerebral artery (11).

The anastomosing vessels have been removed from the base of the brain and spread out in their relative positions.

# Ⓓ *Intracranial endoscopy at the base of the brain*

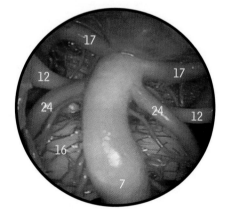

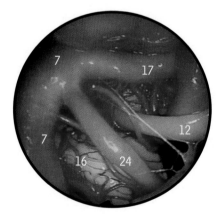

| | |
|---|---|
| **1** Abducent nerve | **8** Filaments of glossopharyngeal, vagus and accessory nerves |
| **2** Anterior cerebral | |
| **3** Anterior choroidal | |
| **4** Anterior communicating | **9** Internal carotid |
| **5** Anterior inferior cerebellar | **10** Medulla oblongata |
| | **11** Middle cerebral |
| **6** Anterior spinal | **12** Oculomotor nerve |
| **7** Basilar with pontine branches | **13** Olfactory tract |
| | **14** Olive |

| | |
|---|---|
| **15** Optic nerve | **23** Spinal part of accessory nerve |
| **16** Pons | |
| **17** Posterior cerebral | **24** Superior cerebellar |
| **18** Posterior communicating | **25** Trigeminal nerve |
| **19** Posterior inferior cerebellar | **26** Unusually large branch of 5 overlying facial and vestibulocochlear nerves |
| **20** Pyramid | |
| **21** Rootlets of first cervical nerve | |
| **22** Spinal cord | **27** Vertebral |

## F Brainstem and floor of the fourth ventricle

In this view of the dorsal surface of the brainstem, it has been cut off from the rest of the brain at the top of the midbrain, just above the superior colliculi (15). The cerebellum has been removed by transecting the superior (14), middle (12) and inferior (6) cerebellar peduncles.

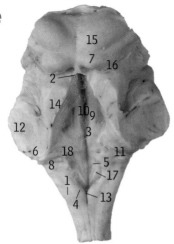

1 Cuneate tubercle
2 Cut edge of superior medullary velum
3 Facial colliculus
4 Gracile tubercle
5 Hypoglossal triangle
6 Inferior cerebellar peduncle
7 Inferior colliculus
8 Lateral recess
9 Medial eminence
10 Median sulcus
11 Medullary striae
12 Middle cerebellar peduncle
13 Obex
14 Superior cerebellar peduncle
15 Superior colliculus
16 Trochlear nerve
17 Vagal triangle
18 Vestibular area

## G Brainstem and upper part of the spinal cord *from behind after removal of vertebrae*

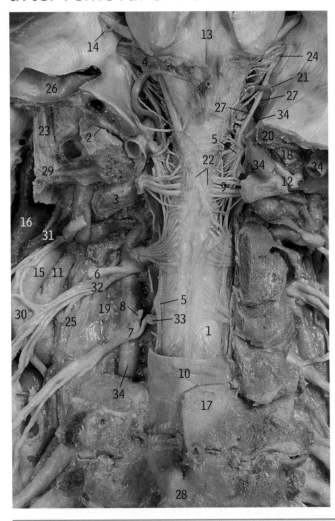

The posterior parts of the skull and upper vertebrae have been removed to show the continuity of the brainstem with the spinal cord, from which dorsal nerve rootlets are seen to emerge (as at 9). The spinal part of the accessory nerve (27) runs up through the foramen magnum (20) to join the cranial part in the jugular foramen (24). Ventral nerve rootlets (as at 33), ventral to the denticulate ligament (5), unite to form a ventral nerve root which joins with a dorsal nerve root (8, whose formative rootlets dorsal to the ligament have been cut off from the cord in order to make the ventral roots visible) to form a spinal nerve immediately beyond the dorsal root ganglion (7). The nerve immediately divides into ventral and dorsal rami (as at 32 and 6).

1 Arachnoid mater
2 Atlanto-occipital joint
3 Capsule of lateral atlanto-axial joint
4 Choroid plexus emerging from lateral recess of fourth ventricle
5 Denticulate ligament
6 Dorsal ramus of third cervical nerve
7 Dorsal root ganglion of fourth cervical nerve
8 Dorsal root of fourth cervical nerve
9 Dorsal rootlets of second cervical nerve
10 Dura mater
11 External carotid artery
12 First cervical nerve and posterior arch of atlas
13 Floor of the fourth vehicle
14 Internal acoustic meatus with facial and vestibulocochlear nerves and labyrinthine artery
15 Internal carotid artery
16 Internal jugular vein
17 Lamina of sixth cervical vertebra
18 Lateral mass of atlas
19 Longus capitis
20 Margin of foramen magnum
21 Posterior inferior cerebellar artery
22 Posterior spinal arteries
23 Rectus capitis lateralis
24 Roots of glossopharyngeal, vagus and cranial part of accessory nerves and jugular foramen
25 Scalenus anterior
26 Sigmoid sinus
27 Spinal part of accessory nerve
28 Spinous process of seventh cervical vertebra
29 Transverse process of atlas
30 Vagus nerve
31 Vein from vertebral venous plexuses
32 Ventral ramus of third cervical nerve
33 Ventral rootlets of fourth cervical nerve
34 Vertebral artery

The lower part of the diamond-shaped floor of the fourth ventricle containing the hypoglossal and vagal triangles (F5 and 17) is part of the medulla oblongata; the rest of the floor is part of the pons.

The gracile and cuneate tubercles (F4 and 1) are caused by the underlying gracile and cuneate nuclei, where the fibres of the gracile and cuneate tracts (posterior white columns) end by synapsing with the cells of the nuclei. The fibres from these cells form the medial lemniscus which runs through the brainstem to the thalamus.

The facial colliculus (F3), at the lower end of the medial eminence (F9) in the floor of the fourth ventricle, is caused by fibres of the facial nerve overlying the abducent nerve nucleus; it is not produced by the facial nerve nucleus, which lies at a deeper level in the pons.

After emerging from the foramen in the transverse process of the atlas the vertebral artery (G34) winds backwards round the lateral mass of the atlas (G18) on its posterior arch before turning upwards to enter the skull.

# Cerebral hemispheres  *sectioned horizontally*  *axial MR image*

Viewed from above, the left cerebral hemisphere has been sectioned on a level with the interventricular foramen (17), and that on the right about 1.5 cm higher. The most important feature seen in the left hemisphere is the internal capsule (3, 13 and 23), situated between the caudate (14) and lentiform (18 and 19) nuclei and the thalamus (25). On the right side, a large part of the corpus callosum (11) has been removed, so opening up the lateral ventricle (6) from above and showing the caudate nucleus (14 and 4) arching backwards over the thalamus (25), with the thalamostriate vein (24) and choroid plexus (9) in the shallow groove between them.

1 Anterior column of fornix
2 Anterior horn of lateral ventricle
3 Anterior limb of internal capsule
4 Body of caudate nucleus
5 Body of fornix
6 Body of lateral ventricle
7 Bulb
8 Calcar avis
9 Choroid plexus
10 Claustrum
11 Corpus callosum
12 Forceps minor (corpus callosum)
13 Genu of internal capsule
14 Head of caudate nucleus
15 Inferior horn of lateral ventricle
16 Insula
17 Interventricular foramen
18 Lentiform nucleus: globus pallidus
19 Lentiform nucleus: putamen
20 Lunate sulcus
21 Optic radiation
22 Posterior horn of lateral ventricle
23 Posterior limb of internal capsule
24 Thalamostriate vein
25 Thalamus
26 Third ventricle
27 Visual area of cortex

The anterior limb of the internal capsule (3) is bounded medially by the head of the caudate nucleus (14) and laterally by the lentiform nucleus (putamen and globus pallidus, 18 and 19).

The genu of the internal capsule (13) lies at the most medial edge of the globus pallidus (18).

The posterior limb of the internal capsule (23) is bounded medially by the thalamus (25) and laterally by the lentiform nucleus (18 and 19).

Corticonuclear fibres (motor fibres from the cerebral cortex to the motor nuclei of cranial nerves) pass through the genu of the internal capsule (13).

Corticospinal fibres (motor fibres from the cerebral cortex to anterior horn cells of the spinal cord) pass through the anterior two-thirds of the posterior limb of the internal capsule (23).

The genu and the posterior limb of the internal capsule, supplied by the striate branches of the anterior and middle cerebral arteries, are of the greatest clinical importance as they are the common sites for cerebral haemorrhage or thrombosis ('stroke').

# Brain Ⓐ *coronal section, from the front* Ⓑ *coronal MR image*

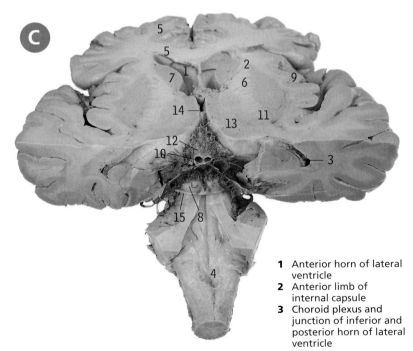

This coronal section is not quite vertical but passes slightly backwards, through the third ventricle (25) and bodies of the lateral ventricles (3) from a level about 0.5 cm behind the interventricular foramina, and down through the pons (17) and the pyramid of the medulla (19). It has been cut in this way to show the path of the important corticospinal (motor) fibres passing down through the internal capsule (11) and pons (17) to form the pyramid of the medulla (19). Compare with features in the MR image.

| | |
|---|---|
| **1** Body of caudate nucleus | **6** Choroid plexus of third ventricle |
| **2** Body of fornix | **7** Choroidal fissure |
| **3** Body of lateral ventricle | **8** Corpus callosum |
| **4** Choroid plexus of inferior horn of lateral ventricle | **9** Hippocampus |
| **5** Choroid plexus of lateral ventricle | **10** Insula |
| | **11** Internal capsule |
| | **12** Interpeduncular cistern |

| | |
|---|---|
| **13** Lentiform nucleus: globus pallidus | **19** Pyramid of medulla oblongata |
| **14** Lentiform nucleus: putamen | **20** Septum pellucidum |
| **15** Olive of medulla oblongata | **21** Substantia nigra |
| **16** Optic tract | **22** Tail of caudate nucleus |
| **17** Pons | **23** Thalamostriate vein |
| **18** Posterior cerebral artery | **24** Thalamus |
| | **25** Third ventricle |

# Ⓒ Sectioned cerebral hemispheres and the brainstem
## *from above and behind*

The cerebral hemispheres have been sectioned horizontally just above the level of the interventricular foramina, and the posterior parts of the hemispheres have been removed, together with the whole of the cerebellum, to show the tela choroidea (12) of the posterior part of the roof of the third ventricle and the underlying internal cerebral veins (10).

| | |
|---|---|
| **1** Anterior horn of lateral ventricle | **4** Floor of fourth ventricle |
| **2** Anterior limb of internal capsule | **5** Forceps minor |
| **3** Choroid plexus and junction of inferior and posterior horn of lateral ventricle | **6** Genu of internal capsule |
| | **7** Head of caudate nucleus |
| | **8** Inferior colliculus |
| | **9** Insula |

| | |
|---|---|
| **10** Internal cerebral vein | |
| **11** Posterior limb of internal capsule | |
| **12** Tela choroidea of roof of third ventricle | |
| **13** Thalamus | |
| **14** Third ventricle | |
| **15** Trochlear nerve | |

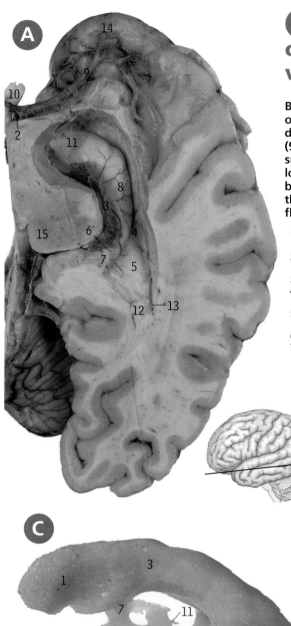

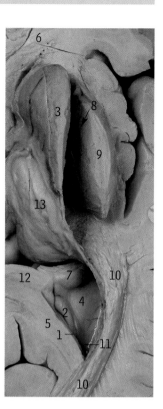

## A Inferior horn of right lateral ventricle

Brain substance above the front part of the lateral sulcus has been removed, displaying the middle cerebral artery (9) running laterally over the upper surface of the front of the temporal lobe (14). Part of the temporal lobe has been opened up from above to show the hippocampus (11 and 8) in the floor of the inferior horn.

| | | | |
|---|---|---|---|
| **1** | Anterior cerebral artery | **8** | Hippocampus |
| **2** | Anterior choroidal artery | **9** | Middle cerebral artery |
| **3** | Choroid plexus | **10** | Optic nerve |
| **4** | Collateral eminence | **11** | Pes hippocampi |
| **5** | Collateral trigone | **12** | Posterior horn |
| **6** | Fimbria | **13** | Tapetum |
| **7** | Fornix | **14** | Temporal pole of temporal lobe |
| | | **15** | Thalamus |

## B Right cerebral hemisphere dissection *from above*

Much of the cerebral substance has been dissected away to show the caudate nucleus (3), thalamus (13) and lentiform nucleus (9). The intervening gap (8) is occupied by the internal capsule. The optic radiation (10) has also been dissected out; it runs backwards lateral to the posterior horn of the lateral ventricle. Compare this three-dimensional view of these structures with the brain sections on page 81.

| | | | | | |
|---|---|---|---|---|---|
| **1** | Bulb | **6** | Forceps minor | **11** | Posterior horn of lateral ventricle |
| **2** | Calcar avis | **7** | Fornix | **12** | Splenium of corpus callosum |
| **3** | Caudate nucleus | **8** | Internal capsule | **13** | Thalamus |
| **4** | Collateral trigone | **9** | Lentiform nucleus | | |
| **5** | Forceps major | **10** | Optic radiation | | |

## C Cast of the cerebral ventricles *from the left*

In this side view, the left lateral ventricle largely overlaps the right one.

| | | | |
|---|---|---|---|
| **1** | Anterior horn of lateral ventricle | **8** | Lateral recess |
| **2** | Aqueduct of midbrain | **9** | Posterior horn of lateral ventricle |
| **3** | Body of lateral ventricle | **10** | Supra-optic recess of third ventricle |
| **4** | Fourth ventricle | **11** | Suprapineal recess of third ventricle |
| **5** | Inferior horn of lateral ventricle | **12** | Third ventricle (with gap for interthalamic connexion) |
| **6** | Infundibular recess of third ventricle | | |
| **7** | Interventricular foramen | | |

The third ventricle (C12) communicates at its upper front end with each lateral ventricle through the interventricular foramen (C7).

The main part of the lateral ventricle is the body (C3). The part in front of the interventricular foramen (C7) is the anterior horn (C1), which extends into the frontal lobe of the brain. At its posterior end, the body divides into the posterior horn (C9), which extends backwards into the occipital lobe, and the inferior horn (C5), which passes downwards and forwards into the temporal lobe.

The lower posterior part of the third ventricle (C12) communicates with the fourth ventricle (C4) through the aqueduct of the midbrain (C2).

The floor of the inferior horn consists of the hippocampus (A11 and 8) medially and the collateral eminence (A4) laterally. At its junction with the posterior horn (A12 and B11) the eminence broadens into the collateral trigone (A5, B4).

The collateral eminence (A4) is produced by the inward projection of the collateral sulcus (page 77, C4).

In the medial wall of the posterior horn, the bulb (B1) is produced by fibres of the corpus callosum, and the calcar avis (B2) by the inward projection of the calcarine sulcus (page 77, C3).

## A Cranial nerve *I – olfactory*

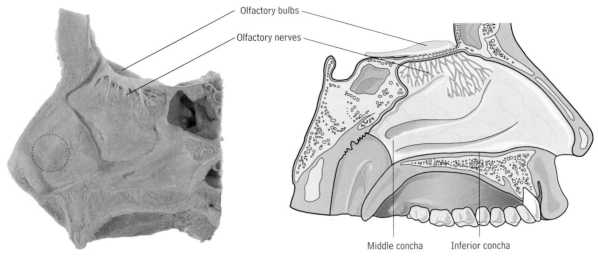

Olfactory bulbs

Olfactory nerves

Middle concha    Inferior concha

**See pages 63, 74 and 75.**

## Endoscopy of olfactory mucosa

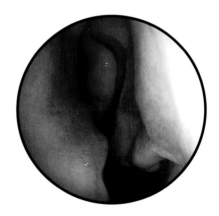

## B Cranial nerve *II – optic*

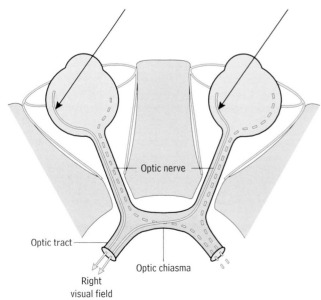

Optic nerve

Optic tract

Optic chiasma

Right
visual field

**See pages 7, 65, 75 and 77.**

## C Fundus of eye
*ophthalmoscopic photograph
of a retina*

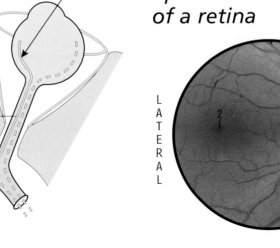

LATERAL

MEDIAL

1 Inferior nasal
branches of
central vein and
artery
2 Macula with
central fovea
3 Optic disc
4 Superior temporal
branches of
central vein and
artery

*Anosmia, epistaxis, tonsillitis, see pages 90, 92.*

# Cranial nerves *III – oculomotor, IV – trochlear, VI – abducens*

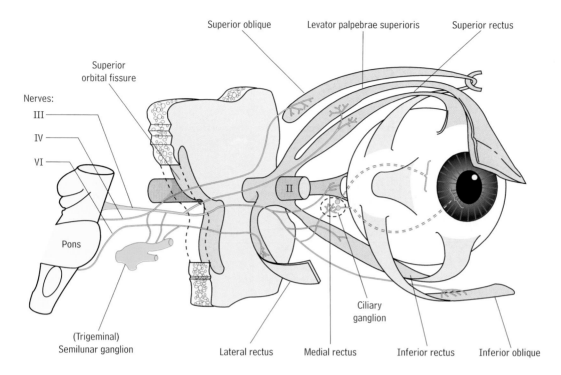

Superior oblique  Levator palpebrae superioris  Superior rectus

Superior orbital fissure

Nerves:
III
IV
VI

Pons

(Trigeminal) Semilunar ganglion

Lateral rectus  Medial rectus  Inferior rectus  Inferior oblique

Ciliary ganglion

**See pages 63–65 for III.**
**See page 63A for IV.**
**See pages 63–67 for VI.**

## Ciliary ganglion

1  Abducent nerve
2  Ciliary ganglion
3  Eyeball
4  Frontal nerve
5  Inferior oblique
6  Inferior rectus
7  Infra-orbital artery
8  Infra-orbital nerve
9  Lacrimal artery
10  Lateral rectus, reflected
11  Levator palpebrae superioris
12  Maxillary artery
13  Maxillary branch of trigeminal nerve
14  Nasociliary nerve
15  Nerve to inferior rectus
16  Oculomotor nerve
17  Ophthalmic artery
18  Optic nerve in anterior cranial fossa
19  Optic nerve in orbit
20  Sensory root to ciliary ganglion
21  Short ciliary arteries
22  Short ciliary nerves
23  Sphenopalatine nerve
24  Superior rectus
25  Supra-orbital nerve
26  Supratrochlear nerve

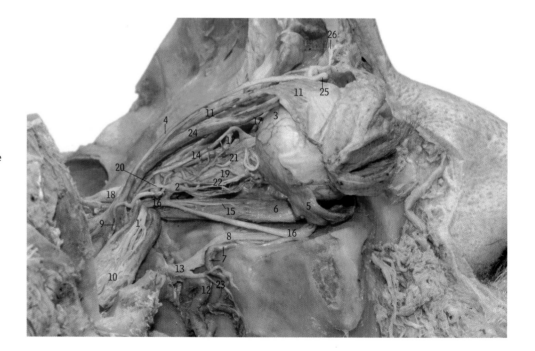

 *Abducent nerve palsy, accommodation reflex, oculomotor nerve palsy, trochlear nerve palsy, see pages 90, 91, 92.*

# Cranial nerve

## A  V – trigeminal (overview)

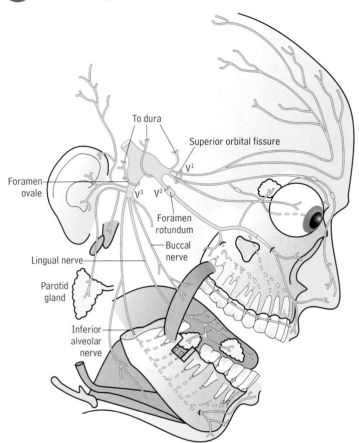

## B  V¹ ophthalmic division of trigeminal

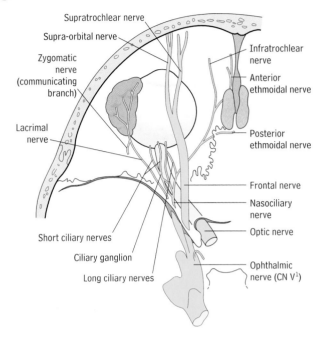

See page 61B for V.
See page 61B for V¹.

## C  V² maxillary division of trigeminal

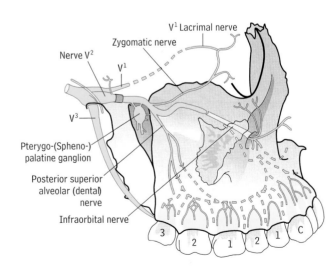

See pages 54, 61 and 69 for V².
See pages 52, 54 and 69 for V³.

## D  V³ mandibular division of trigeminal

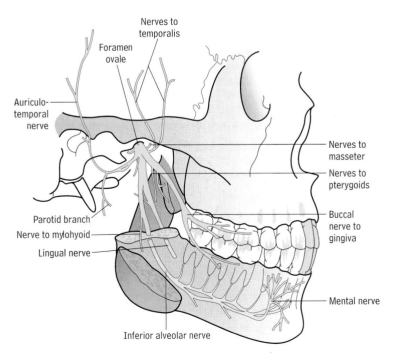

# Trigeminal nerve *branches and associated parasympathetic ganglia*

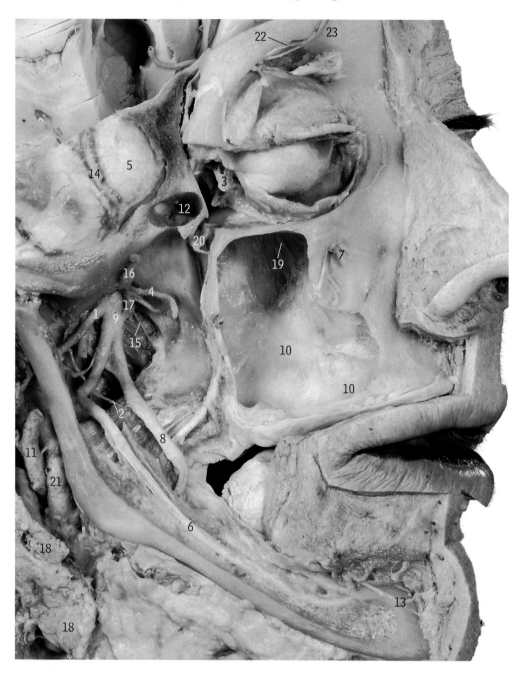

1  Auriculotemporal nerve
2  Chorda tympani
3  Ciliary ganglion
4  Deep temporal nerve
5  Dura mater
6  Inferior alveolar nerve within canal
7  Infra-orbital nerve
8  Lingual nerve
9  Mandibular nerve
10  Maxillary air sinus (opened)
11  Maxillary artery
12  Maxillary nerve
13  Mental nerve
14  Middle meningeal artery
15  Nerve to lateral pterygoid
16  Nerve to masseter
17  Otic ganglion
18  Parotid gland
19  Posterior superior alveolar nerves
20  Pterygopalatine ganglion
21  Retromandibular vein
22  Supra-orbital nerve
23  Supratrochlear nerve

## A    Cranial nerve *VII – facial*

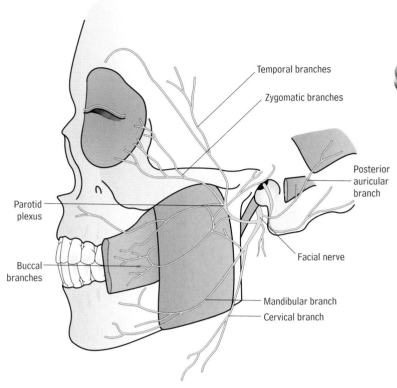

- Temporal branches
- Zygomatic branches
- Posterior auricular branch
- Parotid plexus
- Facial nerve
- Buccal branches
- Mandibular branch
- Cervical branch

## B    Nasal cartilage

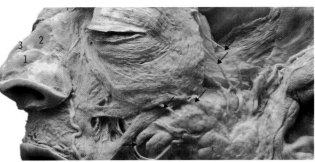

1 Lateral crus of alar cartilage
2 Lateral nasal cartilage
3 Septal angle

**NB: Facial nerve branches exit the parotid gland (arrows).**

**See pages 49, 50, 63, 70 and 71.**

## C    Cranial nerve *VIII – vestibulocochlear*

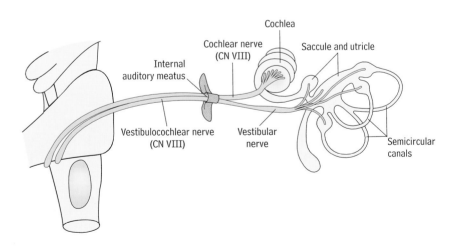

- Cochlea
- Cochlear nerve (CN VIII)
- Saccule and utricle
- Internal auditory meatus
- Vestibulocochlear nerve (CN VIII)
- Vestibular nerve
- Semicircular canals

**See pages 63, 70, 71 and 75.**

*Facial nerve palsy, hyperacuisis, otalgia, see pages 90, 91.*

# Cranial nerve Ⓐ *IX – glossopharyngeal* Ⓑ *X – vagus*

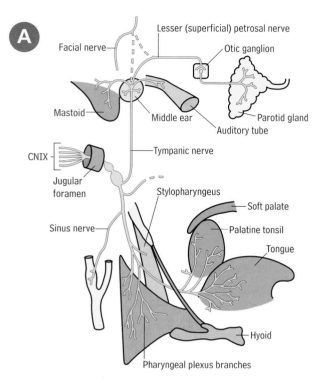

See pages 63, 75, 77 and 79.

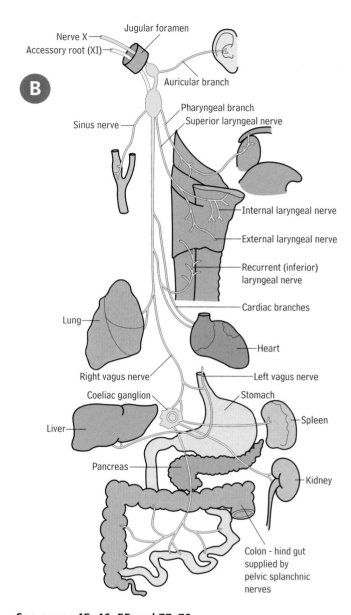

See pages 45, 46, 55 and 77–79.

*Parotid tumours, recurrent laryngeal nerve damage, see pages 91, 92.*

# Cranial nerve (A) *XI – accessory* (B) *XII – hypoglossal*

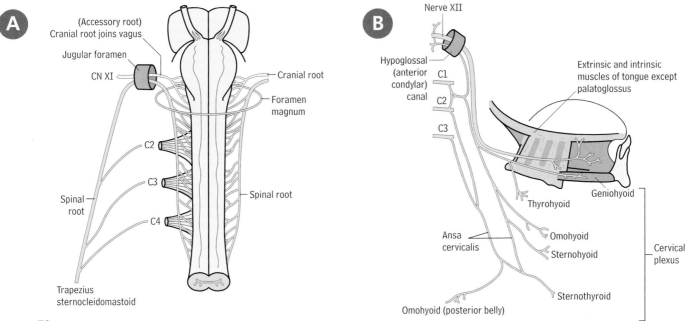

**A**

(Accessory root)
Cranial root joins vagus
Jugular foramen
CN XI
Cranial root
Foramen magnum
C2
C3
C4
Spinal root
Spinal root
Trapezius
sternocleidomastoid

See page 79.

**B**

Nerve XII
Hypoglossal (anterior condylar) canal
C1
C2
C3
Extrinsic and intrinsic muscles of tongue except palatoglossus
Geniohyoid
Thyrohyoid
Ansa cervicalis
Omohyoid
Sternohyoid
Cervical plexus
Sternothyroid
Omohyoid (posterior belly)

See pages 39, 54 and 63.

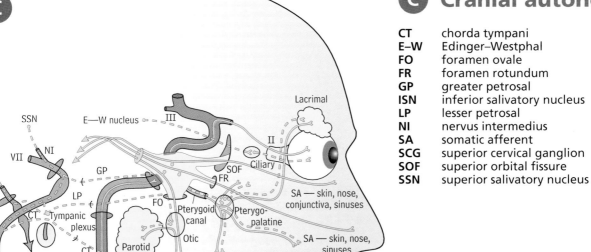

**C**

# Cranial autonomics

SSN
E—W nucleus    III
ISN  VII  NI
IX
GP
LP
CT
Tympanic plexus
CT
Parotid
Otic
FO
Pterygoid canal
Pterygo-palatine
Lingual
Middle meningeal artery
Submandibular
Internal carotid
Facial artery
Sublingual
SCG
Submandibular
II
SOF
FR
Ciliary
Lacrimal
SA — skin, nose, conjunctiva, sinuses
SA — skin, nose, sinuses
CT
SA — mouth, skin

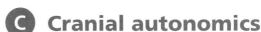

| CT | chorda tympani |
|---|---|
| E–W | Edinger–Westphal |
| FO | foramen ovale |
| FR | foramen rotundum |
| GP | greater petrosal |
| ISN | inferior salivatory nucleus |
| LP | lesser petrosal |
| NI | nervus intermedius |
| SA | somatic afferent |
| SCG | superior cervical ganglion |
| SOF | superior orbital fissure |
| SSN | superior salivatory nucleus |

*Accessory nerve palsy, gag reflex, hypoglossal nerve palsy, see pages 90, 91.*

# Head, neck and brain

Clinical thumbnails, see DVD Head and Neck for details and further clinical images

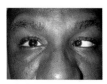

Abducent nerve palsy

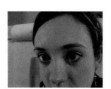

Accessory nerve palsy

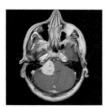

Accommoda-tion reflex

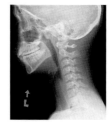

Acoustic neuroma

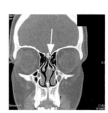

Adenoid enlargement

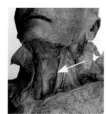

Anosmia

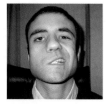

Facial nerve (Bell's) palsy

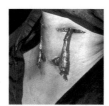

Blow-out fractures of the orbit

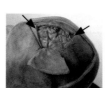

Branchial cleft cysts

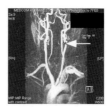

Burr holes

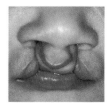

Carotid artery bruits

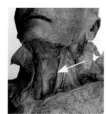

Carotid endarterectomy

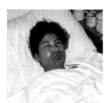

Cavernous sinus thrombosis

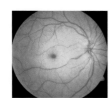

Central retinal artery occlusion

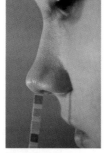

Skull base fracture

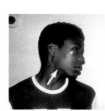

Cervical lymph node enlargement

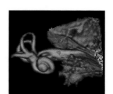

Labyrinthitis

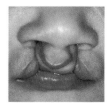

Cleft lip & palate

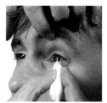

Corneal reflex

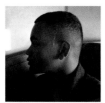

Craniotomy

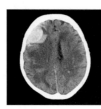

Epistaxis

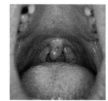

Extradural haemorrhage

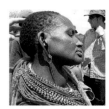

Gag reflex

Goitre

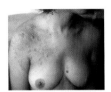

Varicella-zoster virus infection – head and neck

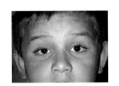

Horner's syndrome

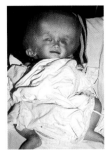

Hydrocephalus

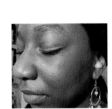

Hyperacuisis

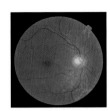

Hypoglossal nerve palsy

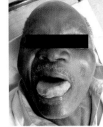

Glaucoma

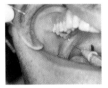

Inferior alveolar nerve block

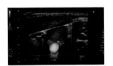

Internal jugular vein catheterisation

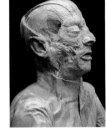

Intracranial spread of infection – face

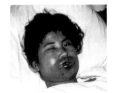

Intracranial spread of infection – scalp

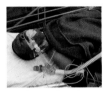

Endotracheal intubation

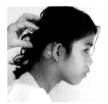

Mastoiditis

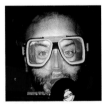

Meibomian cyst (chalazion)

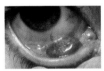

Middle ear pressure equalisation

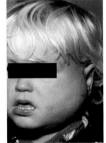

Mumps

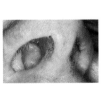

Nasal polyps

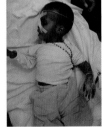

Nasogastric intubation

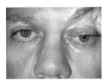

Oculomotor nerve palsy

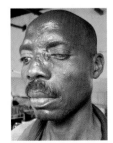

Ophthalmic herpes zoster

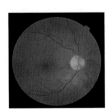

Ophthalmoscopy

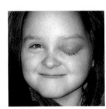

Orbital cellulitis

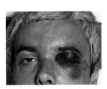

Periorbital & subconjuctival haemorrhage

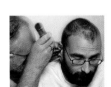

Otalgia

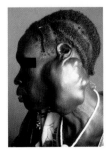

Parotid tumours

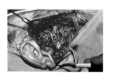

Parotidectomy

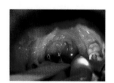

Pharyngitis

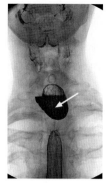

Pharyngeal pouch

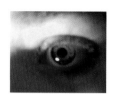

Pituitary tumour

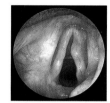

Pupillary reflex

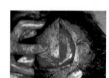

Recurrent laryngeal nerve palsy

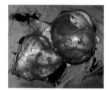

Scalp wounds

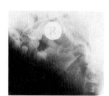

Sialectasis

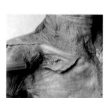

Subarachnoid haemorrhage

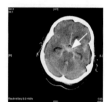

Subclavian vein catheterisation

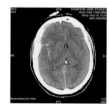

Subdural haemorrhage

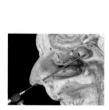

Surgical flaps of scalp

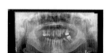

Temporo-mandibular joint dislocation

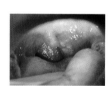

Tonsillitis

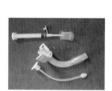

Torticollis

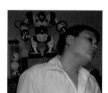

Tracheostomy

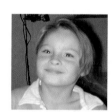

Trochlear nerve palsy

# Vertebral column and spinal cord

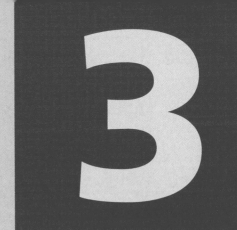

**3**

## Back and vertebral column

**A** *surface anatomy*    **B** *axial skeleton*    **C** *vertebral column*

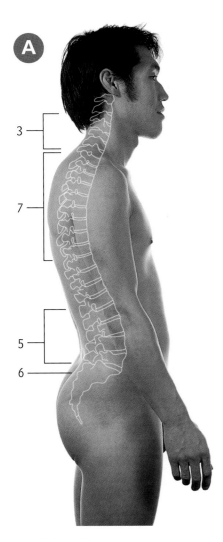

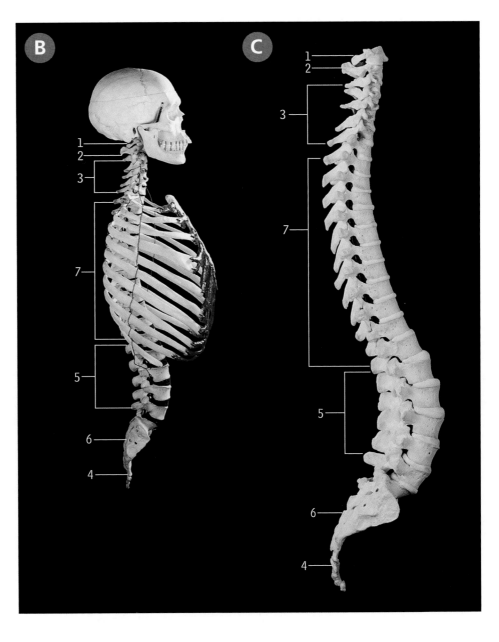

**1** Atlas vertebra
**2** Axis vertebra
**3** Cervical vertebrae, lordosis
**4** Coccyx
**5** Lumbar vertebrae, lordosis
**6** Sacrum
**7** Thoracic vertebrae, kyphosis

# Back and shoulder

 *surface anatomy*     *muscles*

| | | | |
|---|---|---|---|
| **1** | Coccyx | **7** | Medial border scapula (dotted) |
| **2** | Deltoid | **8** | Rhomboid major |
| **3** | External oblique | **9** | Rhomboid minor |
| **4** | Gluteus maximus | **10** | Sacrum |
| **5** | Iliac crest | **11** | Trapezius |
| **6** | Latissimus dorsi | **12** | Thoracolumbar fascia |

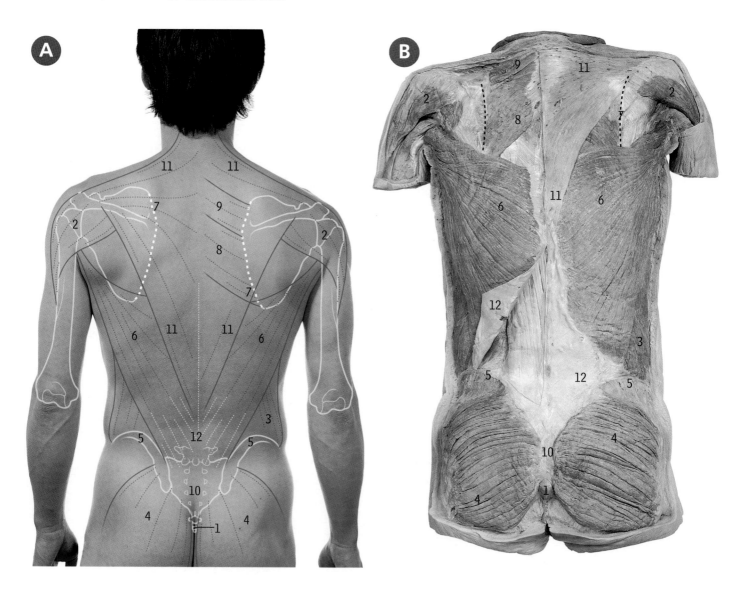

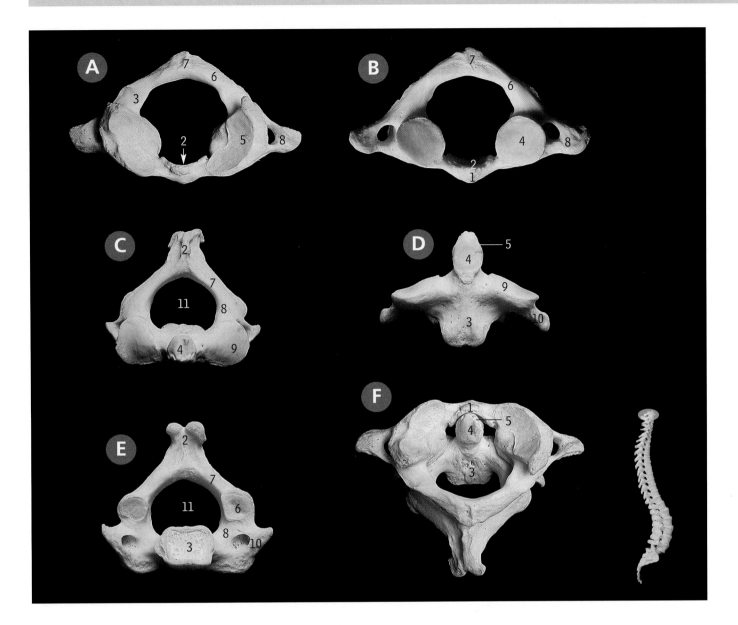

# First cervical vertebra *atlas*

**A** from above

**B** from below

| | |
|---|---|
| **1** Anterior arch and tubercle | **5** Lateral mass with superior |
| **2** Facet for dens of axis | articular facet |
| **3** Groove for vertebral artery | **6** Posterior arch |
| **4** Lateral mass with inferior | **7** Posterior tubercle |
| articular facet | **8** Transverse process and foramen |

The superior articular facets (5) are concave and kidney-shaped.

The inferior articular facets (4) are circular and almost flat.

The anterior arch (1) is straighter and shorter than the posterior arch (6) and contains on its posterior surface the facet for the dens of the axis (2).

The atlas is the only vertebra that has no body.

# Second cervical vertebra *axis*

**C** from above

**D** from the front

**E** from below

**F** articulated with the atlas, from above

| | |
|---|---|
| **1** Anterior arch of atlas | **7** Lamina |
| **2** Bifid spinous process | **8** Pedicle |
| **3** Body | **9** Superior articular surface |
| **4** Dens | **10** Transverse process and |
| **5** Impression for alar ligament | foramen |
| **6** Inferior articular facet | **11** Vertebral foramen |

The axis is unique in having the dens (4) which projects upwards from the body, representing the body of the atlas.

# Fifth cervical vertebra

## a typical cervical vertebra

**A** from above

**B** from the front

**C** from the left

1  Anterior tubercle of transverse process
2  Bifid spinous process
3  Body
4  Foramen of transverse process
5  Inferior articular process
6  Intertubercular lamella of transverse process
7  Lamina
8  Pedicle
9  Posterior tubercle of transverse process
10 Posterolateral lip (uncus)
11 Superior articular process
12 Vertebral foramen

# Seventh cervical vertebra

## vertebra prominens

**D** from above

1  Anterior tubercle of transverse process
2  Body
3  Foramen of transverse process
4  Intertubercular lamella of transverse process
5  Lamina
6  Pedicle
7  Posterior tubercle of transverse process
8  Posterolateral lip (uncus)
9  Spinous process with tubercle
10 Superior articular process
11 Vertebral foramen

All cervical vertebrae (first to seventh) have a foramen in each transverse process (as A4).

Typical cervical vertebrae (third to sixth) have superior articular processes that face backwards and upwards (A11, C11), posterolateral lips on the upper surface of the body (A10), a triangular vertebral foramen (A12) and a bifid spinous process (A2).

The anterior tubercle of the transverse process of the sixth cervical vertebra is large and known as the carotid tubercle.

The seventh cervical vertebra (vertebra prominens) has a spinous process that ends in a single tubercle (D9).

The rib element of a cervical vertebra is represented by the anterior root of the transverse process, the anterior tubercle, the intertubercular lamella (with its groove for the ventral ramus of a spinal nerve) and the anterior part of the posterior tubercle (as at D1, 4 and 7).

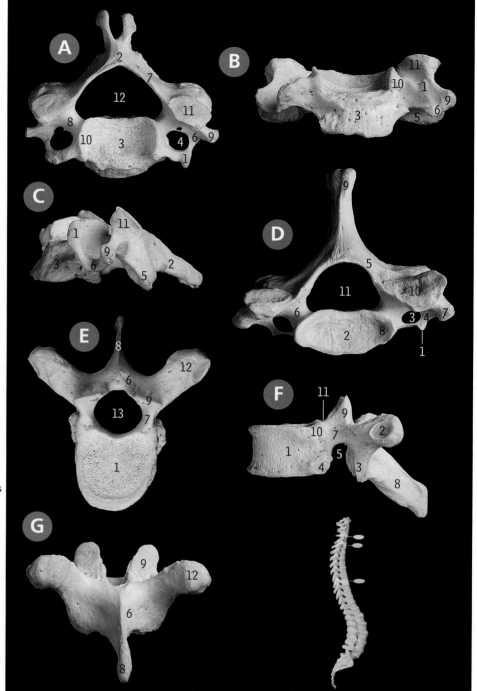

# Seventh thoracic vertebra

## typical

**E** from above

**F** from the left

**G** from behind

1  Body
2  Costal facet of transverse process
3  Inferior articular process
4  Inferior costal facet
5  Inferior vertebral notch
6  Lamina
7  Pedicle
8  Spinous process
9  Superior articular process
10 Superior costal facet
11 Superior vertebral notch
12 Transverse process
13 Vertebral foramen

Typical thoracic vertebrae (second to ninth) are characterised by costal facets on the bodies (F10, 4), costal facets on the transverse processes (F2), a round vertebral foramen (E13), a spinous process that points downwards as well as backwards (F8, G8) and superior articular processes that are vertical, flat and face backwards and laterally (E9, F9, G9).

*Ankylosing spondylosis, see page 116.*

# First thoracic vertebra

**A** from above

**B** from the front and the left

1 Body
2 Inferior articular process
3 Inferior costal facet
4 Lamina
5 Pedicle
6 Posterolateral lip (uncus)
7 Spinous process
8 Superior articular process
9 Superior costal facet
10 Transverse process with costal facet
11 Vertebral foramen

# Tenth and eleventh thoracic vertebrae

**C** tenth thoracic vertebra, from the left

**D** eleventh thoracic vertebra, from the left

1 Body
2 Costal facet
3 Inferior articular process
4 Inferior vertebral notch
5 Pedicle
6 Spinous process
7 Superior articular process
8 Transverse process

# Twelfth thoracic vertebra

**E** from the left

**F** from above

**G** from behind

1 Body
2 Costal facet
3 Inferior articular process
4 Inferior tubercle
5 Lateral tubercle
6 Pedicle
7 Spinous process
8 Superior articular process
9 Superior tubercle

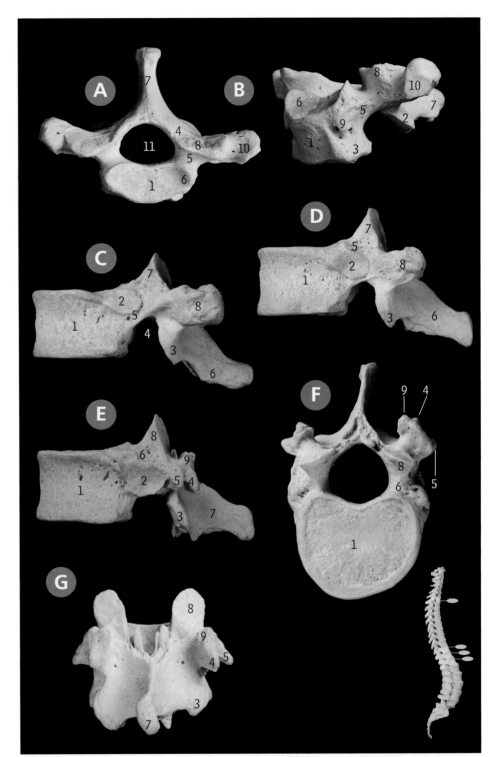

The atypical thoracic vertebrae are the first, tenth, eleventh and twelfth.

The first thoracic vertebra has a posterolateral lip (A6, B6) on each side of the upper surface of the body and a triangular vertebral foramen (features like typical cervical vertebrae), and complete (round) superior costal facets (B9) on the sides of the body.

The tenth, eleventh and twelfth thoracic vertebrae are characterised by a single complete costal facet on each side of the body that in successive vertebrae comes to lie increasingly far from the upper surface of the body and encroaches increasingly onto the pedicle (C2, D2 and E2). There is also no articular facet on the transverse process.

*Spondylolisthesis, see page 116.*

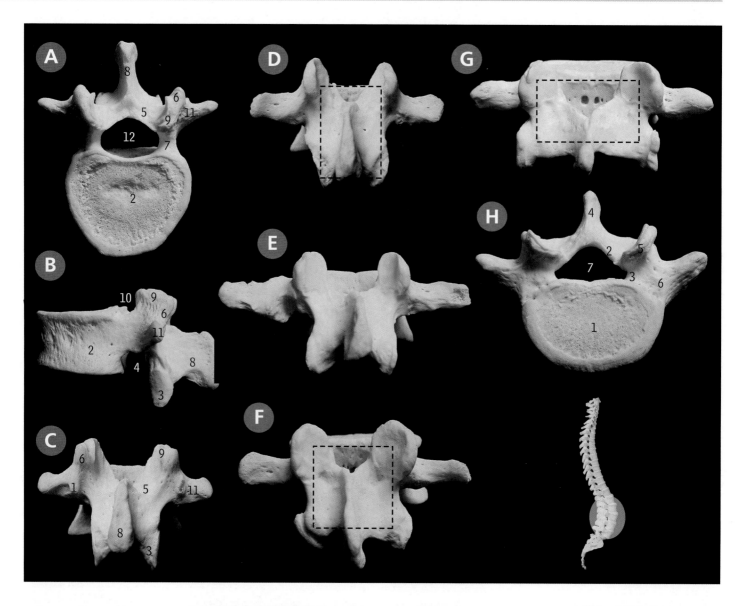

# First lumbar vertebra

**A** from above

**B** from the left

**C** from behind

**1** Accessory process
**2** Body
**3** Inferior articular process
**4** Inferior vertebral notch
**5** Lamina
**6** Mamillary process
**7** Pedicle
**8** Spinous process
**9** Superior articular process
**10** Superior vertebral notch
**11** Transverse process
**12** Vertebral foramen

Lumbar vertebrae are characterized by the large size of the bodies, the absence of costal facets on the bodies and the transverse processes, a triangular vertebral foramen (A12), a spinous process that points backwards and is quadrangular or hatchet-shaped (B8) and superior articular processes that are vertical, curved, face backwards and medially (A9) and possess a mamillary process at their posterior rim (A6).

The rib element of a lumbar vertebra is represented by the transverse process (A11).

The level at which facet joint orientation changes between the thoracic and lumbar regions is variable.

## Posterior view

**D** second lumbar vertebra

**E** third lumbar vertebra

**F** fourth lumbar vertebra

**G** fifth lumbar vertebra

## View from above

**H** fifth lumbar vertebra

**1** Body
**2** Lamina
**3** Pedicle
**4** Spinous process
**5** Superior articular process
**6** Transverse process fusing with pedicle and body
**7** Vertebral foramen

Viewed from behind, the four articular processes of the first and second lumbar vertebrae make a pattern (indicated by the interrupted line) of a vertical rectangle; those of the third or fourth vertebra make a square, and those of the fifth lumbar vertebra make a horizontal rectangle.

The fifth lumbar vertebra is unique in that the transverse process (H6) unites directly with the side of the body (H1) as well as with the pedicle (H3).

*Laminectomy, see page 116.*

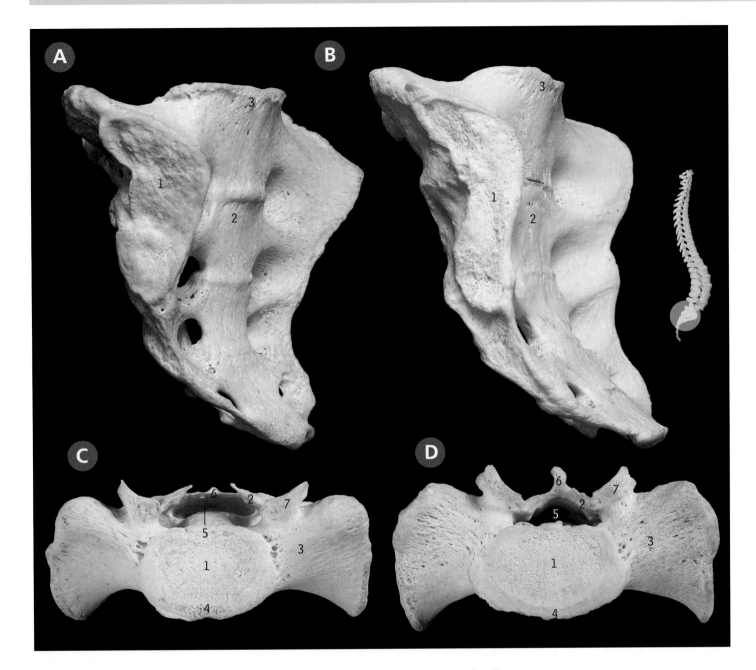

## Sacrum *from the front and the right*

**A** in the female

**B** in the male

1 Auricular surface
2 Pelvic surface
3 Promontory

---

In the female, the pelvic surface is relatively straight over the first three sacral vertebrae and becomes more curved below. In the male, the pelvic surface is more uniformly curved.

The capsule of the sacro-iliac joint is attached to the margin of the auricular (articular) surface (A1, B1).

## Base of the sacrum *upper surface*

**C** in the female   **D** in the male

1 Body of first sacral vertebra
2 Lamina
3 Lateral part (ala)
4 Promontory

5 Sacral canal
6 Spinous tubercle of median sacral crest
7 Superior articular process

---

In the male, the body of the first sacral vertebra (judged by its transverse diameter) forms a greater part of the base of the sacrum than in the female (compare D1 with C1).

In C, there is some degree of spina bifida (non-fusion of the laminae, 2, in the vertebral arch of the first sacral vertebra). Compare with the complete arch in D.

# Sacrum and coccyx

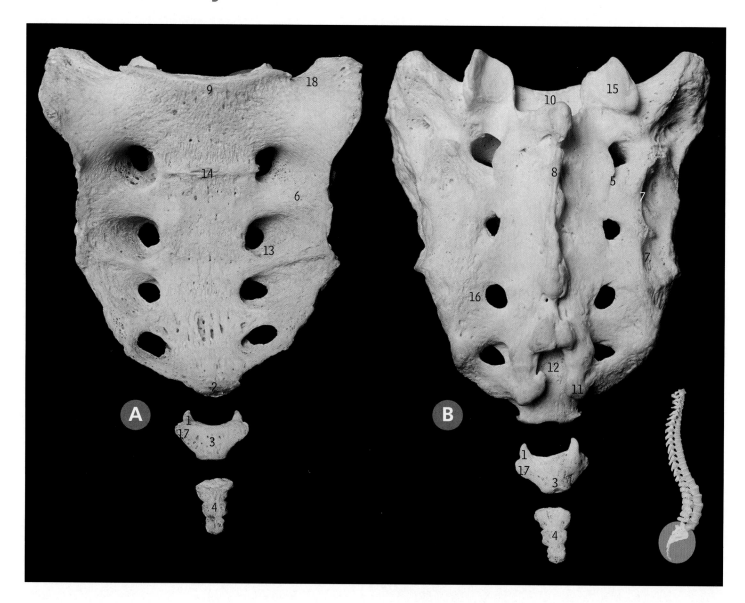

**A** pelvic surface

1. Coccygeal cornu
2. Facet for coccyx
3. First coccygeal vertebra
4. Fused second to fourth vertebrae
5. Intermediate sacral crest
6. Lateral part
7. Lateral sacral crest
8. Median sacral crest
9. Promontory
10. Sacral canal

**B** dorsal surface

11. Sacral cornu
12. Sacral hiatus
13. Second pelvic sacral foramen
14. Site of fusion of first and second sacral vertebrae
15. Superior articular process
16. Third dorsal sacral foramen
17. Transverse process
18. Upper surface of lateral part (ala)

The sacrum is formed by the fusion of the five sacral vertebrae. The median sacral crest (B8) represents the fused spinous processes, the intermediate crest (B5) the fused articular processes, and the lateral crest (B7) the fused transverse processes.

The sacral hiatus (B12) is the lower opening of the sacral canal (B10).

The coccyx is usually formed by the fusion of four rudimentary vertebrae but the number varies from three to five. In this specimen, the first piece of the coccyx (3) is not fused with the remainder (4).

*Coccydynia, see page 116.*

# Sacrum *with sacralization of the fifth lumbar vertebra*

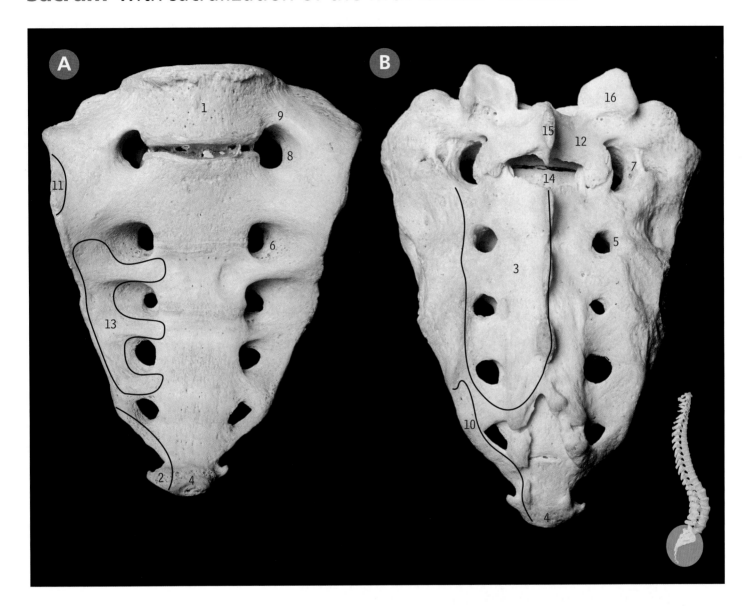

### A pelvic surface

### B dorsal surface, and sacral muscle attachments

| | |
|---|---|
| **1** Body of fifth lumbar vertebra | **9** Fusion of transverse process and lateral part of sacrum |
| **2** Coccygeus | **10** Gluteus maximus |
| **3** Erector spinae | **11** Iliacus |
| **4** First coccygeal vertebra fused to apex of sacrum | **12** Lamina |
| **5** First dorsal sacral foramen | **13** Piriformis |
| **6** First pelvic sacral foramen | **14** Sacral canal |
| **7** Foramen for dorsal ramus of fifth lumbar nerve | **15** Spinous process of fifth lumbar vertebra |
| **8** Foramen for ventral ramus of fifth lumbar nerve | **16** Superior articular process of fifth lumbar vertebra |

In sacralization of the fifth lumbar vertebra, that vertebra (A1) is (usually incompletely) fused with the sacrum. In the more rare condition of lumbarization of the first sacral vertebra (not illustrated) the first piece of the sacrum is incompletely fused with the remainder.

In this specimen, as well as fusion of the fifth lumbar vertebra with the top of the sacrum, the body of the first coccygeal vertebra (4) is fused with the apex of the sacrum.

*Caudal anaesthesia, see page 116.*

# Bony pelvis *from in front and above*

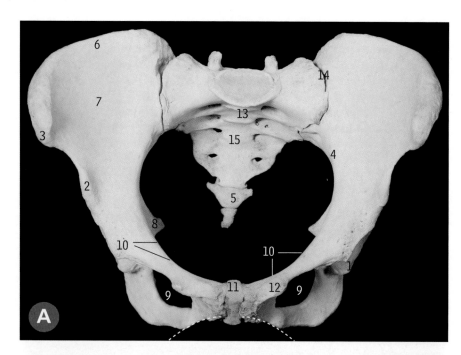

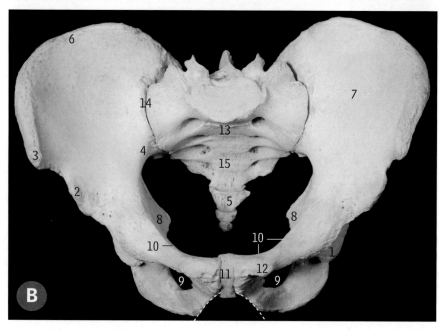

**A** female

**B** male

1 Acetabulum
2 Anterior inferior iliac spine
3 Anterior superior iliac spine
4 Arcuate line
5 Coccyx
6 Iliac crest
7 Iliac fossa
8 Ischial spine
9 Obturator foramen
10 Pectineal line
11 Pubic symphysis
12 Pubic tubercle
13 Sacral promontory
14 Sacro-iliac joint
15 Sacrum

The pelvic inlet (brim) is bounded by the sacral promontory (13), arcuate and pectineal lines (4 and 10), the crest of the pubic bones and anteriorly the pubic symphysis (11).

The female brim is more circular, the male more heart-shaped.

The female sacrum is wider, shorter and less curved.

The female ischial spines are further apart.

The female subpubic angle (white dotted line on A) is wide (90–120°) and the male subpubic angle (white dotted line on B) only 60–90°.

# Vertebrae, ribs and sternum *ossification*

**A** typical vertebra in a 6-month fetus

**B** at 4 years of age

**C D** during puberty

**E** atlas at 4 years of age

**F** axis, primary and secondary centres

**G** typical rib, secondary centres

**H** sternum at birth, with primary centres

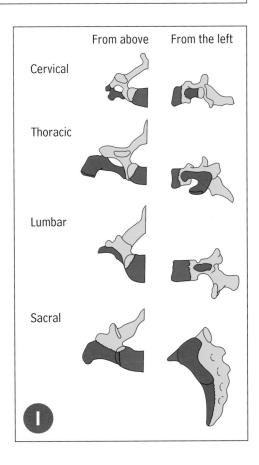

A
From above
1
2

B
From above
3
4
5

C
From the front
6

D
From above
6

E
From above
7
8

F
From behind
12
8
9
10
11

G
From behind
13
14
15

H
From the front
16

A typical vertebra, which is first cartilaginous, ossifies in early fetal life from three primary centres – one for most of the body (the centrum, A2) and one for each half of the neural arch (A1). The part of the adult body to which the pedicle is attached (B4) is part of the centre for the arch; the site in the developing vertebra where they meet is the neurocentral junction (B5). The two halves of the arch and the neurocentral junctions unite at variable times between birth and 6 years. Ossification spreads into the transverse processes and spine which grow out from the arch, but secondary centres (B3) appear at their tips during puberty and become fused at about 25 years of age. (Lumbar vertebrae have similar additional secondary centres for the mamillary processes.) There are also ring-like epiphyses on the periphery of the upper and lower surfaces of the vertebral bodies (C6 and D6).

The atlas has a primary centre (E7) for each lateral mass and the adjacent half of the posterior arch, and one for the anterior arch (E8). Fusion is complete by about 8 years.

The axis has five primary centres – one for most of the body (F10), one for each lateral mass (F9), and one for each half of the dens and adjacent part of the body (F8). They should all fuse by about 3 years. There are secondary centres for the tip of the dens (F12, appearing by about 2 years and fusing at 12) and the lower surface of the body (F11, appearing during puberty and fusing at about 25 years).

The sacrum, representing five fused sacral vertebrae, has many ossification centres, corresponding to the centrum, neural arch halves and costal elements of each vertebra, as well as ring epiphyses for the vertebral bodies and for the auricular surfaces. Most have fused by about 20 years, but some not until middle-age or later.

A typical rib has a primary centre for the body with secondary centres for the head (G13) and the articular and non-articular parts of the tubercle (G14 and 15), appearing during puberty and uniting at about 20 years.

The sternum has a variable number of primary centres (H16), one or two in the manubrium and in each of the four pieces of the body. Fusion occurs between puberty and 25 years of age. 'Bullet holes' in the sternum (sternal foramina) may occur when fusion is incomplete.

## **I** Vertebrae *developmental origins*

**Red, costal elements; green, centrum; yellow, neural arch**

Parts of the cervical, lumbar and sacral vertebrae represent the ribs that articulate with thoracic vertebrae. These costal elements are indicated here in red.

*Cervical*: anterior and posterior tubercles and the intertubercular lamella.

*Thoracic*: the true rib articulates with the vertebra.

*Lumbar*: the anterior part of the transverse process.

*Sacral*: the lateral part, including the auricular surface.

From above    From the left

Cervical

Thoracic

Lumbar

Sacral

I

# Vertebral column and spinal cord

**A** *cervical region, from the front*

**B** *cervical region, from behind*

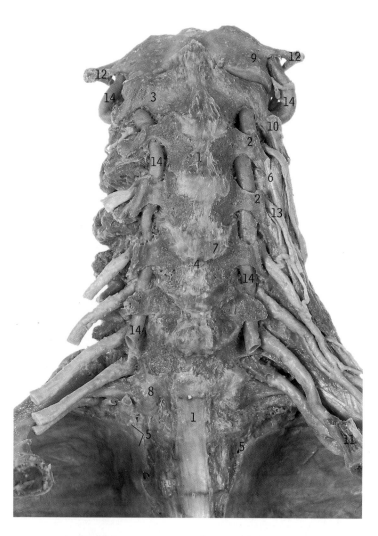

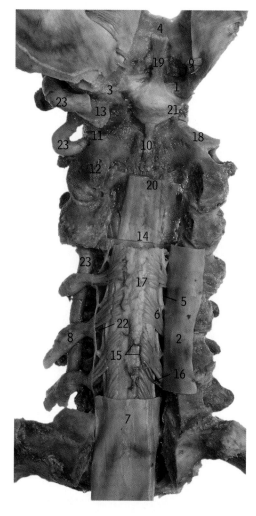

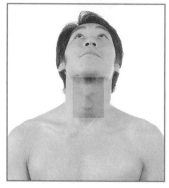

The vertebral artery (14) is seen within foramina of cervical transverse processes.

| | |
|---|---|
| **1** | Anterior longitudinal ligament |
| **2** | Anterior tubercle of transverse process |
| **3** | Axis |
| **4** | Body of the fifth cervical vertebra |
| **5** | Cut edge of the pleura |
| **6** | Intertubercular lamella of transverse process |
| **7** | Intervertebral disc |
| **8** | Joint of head of first rib |
| **9** | Lateral mass of atlas |
| **10** | Posterior tubercle of transverse process |
| **11** | Scalenus anterior muscle |
| **12** | Transverse process of atlas |
| **13** | Ventral ramus of third cervical nerve |
| **14** | Vertebral artery |

Much of the skull, the vertebral arches, brainstem and the upper part of the spinal cord have been removed to show the cruciform, transverse and alar ligaments (19, 10, 21 and 1). Lower down, the arachnoid and dura mater (2) have been reflected to show dorsal and ventral nerve roots (as at 6 and 22).

| | | | |
|---|---|---|---|
| **1** | Alar ligament | **12** | Pedicle of axis |
| **2** | Arachnoid and dura mater (reflected) | **13** | Posterior arch of atlas |
| **3** | Atlanto-occipital joint | **14** | Posterior longitudinal ligament |
| **4** | Basilar part of occipital bone and position of attachment of tectorial membrane | **15** | Posterior spinal arteries |
| | | **16** | Radicular artery |
| | | **17** | Spinal cord |
| **5** | Denticulate ligament | **18** | Superior articular surface of axis |
| **6** | Dorsal rootlets of spinal nerve | **19** | Superior longitudinal band of cruciform ligament |
| **7** | Dura mater | **20** | Tectorial membrane |
| **8** | Dural sheath over dorsal root ganglion | **21** | Transverse ligament of atlas (transverse part of cruciform ligament) |
| **9** | Hypoglossal nerve and canal | | |
| **10** | Inferior longitudinal band of cruciform ligament | **22** | Ventral rootlets of spinal nerve |
| **11** | Lateral atlanto-axial joint | **23** | Vertebral artery |

# Vertebral column and spinal cord

## C cervical and upper thoracic regions, from the right

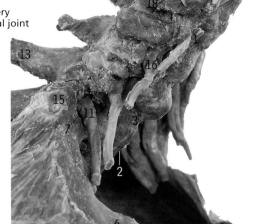

Ventral and dorsal rami of spinal nerves (as at 16 and 4) are seen emerging from intervertebral foramina (as at 7).

| | | |
|---|---|---|
| 1 Anterior tubercle of transverse process of fifth cervical vertebra | 5 First cervical nerve | 13 Spinous process of seventh cervical vertebra |
| | 6 First rib | 14 Transverse process of atlas |
| | 7 Intervertebral foramen | |
| 2 Body of first thoracic vertebra | 8 Lateral atlanto-axial joint | 15 Tubercle of first rib |
| | 9 Lateral mass of atlas | 16 Ventral ramus of fifth cervical nerve |
| 3 Body of seventh cervical vertebra | 10 Posterior arch of atlas | |
| | 11 Seventh cervical nerve | 17 Vertebral artery |
| 4 Dorsal ramus of first cervical nerve | 12 Spinous process of second cervical vertebra | 18 Zygapophyseal joint |

> The first and second spinal nerves pass, respectively, above and below the posterior arch of the atlas.

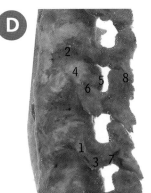

## D Cervical region, from the left

Soft tissue has been removed to show the boundaries of intervertebral foramina (as at 5). Compare with the cleared specimens of thoracic vertebrae on page 108, A.

1 Anterior tubercle of transverse process of fifth cervical vertebra
2 Body of third cervical vertebra
3 Intertubercular lamella of transverse process of fifth cervical vertebra
4 Intervertebral disc
5 Intervertebral foramen
6 Pedicle
7 Posterior tubercle of transverse process of fifth cervical vertebra
8 Zygapophyseal joint

> Each intervertebral foramen (as at D5) is bounded in front by a vertebral body and intervertebral disc (D2 and 4), above and below by pedicles (D6), and behind by a zygapophyseal joint (D8).
>
> In the thoracic and lumbar regions there are the same number of pairs of spinal nerves as there are vertebrae (twelve thoracic and five lumbar), and spinal nerves are numbered from the vertebra beneath whose pedicles they emerge. In the cervical region, there are seven cervical vertebrae and eight cervical nerves. The first nerve emerges between the occipital bone of the skull and the atlas, and the eighth below the pedicle of the seventh cervical vertebra.

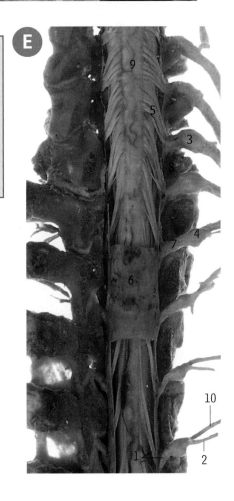

## E Lower cervical and upper thoracic regions, from behind

The vertebral arches and most of the dura mater and arachnoid have been removed, to show dorsal nerve rootlets (5) emerging from the spinal cord (9) to unite as a dorsal nerve root and enter the dural sheath (as at 7). Ventral nerve roots do the same from the ventral aspect of the cord but are not seen in this view as they are obscured by the dorsal roots.

1 Angulation of nerve roots entering dural sheath
2 Dorsal ramus of fifth thoracic nerve
3 Dorsal root ganglion of eighth cervical nerve
4 Dorsal root ganglion of second thoracic nerve
5 Dorsal rootlets of eighth cervical nerve
6 Dura mater
7 Dural sheath of second thoracic nerve
8 Pedicle of first thoracic vertebra
9 Spinal cord and posterior spinal vessels
10 Ventral ramus of fifth thoracic nerve

## A Vertebral column and spinal cord
### *cervical and upper thoracic regions, from the left*

1  Arachnoid mater
2  Body of first thoracic vertebra
3  Denticulate ligament
4  Dorsal ramus of fifth cervical nerve
5  Dorsal root ganglion of eighth cervical nerve
6  Dorsal root ganglion of fifth cervical nerve
7  Dorsal rootlets of fifth cervical nerve
8  Dura mater
9  Foramen magnum
10  Medulla oblongata
11  Occipital bone
12  Posterior arch of atlas
13  Spinal cord
14  Spinal part of accessory nerve
15  Spinous process of axis (abnormally large)
16  Spinous process of seventh cervical vertebra
17  Sympathetic trunk
18  Ventral ramus of fifth cervical nerve
19  Ventral rootlets of fifth cervical nerve

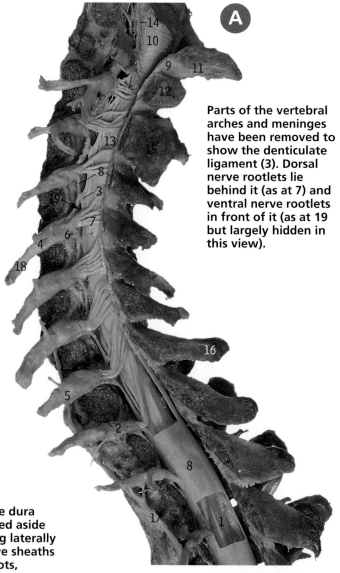

A

Parts of the vertebral arches and meninges have been removed to show the denticulate ligament (3). Dorsal nerve rootlets lie behind it (as at 7) and ventral nerve rootlets in front of it (as at 19 but largely hidden in this view).

Each spinal nerve is formed by the union of ventral and dorsal nerve roots.

Each nerve root is formed by the union of several rootlets (as at A7).

The union of ventral and dorsal nerve roots to form a spinal nerve occurs immediately distal to the ganglion on the dorsal root (as at A6), within the intervertebral foramen, and the nerve at once divides into a ventral and a dorsal ramus (formerly called ventral and dorsal primary rami) (as at A18 and 4). The spinal nerve proper is thus only 1–2 mm in length, but is often so short that the rami appear to be branches of the ganglion itself.

The lowest cervical and upper thoracic nerve roots become acutely angled in order to enter their dural sheaths.

## B Spinal cord
### *cervical region, from the front*

**For this ventral view of the upper part of the spinal cord (6), the dura and arachnoid mater have been incised longitudinally and turned aside (2) to show the ventral nerve rootlets and roots (as at 7) passing laterally in front of the denticulate ligament (3) to enter meningeal nerve sheaths with dorsal roots (as at 4) and form a spinal nerve. On some roots, branches of radicular vessels (as at 5) are seen anastomosing with anterior spinal vessels (1).**

1  Anterior spinal vessels
2  Arachnoid and dura mater
3  Denticulate ligament
4  Dorsal root of sixth cervical nerve
5  Radicular vessels
6  Spinal cord
7  Ventral root of seventh cervical nerve entering dural sheath

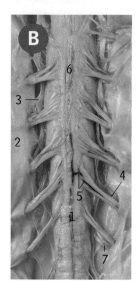

B

The denticulate ligament (B3) is composed of pia mater. The ventral and dorsal nerve roots pass, respectively, ventral and dorsal to the ligament, which extends laterally from the side of the cord and is attached by its spiky denticulations (as at B3) to the arachnoid and dura mater in the intervals between dural nerve sheaths. The highest denticulation is above the first cervical nerve and the lowest below the twelfth thoracic nerve.

# Vertebral column and spinal cord

## C *lumbar and sacral regions, from behind*  D *lumbar radiculogram*

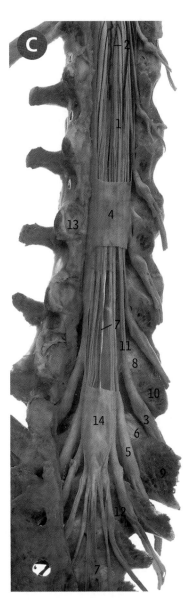

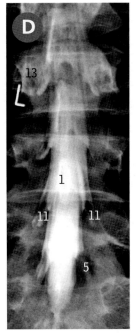

Parts of the vertebral arches and meninges have been removed, to show the cauda equina (1) and nerve roots entering their meningeal sheaths (as at 11), outlined as linear bands by contrast medium in the radiculogram.

1  Cauda equina
2  Conus medullaris of spinal cord
3  Dorsal root ganglion of fifth lumbar nerve
4  Dura mater
5  Dural sheath of first sacral nerve roots
6  Fifth lumbar (lumbosacral) intervertebral disc
7  Filum terminale
8  Fourth lumbar intervertebral disc
9  Lateral part of sacrum
10  Pedicle of fifth lumbar vertebra
11  Roots of fifth lumbar nerve
12  Second sacral vertebra
13  Superior articular process of third lumbar vertebra
14  Thecal sac

The spinal cord usually ends at the level of the first lumbar vertebra.

The subarachnoid space ends at the level of the second sacral vertebra.

The conus medullaris (C2) is the lower, pointed end of the spinal cord.

The cauda equina (C1) consists of the dorsal and ventral roots of the lumbar, sacral and coccygeal nerves. Note that it is nerve roots which form the cauda, not the spinal nerves themselves; these are not formed until ventral and dorsal roots unite at the level of an intervertebral foramen, immediately distal to the dorsal root ganglion (as at C3).

## E *Coronal lumbar MR image*

## F *Lower thoracic and upper lumbar regions*

The specimen is seen from the left with parts of the vertebral arches and meninges removed, to show (at the front) part of the sympathetic trunk (13) on the vertebral bodies and (at the back) the spinous ligaments (7 and 11).

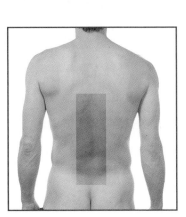

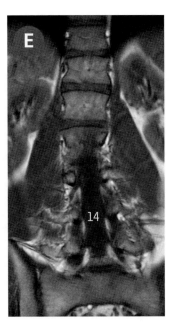

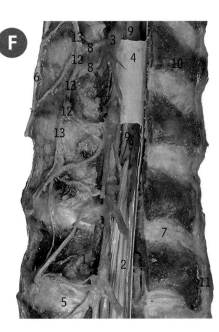

1  Body of first lumbar vertebra
2  Cauda equina
3  Dorsal root ganglion of tenth thoracic nerve
4  Dura mater
5  First lumbar intervertebral disc
6  Greater splanchnic nerve
7  Interspinous ligament
8  Rami communicantes
9  Spinal cord
10  Spinous process of tenth thoracic vertebra
11  Supraspinous ligament
12  Sympathetic ganglion
13  Sympathetic trunk
14  Thecal sac

*Epidural anaesthesia, spinal anaesthesia, see page 116.*

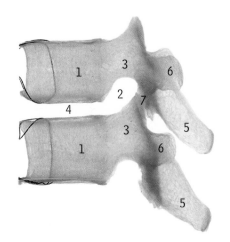

## A Thoracic vertebrae *cleared specimens*

**The pairs of vertebrae are seen from the side and articulated to show the boundaries of an intervertebral foramen (2).**

1 Body
2 Intervertebral foramen
3 Pedicle
4 Space for intervertebral disc
5 Spinous process
6 Transverse process
7 Zygapophyseal joint

> The intervertebral foramen (A2) is bounded in front by the lower part of the vertebral body (A1) and the intervertebral disc (A4), above and below by the pedicles (A3), and behind by the zygapophyseal joint (A7).
>
> The posterior longitudinal ligament is broad where it is firmly attached to the intervertebral discs, but narrow and less firmly attached to the vertebral bodies, leaving vascular foramina patent and allowing the basivertebral veins which emerge from them to enter the internal vertebral venous plexus.
>
> The anterior longitudinal ligament (B1) is uniformly broad and firmly attached to discs and vertebral bodies.

## B Vertebral column
### *lower lumbar region, from the front*

**At the top the anterior longitudinal ligament (1) has a marker behind it, and part of it lower down has been reflected off an intervertebral disc (4) and vertebral bodies (2 and 3).**

1 Anterior longitudinal ligament
2 Body of fifth lumbar vertebra
3 Body of fourth lumbar vertebra
4 Fourth lumbar intervertebral disc
5 Lateral part of sacrum
6 Ventral ramus of fifth lumbar nerve

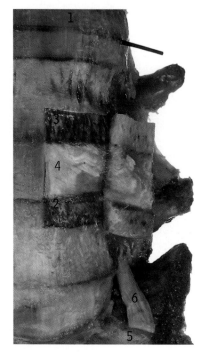

## C Vertebral column
### *upper lumbar region, from the right*

**The side view shows lumbar nerves emerging from intervertebral foramina (as at 5).**

1 Anterior longitudinal ligament
2 Dorsal ramus of first lumbar nerve
3 Dorsal ramus of second lumbar nerve
4 First lumbar intervertebral disc
5 First lumbar nerve emerging from intervertebral foramen
6 First lumbar vertebra
7 Interspinous ligament
8 Rami communicantes
9 Spinous process of second lumbar vertebra
10 Supraspinous ligament
11 Sympathetic trunk ganglion
12 Twelfth rib
13 Ventral ramus of first lumbar nerve
14 Ventral ramus of second lumbar nerve
15 Zygapophyseal joint

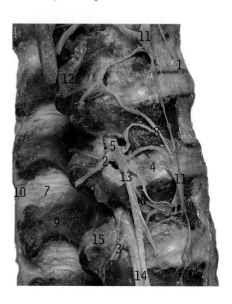

*Compression of spinal nerve, vertebral venous plexus, see page 116.*

# A Vertebral column
## *lumbar region, from the right and behind*

This posterolateral view of the right side of some lumbar vertebrae shows ligamenta flava (as at 4), which pass between the laminae of adjacent vertebrae (as at 2 and 3).

1 Interspinous ligament
2 Lamina of second lumbar vertebra
3 Lamina of third lumbar vertebra
4 Ligamentum flavum
5 Spinous process of second lumbar vertebra
6 Supraspinous ligament
7 Transverse process of third lumbar vertebra
8 Zygapophyseal joint

# B The lumbar intervertebral disc
## *from above, in situ*

1 Annulus fibrosus
2 Aorta
3 Extraperitoneal fat
4 Inferior vena cava
5 Laminations of annulus
6 Nucleus pulposus
7 Ovarian artery
8 Ovarian vein
9 Peritoneum, posterior abdominal wall
10 Psoas muscle
11 Thoracolumbar fascia, anterior layer
12 Ureter

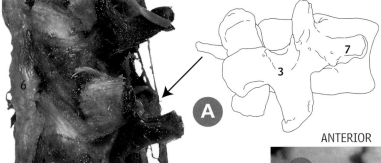

ANTERIOR

The nucleus pulposus of an intervertebral disc represents the remains of the notochord.

The annulus fibrosus of an intervertebral disc is derived from the mesenchyme between adjacent vertebral bodies.

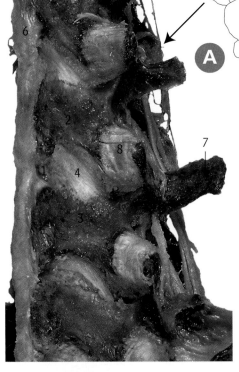

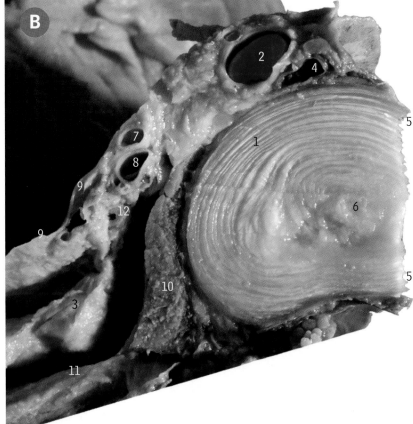

POSTERIOR

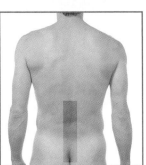

 *Lumbar puncture, spinal malformations (meningocoele), see page 116.*

# Back *surface anatomy*

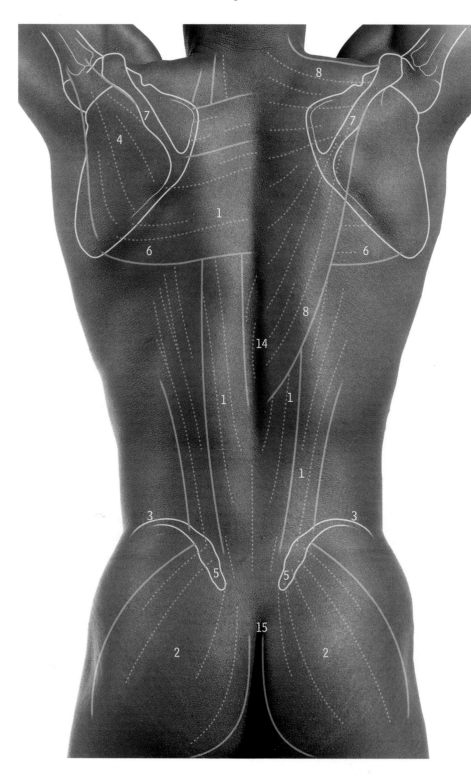

1 Erector spinae
2 Gluteus maximus
3 Iliac crest
4 Infraspinatus
5 Posterior superior iliac spine
6 Rhomboids
7 Spine of scapula
8 Trapezius

# Back

Superficial musculature on left, deeper dissection on right

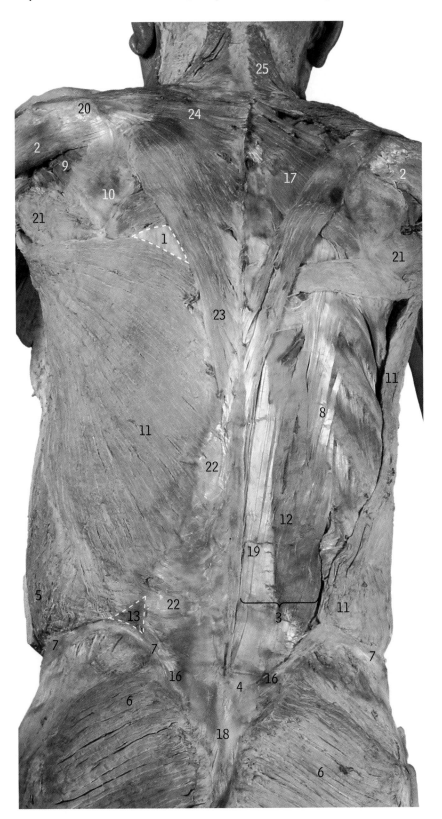

1. Auscultation triangle
2. Deltoid
3. Erector spinae
4. Erector spinae, tendon
5. External oblique muscle of the abdomen
6. Gluteus maximus
7. Iliac crest
8. Iliocostalis
9. Infraspinatus
10. Infraspinatus fascia
11. Latissimus dorsi
12. Longissimus
13. Lumbar triangle
14. Median furrow – see surface
15. Natal cleft – see surface
16. Posterior superior iliac spine
17. Rhomboid major
18. Sacrum
19. Spinalis
20. Spine of scapula
21. Teres major
22. Thoracolumbar fascia
23. Trapezius, lower fibres
24. Trapezius, middle fibres
25. Trapezius, upper fibres

# Back

 **A** *close up left side*

**B** *close up right side*

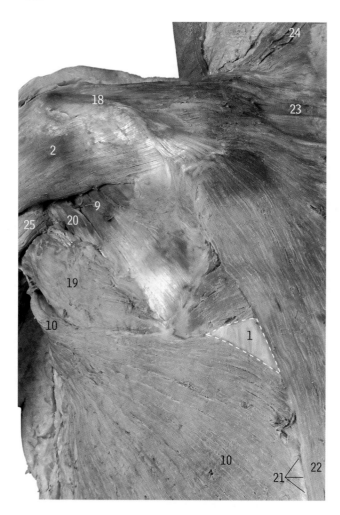

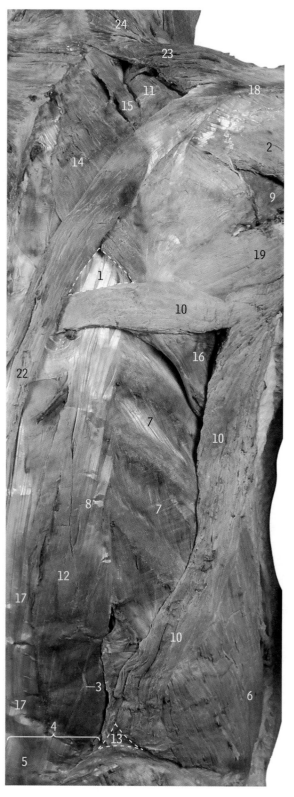

**Windows cut in latissimus dorsi and trapezius muscles to reveal deeper layer of back musculature**

| | | | |
|---|---|---|---|
| **1** | Auscultation triangle | **13** | Lumbar triangle |
| **2** | Deltoid | **14** | Rhomboid major |
| **3** | Dorsal ramus, lumbar spinal nerve | **15** | Rhomboid minor |
| **4** | Erector spinae | **16** | Serratus anterior |
| **5** | Erector spinae, tendon | **17** | Spinalis |
| **6** | External oblique muscle of the abdomen | **18** | Spine of scapula |
| **7** | External intercostal | **19** | Teres major |
| **8** | Iliocostalis | **20** | Teres minor |
| **9** | Infraspinatus | **21** | Thoracolumbar fascia |
| **10** | Latissimus dorsi | **22** | Trapezius, lower fibres |
| **11** | Levator scapulae | **23** | Trapezius, middle fibres |
| **12** | Longissimus | **24** | Trapezius, upper fibres |
| | | **25** | Triceps, long head |

# Back

**A** *close up right side*

Note windows cut in latissimus dorsi and trapezius.

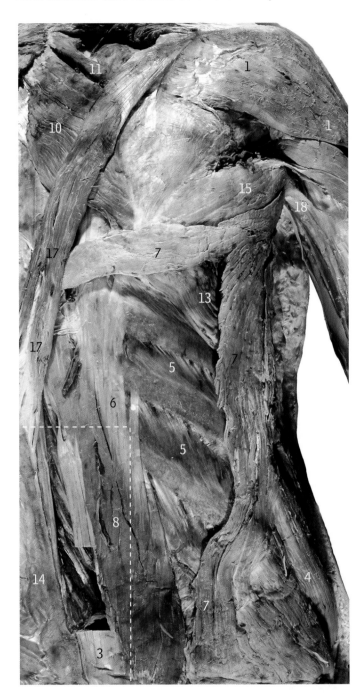

**B** *close up right side*

Note resection of upper lumbar and lower thoracic spinalis and part of longissimus muscles to reveal the transversospinalis group of muscles – the deepest components of erector spinae.

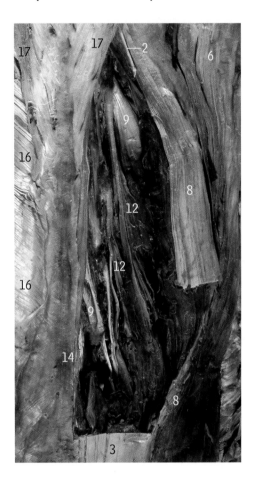

| | | | |
|---|---|---|---|
| **1** | Deltoid | **9** | Multifidus |
| **2** | Dorsal ramus, thoracic spinal nerve | **10** | Rhomboid major |
| | | **11** | Rhomboid minor |
| **3** | Erector spinae, tendon | **12** | Semispinalis |
| **4** | External oblique muscle of the abdomen | **13** | Serratus anterior |
| | | **14** | Spinalis |
| **5** | External intercostal | **15** | Teres major |
| **6** | Iliocostalis | **16** | Thoracolumbar fascia |
| **7** | Latissimus dorsi | **17** | Trapezius, lower fibres |
| **8** | Longissimus | **18** | Triceps, long head |

## A Upper cervical vertebrae

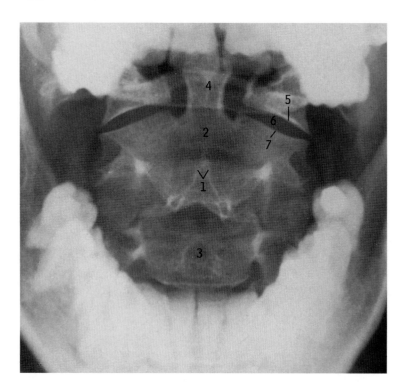

This is a standard radiographic view of the axis and its dens (4). The correct angle must be chosen with the mouth open to avoid overlying shadows of the teeth and jaws. The surfaces of the lateral atlanto-axial joints (5 and 7) do not appear congruent because the hyaline cartilage which covers the bony surfaces is not radio-opaque (this applies to any synovial joint). The outlines of the arches of the atlas are seen faintly between the sides of the shadow of the dens (4) and the lateral masses of the atlas (5).

1  Bifid spinous process of axis
2  Body of axis
3  Body of third cervical vertebra
4  Dens of axis
5  Inferior articular surface of lateral mass of atlas
6  Lateral atlanto-axial joint
7  Superior articular surface of axis

## B Lower cervical and upper thoracic vertebrae *from the front*

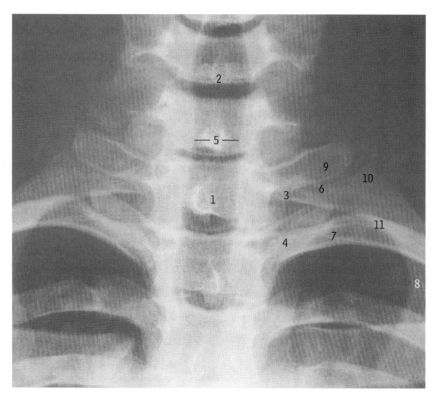

Note the tracheal shadow produced by the translucency of its contained air.

1  Body of first thoracic vertebra
2  Body of sixth cervical vertebra
3  Head of first rib
4  Head of second rib
5  Margin of tracheal shadow
6  Neck of first rib
7  Neck of second rib
8  Shaft of first rib
9  Transverse process of first thoracic vertebra
10  Tubercle of first rib
11  Tubercle of second rib

*Cervical spinal immobilisation, see page 116.*

# Spine

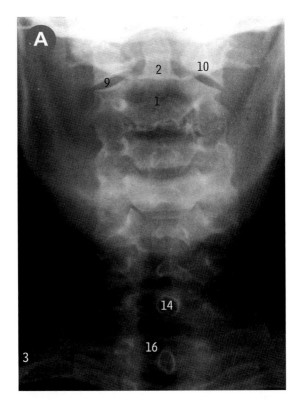

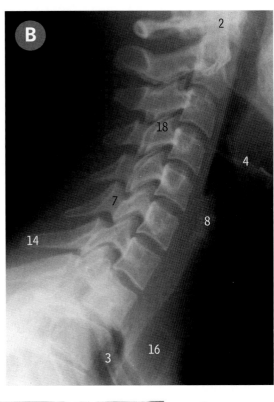

1  Body of axis
2  Dens of axis
3  First rib
4  Hyoid bone
5  Inferior articular process of first lumbar vertebra
6  Intervertebral disc space L2/3 level
7  Lamina of sixth cervical vertebra
8  Larynx
9  Lateral atlanto-axial joint
10 Lateral mass of atlas
11 Pars interarticularis of second lumbar vertebra
12 Pedicle of third lumbar vertebra
13 Spinous process of second lumbar vertebra
14 Spinous process of seventh cervical vertebra
15 Superior articular process of second lumbar vertebra
16 Trachea
17 Transverse process of third lumbar vertebra
18 Zygapophyseal joint

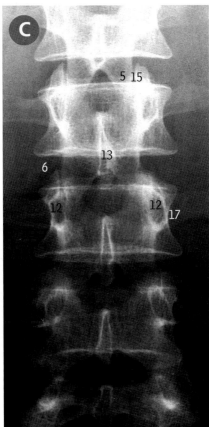

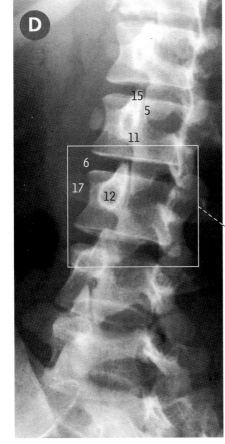

**A** cervical spine, anteroposterior projection

**B** cervical spine, lateral projection

**C** lumbar spine, anteroposterior projection

**D** lumbar spine, oblique projection

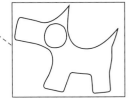

The Scottie dog is seen on the oblique projection lumbar spine. The nose (17) is the transverse process, the ear (15) is the superior articular process, the eye (12) is the pedicle and the neck (11) is the pars interarticularis which may be incomplete in spondylolysis.

*Vertebral fractures, see page 116.*

# Vertebral column and spinal cord

Clinical thumbnails, see DVD for details and further clinical images.

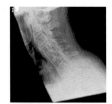

Ankylosing
spondylitis

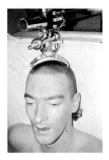

Caudal
anaesthesia

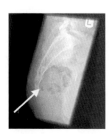

Cervical spinal
immobilisation

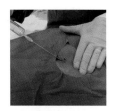

Coccydynia

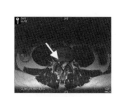

Compression of
spinal nerve

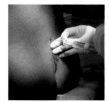

Epidural
anaesthesia

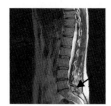

Laminectomy

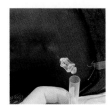

Lumbar
puncture

Spinal
anaesthesia

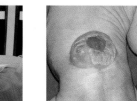

Spinal
malformations

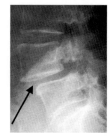

Spondylolisthesis

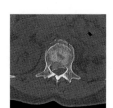

Vertebral
fracture

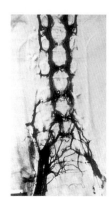

Vertebral venous
plexus

# Upper limb

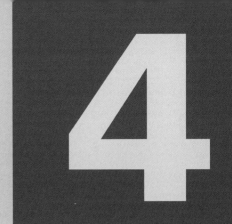

**4**

## Upper limb

**A** *surface anatomy*  **B** *muscles*  **C** *bones*

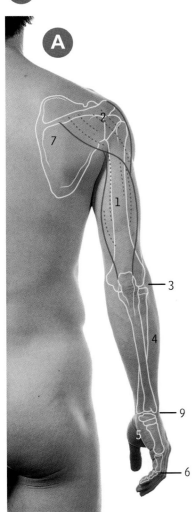

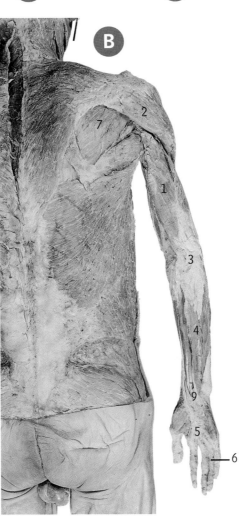

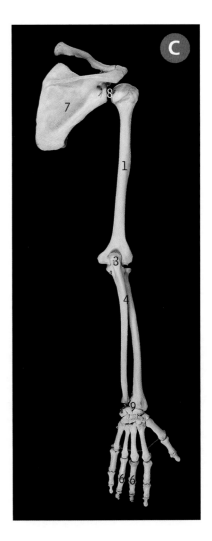

| | |
|---|---|
| **1** Arm | **6** Interphalangeal |
| **2** Deltoid | joint |
| **3** Elbow joint | **7** Scapula |
| **4** Forearm | **8** Shoulder joint |
| **5** Hand | **9** Wrist joint |

# Left scapula

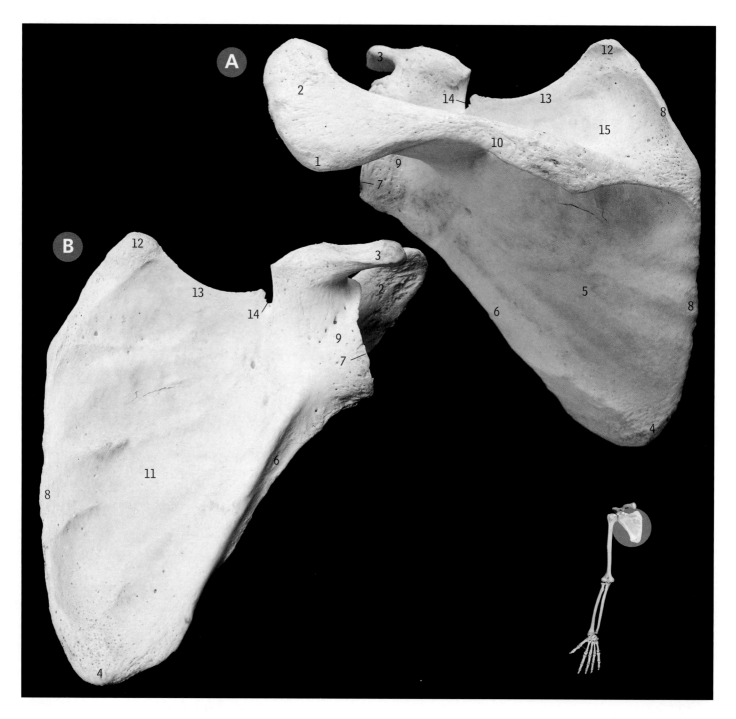

**A** dorsal surface

**B** costal surface

| | |
|---|---|
| **1** Acromial angle | **9** Neck (and spinoglenoid notch on dorsal surface) |
| **2** Acromion | |
| **3** Coracoid process | **10** Spine |
| **4** Inferior angle | **11** Subscapular fossa |
| **5** Infraspinous fossa | **12** Superior angle |
| **6** Lateral border | **13** Superior border |
| **7** Margin of glenoid cavity | **14** Suprascapular notch |
| **8** Medial border | **15** Supraspinous fossa |

The spine (A10) of the scapula projects from its dorsal surface with the acromion (A2) at the lateral end of the spine.

# Left scapula *attachments*

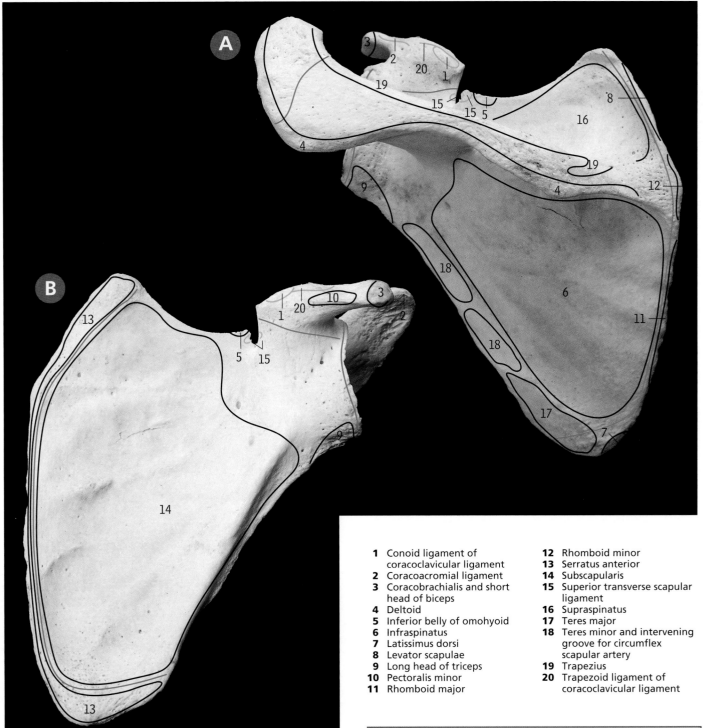

1  Conoid ligament of
   coracoclavicular ligament
2  Coracoacromial ligament
3  Coracobrachialis and short
   head of biceps
4  Deltoid
5  Inferior belly of omohyoid
6  Infraspinatus
7  Latissimus dorsi
8  Levator scapulae
9  Long head of triceps
10 Pectoralis minor
11 Rhomboid major

12 Rhomboid minor
13 Serratus anterior
14 Subscapularis
15 Superior transverse scapular
   ligament
16 Supraspinatus
17 Teres major
18 Teres minor and intervening
   groove for circumflex
   scapular artery
19 Trapezius
20 Trapezoid ligament of
   coracoclavicular ligament

**A** **dorsal surface**          **B** **costal surface**

Blue lines, epiphysial lines; green lines, capsular
attachments of shoulder joint; pale green lines, ligament
attachments

The suprascapular notch is bridged by the superior transverse
scapular ligament (15).

The conoid (1) and trapezoid (20) ligaments together form the
coracoclavicular ligament, which attaches the coracoid process of
the scapula to the under-surface of the lateral end of the clavicle.

The coracoacromial ligament (2) passes between the coracoid
process and the acromion, forming with these bony processes an
arch above the shoulder joint.

## A Left scapula *from the lateral side*

| | | | |
|---|---|---|---|
| **1** | Acromion | **6** | Infraspinous fossa |
| **2** | Coracoid process | **7** | Lateral border |
| **3** | Glenoid cavity | **8** | Spine |
| **4** | Inferior angle | **9** | Supraglenoid tubercle |
| **5** | Infraglenoid tubercle | **10** | Supraspinous fossa |

## B Left scapula and clavicle *articulation, from above*

| | | | |
|---|---|---|---|
| **1** | Acromial end of clavicle | **5** | Shaft of clavicle |
| **2** | Acromioclavicular joint | **6** | Spine of scapula |
| **3** | Acromion | **7** | Sternal end of clavicle |
| **4** | Coracoid process | **8** | Supraspinous fossa |

## C Left clavicle *from below*

**1** Acromial end with articular surface (arrow)
**2** Conoid tubercle
**3** Groove for subclavius muscle
**4** Impression for costoclavicular ligament
**5** Sternal end with articular surface (arrow)
**6** Trapezoid line

The sternal end of the clavicle (B7, C5) is bulbous; the acromial end (B1, C1) is flattened. The shaft is convex towards the front in its medial two-thirds, and the groove for the subclavius muscle is on the inferior surface (C3).

*Acromioclavicular separation, see page 174.*

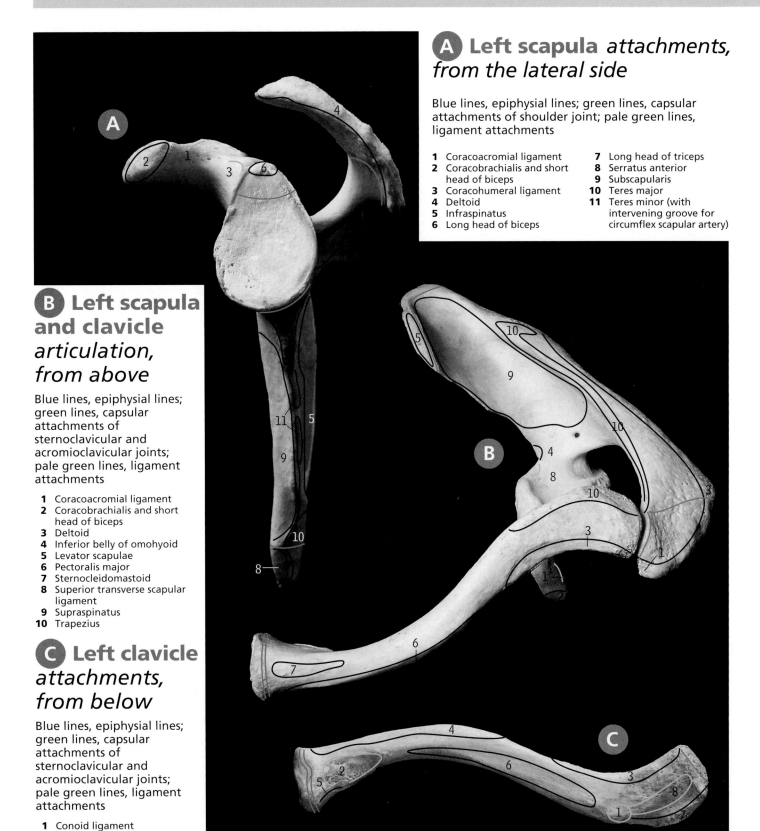

### A Left scapula *attachments, from the lateral side*

Blue lines, epiphysial lines; green lines, capsular attachments of shoulder joint; pale green lines, ligament attachments

1 Coracoacromial ligament
2 Coracobrachialis and short head of biceps
3 Coracohumeral ligament
4 Deltoid
5 Infraspinatus
6 Long head of biceps
7 Long head of triceps
8 Serratus anterior
9 Subscapularis
10 Teres major
11 Teres minor (with intervening groove for circumflex scapular artery)

### B Left scapula and clavicle *articulation, from above*

Blue lines, epiphysial lines; green lines, capsular attachments of sternoclavicular and acromioclavicular joints; pale green lines, ligament attachments

1 Coracoacromial ligament
2 Coracobrachialis and short head of biceps
3 Deltoid
4 Inferior belly of omohyoid
5 Levator scapulae
6 Pectoralis major
7 Sternocleidomastoid
8 Superior transverse scapular ligament
9 Supraspinatus
10 Trapezius

### C Left clavicle *attachments, from below*

Blue lines, epiphysial lines; green lines, capsular attachments of sternoclavicular and acromioclavicular joints; pale green lines, ligament attachments

1 Conoid ligament
2 Costoclavicular ligament
3 Deltoid
4 Pectoralis major
5 Sternohyoid
6 Subclavius and clavipectoral fascia
7 Trapezius
8 Trapezoid ligament

# Right humerus *upper end*

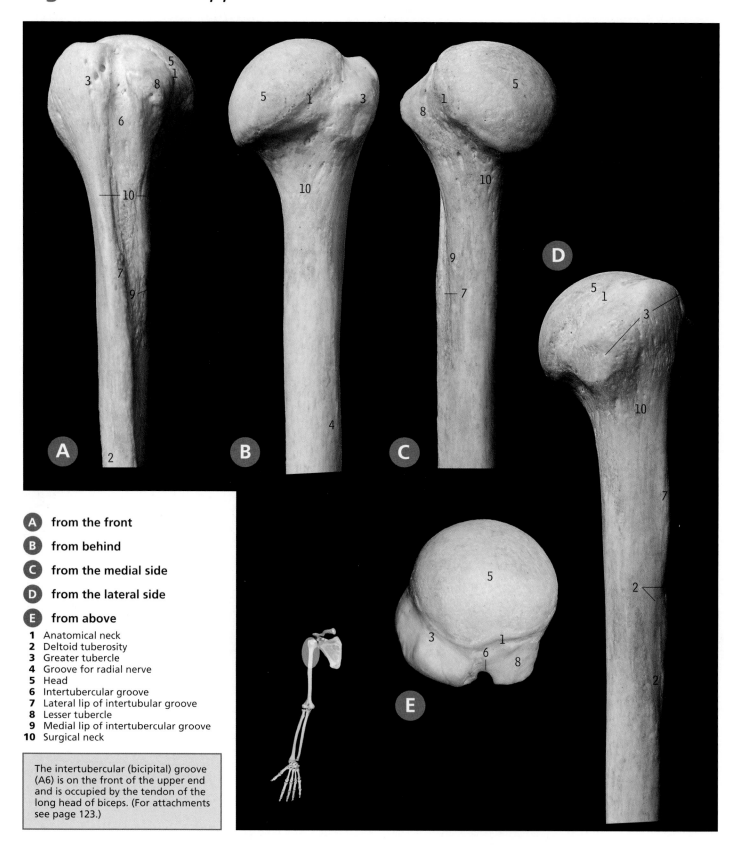

A **from the front**

B **from behind**

C **from the medial side**

D **from the lateral side**

E **from above**

**1** Anatomical neck
**2** Deltoid tuberosity
**3** Greater tubercle
**4** Groove for radial nerve
**5** Head
**6** Intertubercular groove
**7** Lateral lip of intertubular groove
**8** Lesser tubercle
**9** Medial lip of intertubercular groove
**10** Surgical neck

The intertubercular (bicipital) groove (A6) is on the front of the upper end and is occupied by the tendon of the long head of biceps. (For attachments see page 123.)

*Dislocation of the humerus, see page 174.*

# Right humerus *attachments, upper end*

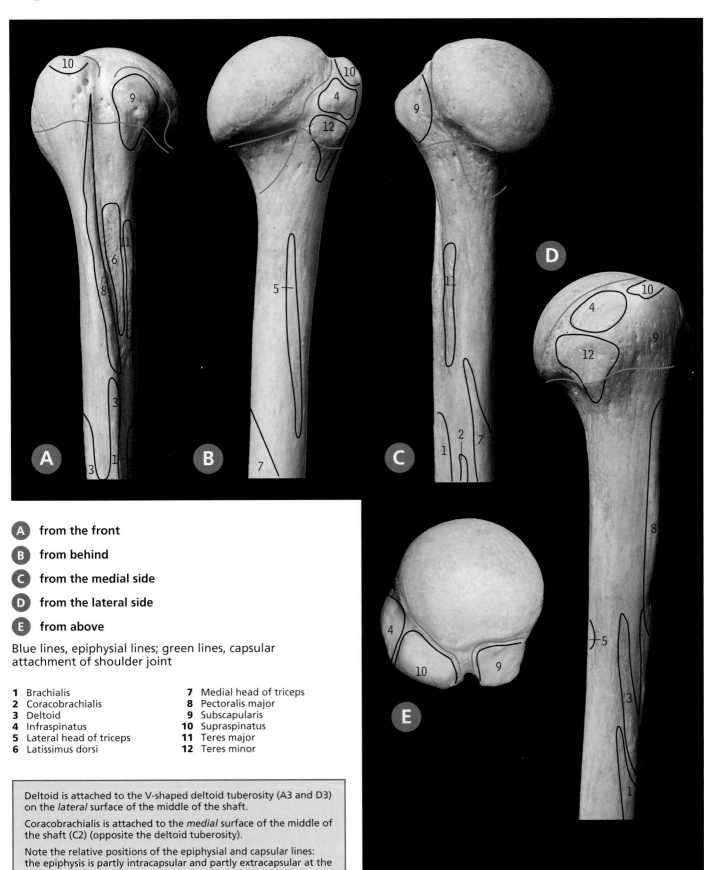

**A** from the front

**B** from behind

**C** from the medial side

**D** from the lateral side

**E** from above

Blue lines, epiphysial lines; green lines, capsular attachment of shoulder joint

| | | | |
|---|---|---|---|
| **1** | Brachialis | **7** | Medial head of triceps |
| **2** | Coracobrachialis | **8** | Pectoralis major |
| **3** | Deltoid | **9** | Subscapularis |
| **4** | Infraspinatus | **10** | Supraspinatus |
| **5** | Lateral head of triceps | **11** | Teres major |
| **6** | Latissimus dorsi | **12** | Teres minor |

Deltoid is attached to the V-shaped deltoid tuberosity (A3 and D3) on the *lateral* surface of the middle of the shaft.

Coracobrachialis is attached to the *medial* surface of the middle of the shaft (C2) (opposite the deltoid tuberosity).

Note the relative positions of the epiphysial and capsular lines: the epiphysis is partly intracapsular and partly extracapsular at the upper end of the humerus.

# Right humerus *lower end*

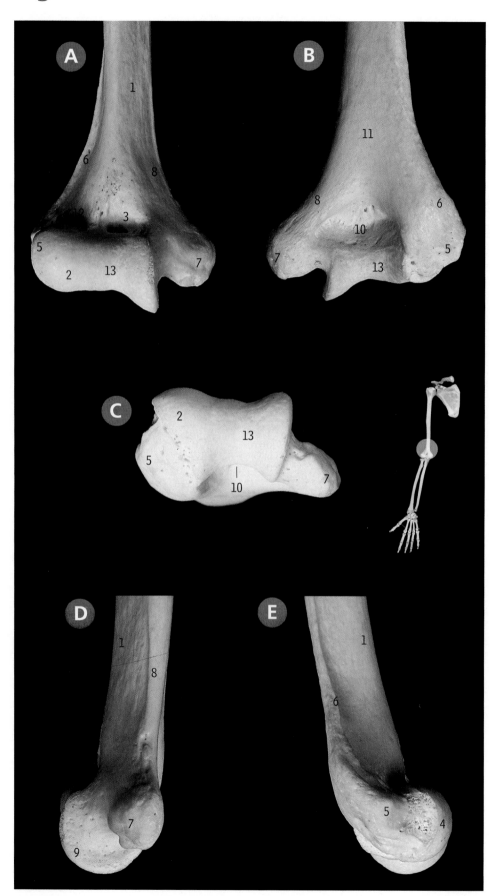

**A** from the front
**B** from behind
**C** from below
**D** from the medial side
**E** from the lateral side

1 Anterior surface
2 Capitulum
3 Coronoid fossa
4 Lateral edge of capitulum
5 Lateral epicondyle
6 Lateral supracondylar ridge
7 Medial epicondyle
8 Medial supracondylar ridge
9 Medial surface of trochlea
10 Olecranon fossa
11 Posterior surface
12 Radial fossa
13 Trochlea

The medial epicondyle (7) is more prominent than the lateral (5).

The medial part of the trochlea (13) is more prominent than the lateral part.

The olecranon fossa (10) on the posterior surface is deeper than the radial and coronoid fossae on the anterior surface (12 and 3).

# Right humerus *attachments, lower end*

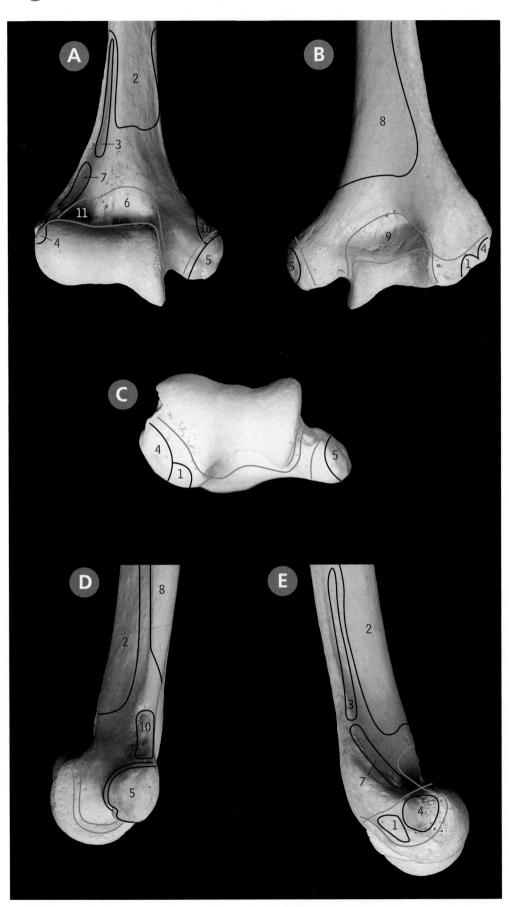

A from the front

B from behind

C from below

D from the medial side

E from the lateral side

Blue lines, epiphysial lines; green lines, capsular attachment of elbow joint

1 Anconeus
2 Brachialis
3 Brachioradialis
4 Common extensor origin
5 Common flexor origin
6 Coronoid fossa
7 Extensor carpi radialis longus
8 Medial head of triceps
9 Olecranon fossa
10 Pronator teres, humeral head
11 Radial fossa

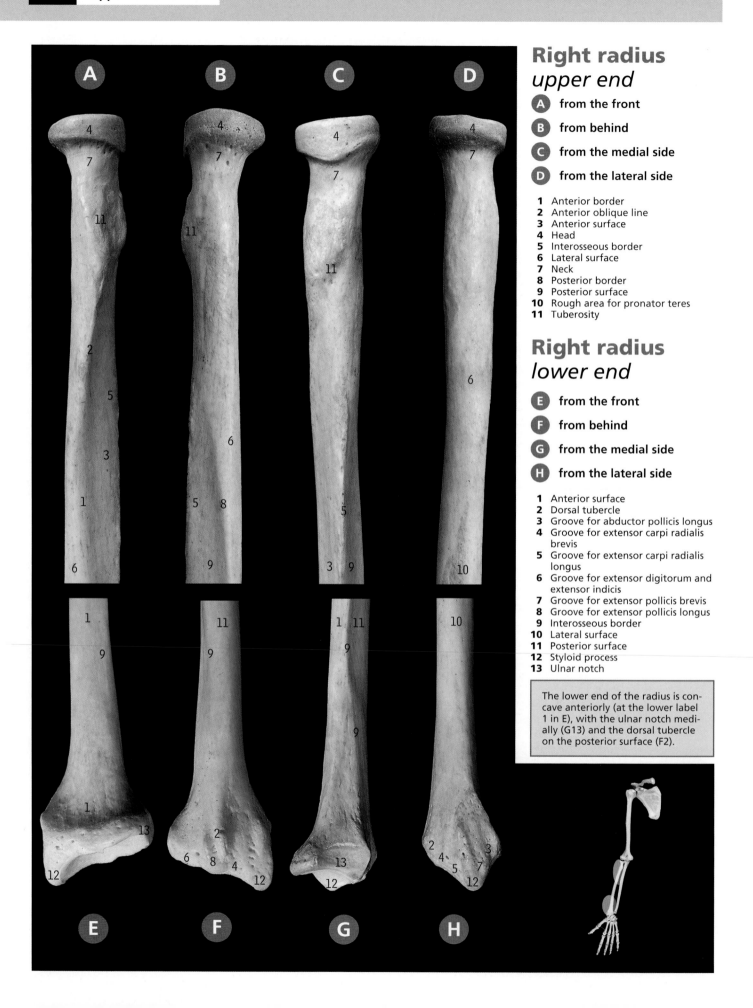

### Right radius
*upper end*

**A** from the front

**B** from behind

**C** from the medial side

**D** from the lateral side

1  Anterior border
2  Anterior oblique line
3  Anterior surface
4  Head
5  Interosseous border
6  Lateral surface
7  Neck
8  Posterior border
9  Posterior surface
10  Rough area for pronator teres
11  Tuberosity

### Right radius
*lower end*

**E** from the front

**F** from behind

**G** from the medial side

**H** from the lateral side

1  Anterior surface
2  Dorsal tubercle
3  Groove for abductor pollicis longus
4  Groove for extensor carpi radialis brevis
5  Groove for extensor carpi radialis longus
6  Groove for extensor digitorum and extensor indicis
7  Groove for extensor pollicis brevis
8  Groove for extensor pollicis longus
9  Interosseous border
10  Lateral surface
11  Posterior surface
12  Styloid process
13  Ulnar notch

The lower end of the radius is concave anteriorly (at the lower label 1 in E), with the ulnar notch medially (G13) and the dorsal tubercle on the posterior surface (F2).

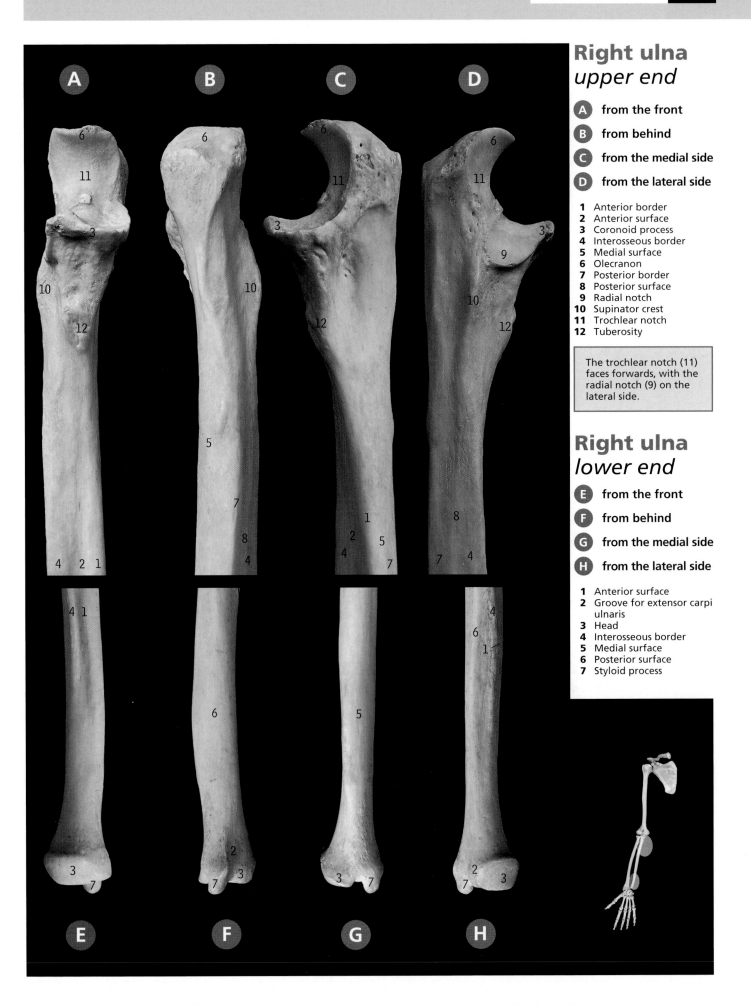

## Right ulna
### *upper end*

**A** from the front

**B** from behind

**C** from the medial side

**D** from the lateral side

1 Anterior border
2 Anterior surface
3 Coronoid process
4 Interosseous border
5 Medial surface
6 Olecranon
7 Posterior border
8 Posterior surface
9 Radial notch
10 Supinator crest
11 Trochlear notch
12 Tuberosity

The trochlear notch (11) faces forwards, with the radial notch (9) on the lateral side.

## Right ulna
### *lower end*

**E** from the front

**F** from behind

**G** from the medial side

**H** from the lateral side

1 Anterior surface
2 Groove for extensor carpi ulnaris
3 Head
4 Interosseous border
5 Medial surface
6 Posterior surface
7 Styloid process

E F G H

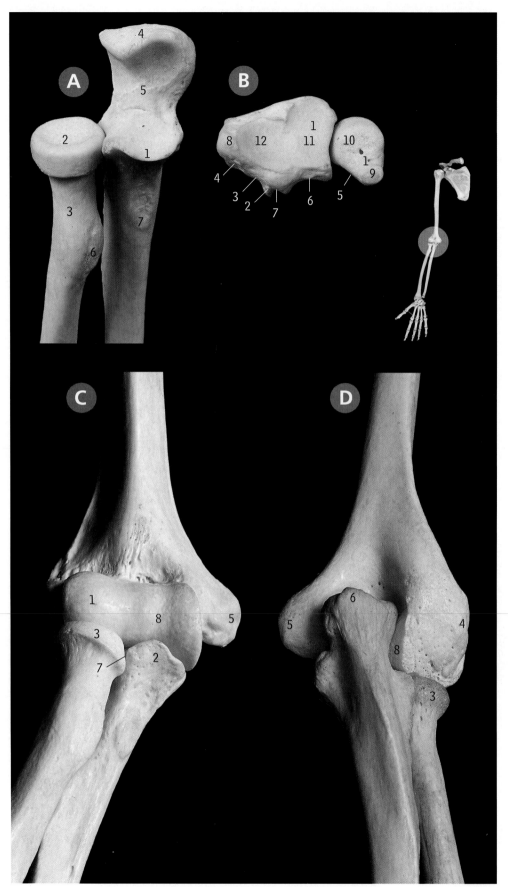

## A Right radius and ulna
*upper ends, from above and in front*

1 Coronoid process of ulna
2 Head of radius
3 Neck of radius
4 Olecranon of ulna
5 Trochlear notch of ulna
6 Tuberosity of radius
7 Tuberosity of ulna

## B Right radius and ulna *lower ends, from below*

1 Attachment of articular disc
2 Dorsal tubercle
3 Groove for extensor carpi radialis brevis
4 Groove for extensor carpi radialis longus
5 Groove for extensor carpi ulnaris
6 Groove for extensor digitorum and extensor indicis
7 Groove for extensor pollicis longus
8 Styloid process of radius
9 Styloid process of ulna
10 Surface for disc
11 Surface for lunate
12 Surface for scaphoid

## Right humerus, radius and ulna *articulation*

**C** from the front

**D** from behind

1 Capitulum of humerus
2 Coronoid process of ulna
3 Head of radius
4 Lateral epicondyle of humerus
5 Medial epicondyle of humerus
6 Olecranon of ulna
7 Radial notch of ulna
8 Trochlea of humerus

The elbow joint and the proximal radio-ulnar joint share a common synovial cavity.

*Dislocation of the elbow, supracondylar fracture of the humerus, see pages 174, 175.*

# Right radius and ulna *attachments*

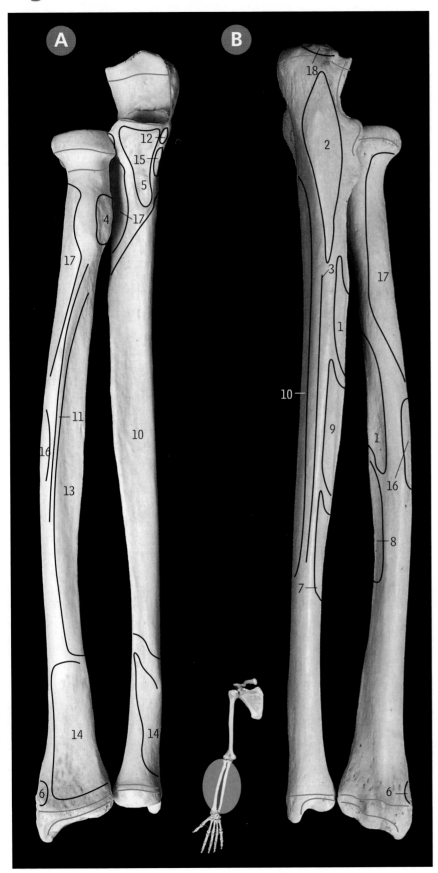

**A** from the front

**B** from behind

Blue lines, epiphysial lines; green lines, capsular attachments of elbow and wrist joints

1 Abductor pollicis longus
2 Anconeus
3 Aponeurotic attachment of flexor digitorum profundus, flexor carpi ulnaris and extensor carpi ulnaris
4 Biceps
5 Brachialis
6 Brachioradialis
7 Extensor indicis
8 Extensor pollicis brevis
9 Extensor pollicis longus
10 Flexor digitorum profundus
11 Flexor digitorum superficialis, radial head
12 Flexor digitorum superficialis, ulnar head
13 Flexor pollicis longus
14 Pronator quadratus
15 Pronator teres, ulnar head
16 Pronator teres
17 Supinator
18 Triceps

Abductor pollicis longus (1) and extensor pollicis brevis (8) are the only two muscles to have an origin from the posterior surface of the radius (although both extend on to the interosseous membrane and the abductor also has an origin from the posterior surface of the ulna). These muscles remain companions as they wind round the lateral side of the radius (page 157) and form the radial boundary of the anatomical snuffbox (page 158B).

In the young subject, the radius sometimes fractures across the lower epiphysis following an injury to the wrist. In the adult the term "Colles' fracture" (pages 131, 174) refers to a transverse break across the lower radius within about 2.5 cm of the lower end of the bone. The ulnar styloid process is also often fractured.

*Traction of forearm fractures, see page 176.*

# Bones of the right hand

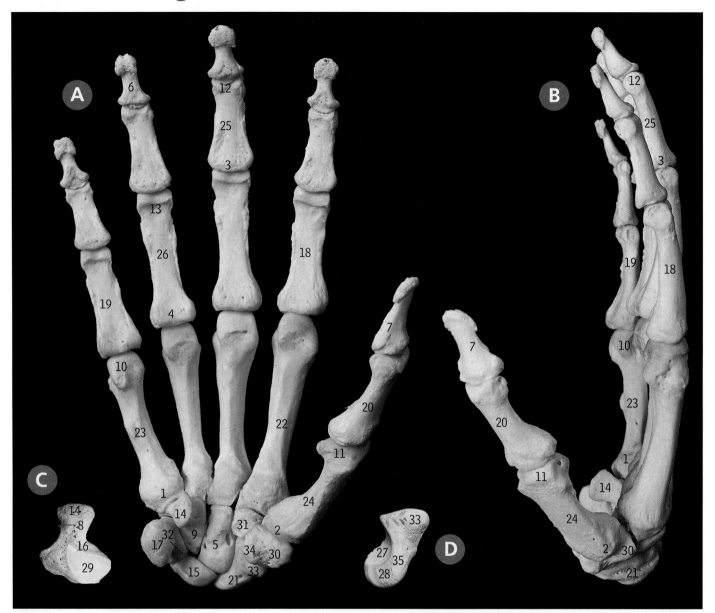

A palmar surface

B from the lateral side

C hamate from the medial side

D scaphoid, palmar surface

The scaphoid, lunate, triquetral and pisiform bones form the proximal row of carpal bones.

The trapezium, trapezoid, capitate and hamate bones form the distal row of carpal bones.

The tubercle (33) and waist (35) are the non-articular parts of the scaphoid and therefore contain nutrient foramina. A fracture across the waist may therefore interfere with the blood supply of the proximal pole of the bone and lead to avascular necrosis (see page 174). The waist of the scaphoid lies in the anatomical snuff-box; the tubercle may be palpated in front of the radial boundary of the snuffbox.

1 Base of fifth metacarpal
2 Base of first metacarpal
3 Base of middle phalanx of middle finger
4 Base of proximal phalanx of ring finger
5 Capitate
6 Distal phalanx of ring finger
7 Distal phalanx of thumb
8 Groove for deep branch of ulnar nerve
9 Hamate
10 Head of fifth metacarpal
11 Head of first metacarpal
12 Head of middle phalanx of middle finger
13 Head of proximal phalanx of ring finger
14 Hook of hamate
15 Lunate
16 Palmar surface, hamate
17 Pisiform

18 Proximal phalanx of index finger
19 Proximal phalanx of little finger
20 Proximal phalanx of thumb
21 Scaphoid
22 Shaft of second metacarpal
23 Shaft of fifth metacarpal
24 Shaft of first metacarpal
25 Shaft of middle phalanx of middle finger
26 Shaft of proximal phalanx of ring finger
27 Surface for capitate
28 Surface for lunate
29 Surface for triquetral
30 Trapezium
31 Trapezoid
32 Triquetral
33 Tubercle of scaphoid
34 Tubercle of trapezium
35 Waist of scaphoid

# Bones of the right hand *dorsal surface*

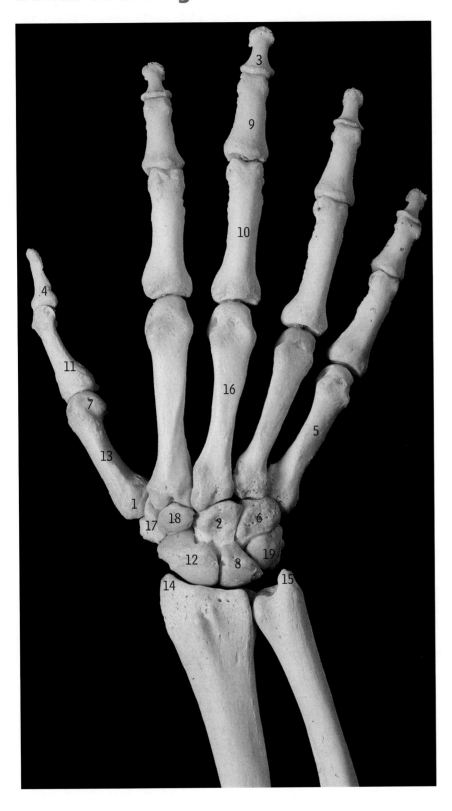

1 Base of first metacarpal
2 Capitate
3 Distal phalanx of middle finger
4 Distal phalanx of thumb
5 Fifth metacarpal
6 Hamate
7 Head of first metacarpal
8 Lunate
9 Middle phalanx of middle finger
10 Proximal phalanx of middle finger
11 Proximal phalanx of thumb
12 Scaphoid
13 Shaft of first metacarpal
14 Styloid process of radius
15 Styloid process of ulna
16 Third metacarpal
17 Trapezium
18 Trapezoid
19 Triquetral

The wrist joint (properly called the radiocarpal joint) is the joint between (proximally) the lower end of the radius and the interarticular disc which holds the lower ends of the radius and the ulna together, and (distally) the scaphoid, lunate and triquetral bones.

The midcarpal joint is the joint between the proximal and distal rows of carpal bones (see the note on page 130).

The carpometacarpal joint of the thumb is the joint between the trapezium and the base of the first metacarpal.

*Colles' fracture, dislocation of the finger, see page 174.*

# Bones of the right hand *attachments*

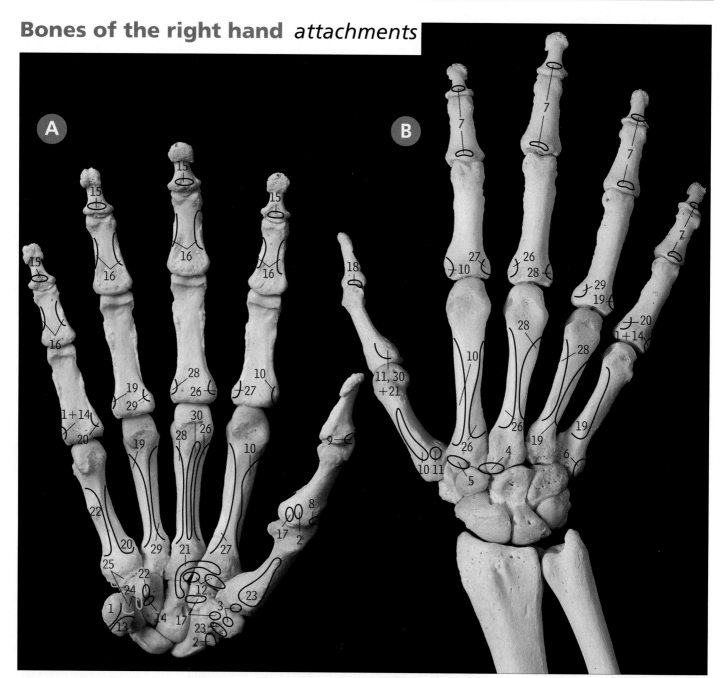

**A** palmar surface     **B** dorsal surface

Pale green lines, ligament attachments

| | |
|---|---|
| **1** Abductor digiti minimi | **17** Flexor pollicis brevis |
| **2** Abductor pollicis brevis | **18** Flexor pollicis longus |
| **3** Abductor pollicis longus | **19** Fourth dorsal interosseous |
| **4** Extensor carpi radialis brevis | **20** Fourth palmar interosseous |
| **5** Extensor carpi radialis longus | **21** Oblique head of adductor pollicis |
| **6** Extensor carpi ulnaris | **22** Opponens digiti minimi |
| **7** Extensor expansion | **23** Opponens pollicis |
| **8** Extensor pollicis brevis | **24** Pisohamate ligament |
| **9** Extensor pollicis longus | **25** Pisometacarpal ligament |
| **10** First dorsal interosseous | **26** Second dorsal interosseous |
| **11** First palmar interosseous | **27** Second palmar interosseous |
| **12** Flexor carpi radialis | **28** Third dorsal interosseous |
| **13** Flexor carpi ulnaris | **29** Third palmar interosseous |
| **14** Flexor digiti minimi brevis | **30** Transverse head of adductor pollicis |
| **15** Flexor digitorum profundus | |
| **16** Flexor digitorum superficialis | |

The metacarpophalangeal joints are the joints between the heads of the metacarpals and the bases of the proximal phalanges.

The interphalangeal joints are the joints between the head of one phalanx and the base of the adjoining phalanx.

The pisiform is a sesamoid bone in the tendon of flexor carpi ulnaris and is anchored by the pisohamate and pisometacarpal ligaments (24 and 25).

Dorsal interossei arise from the sides of two adjacent metacarpal bones (as at 26, from the sides of the second and third metacarpals); palmar interossei arise only from the metacarpal of their own finger (as at 27, from the second metacarpal). Compare with dissection B on page 166 and note that when looking at the palm, parts of the dorsal interossei can be seen as well as the palmar interossei, but when looking at the dorsum of the hand (as on page 170A) only dorsal interossei are seen.

# Right upper limb bones *secondary centres of ossification*

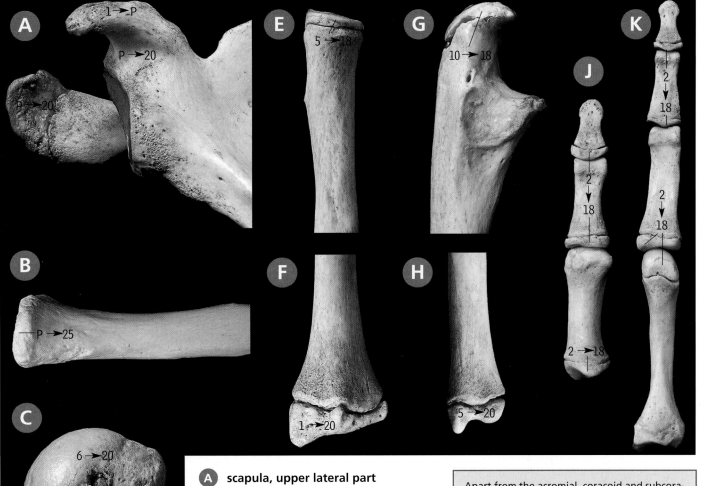

A    scapula, upper lateral part

B    clavicle, sternal end

C D    humerus, upper and lower ends

E F    radius, upper and lower ends

G H    ulna, upper and lower ends

J    first metacarpal and phalanges of thumb

K    second metacarpal and phalanges of index finger

Figures in years after birth, commencement of ossification → fusion. (P, puberty)

The first figure indicates the approximate date when ossification begins in the secondary centre, and the second figure (beyond the arrowhead) when the centre finally becomes fused with the rest of the bone. Single average dates have been given (both here and for the lower limb bone centres on pages 314 and 315) and although there may be considerable individual variations, the 'growing end' of the bone (when fusion occurs last) is constant. The dates in females are often a year or more earlier than in males.

Apart from the acromial, coracoid and subcoracoid centres illustrated (A), the scapula usually has other centres for the inferior angle, medial border, and the lower part of the rim of the glenoid cavity (all P → 20; see pages 119 and 121).

The clavicle is the first bone in the body to start to ossify (fifth week of gestation). It ossifies in membrane, but the ends of the bone have a cartilaginous phase of ossification; a secondary centre appearing at the sternal end (B) unites with the body at about the 25th year.

The centre illustrated at the upper end of the humerus (C) is the result of the union at 6 years of centres for the head (1 year), greater tubercle (3 years) and lesser tubercle (5 years).

At the lower end of the humerus (D) the centres for the capitulum, trochlea and lateral epicondyle fuse together before uniting with the shaft.

All the phalanges (as in K), and the first metacarpal (J) have a secondary centre at their proximal ends; the other metacarpals (as in K) have one at their distal ends.

All the carpal bones are cartilaginous at birth and none has a secondary centre. The largest, the capitate, is the first to begin to ossify (in the second month after birth), followed in a month or so by the hamate, with the triquetral at 3 years, lunate at 4 years, scaphoid, trapezoid and trapezium at 5 years and the pisiform last at 9 years or later. There are often variations in the above common pattern.

# Right shoulder
*surface markings, from the front*

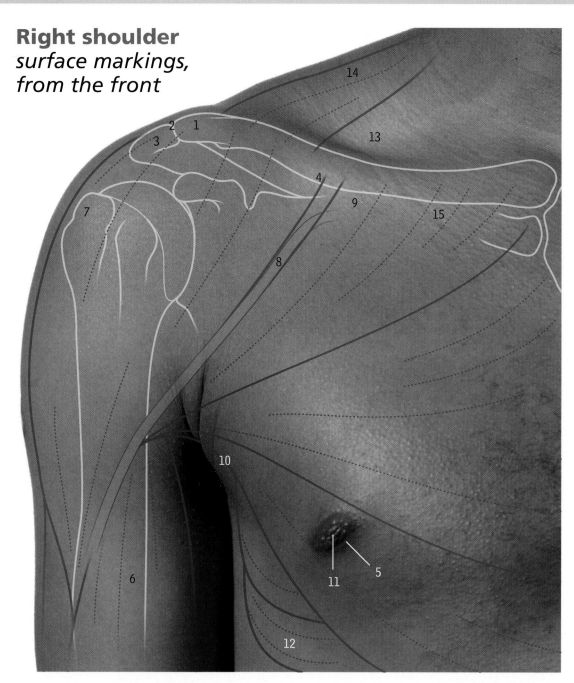

1 Acromial end of clavicle
2 Acromioclavicular joint
3 Acromion
4 Anterior margin of deltoid
5 Areola
6 Biceps
7 Deltoid overlying greater tubercle of humerus
8 Deltopectoral groove and cephalic vein
9 Infraclavicular fossa
10 Lower margin of pectoralis major
11 Nipple
12 Serratus anterior
13 Supraclavicular fossa
14 Trapezius
15 Upper margin of pectoralis major

The nipple in the male (11) normally lies at the level of the fourth intercostal space.

The lower border of pectoralis major (10) forms the anterior axillary fold.

Note that the most lateral bony point in the shoulder is the greater tubercle (7).

The clavicle is subcutaneous throughout its length. Its acromial end (1) at the acromioclavicular joint (2) lies at a slightly higher level than the acromion of the scapula (3). At the most lateral part of the shoulder, the deltoid overlies the humerus; the acromion of the scapula does not extend so far laterally. Compare the positions of the features noted here with the dissection on the next page.

*Dislocation of humerus, see page 174.*

# Right shoulder
*superficial
dissection*

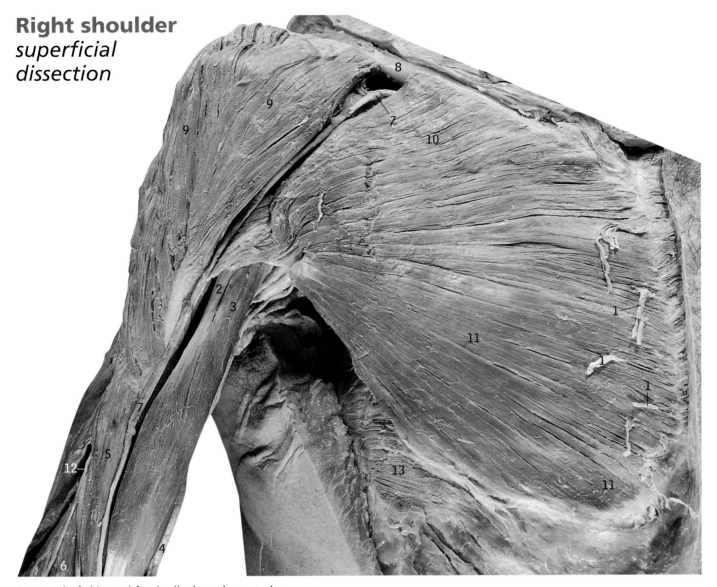

**Removal of skin and fascia displays the anterior
musculature of the shoulder and thoracic wall.**

1   Anterior perforating
    branches of intercostal
    neurovascular bundle
2   Biceps brachii, long head
3   Biceps brachii, short head
4   Brachial artery
5   Brachialis
6   Brachioradialis

7   Cephalic vein
8   Clavicle
9   Deltoid
10  Pectoralis major, clavicular
    head
11  Pectoralis major, sternal head
12  Radial nerve
13  Serratus anterior

# Right shoulder
## *superficial dissection, from the front*

Removal of skin and fascia displays branches of the
supraclavicular nerve (6) crossing the clavicle (9), and the
cephalic vein (7) lying in the deltopectoral groove
between deltoid (13) and pectoralis major (11).

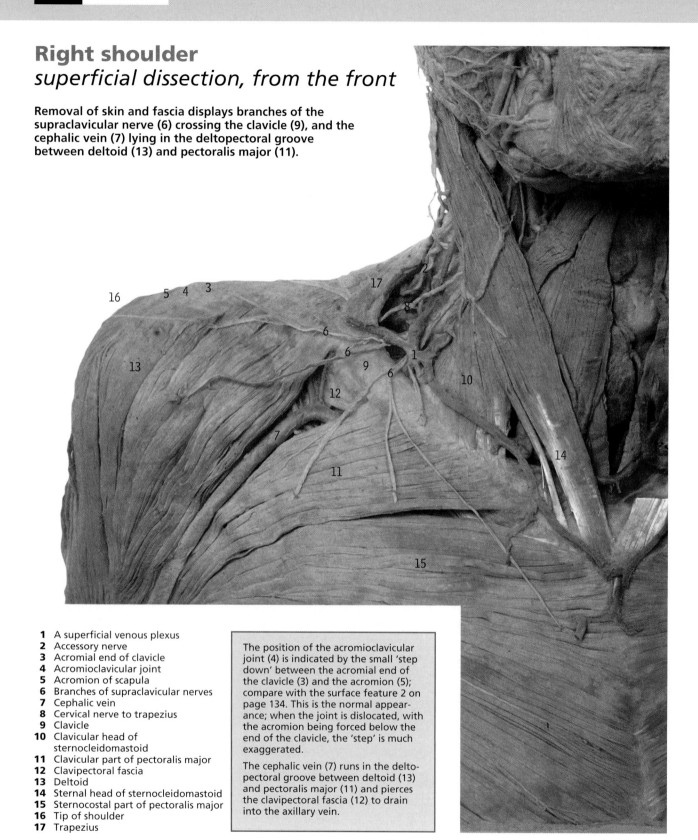

1. A superficial venous plexus
2. Accessory nerve
3. Acromial end of clavicle
4. Acromioclavicular joint
5. Acromion of scapula
6. Branches of supraclavicular nerves
7. Cephalic vein
8. Cervical nerve to trapezius
9. Clavicle
10. Clavicular head of
    sternocleidomastoid
11. Clavicular part of pectoralis major
12. Clavipectoral fascia
13. Deltoid
14. Sternal head of sternocleidomastoid
15. Sternocostal part of pectoralis major
16. Tip of shoulder
17. Trapezius

The position of the acromioclavicular
joint (4) is indicated by the small 'step
down' between the acromial end of
the clavicle (3) and the acromion (5);
compare with the surface feature 2 on
page 134. This is the normal appearance; when the joint is dislocated, with
the acromion being forced below the
end of the clavicle, the 'step' is much
exaggerated.

The cephalic vein (7) runs in the deltopectoral groove between deltoid (13)
and pectoralis major (11) and pierces
the clavipectoral fascia (12) to drain
into the axillary vein.

# Right shoulder *deeper dissection, from the front*

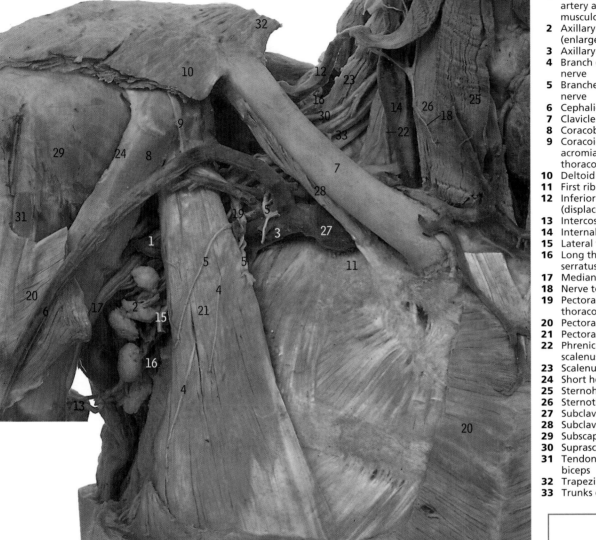

1 Anterior circumflex humeral artery and musculocutaneous nerve
2 Axillary lymph nodes (enlarged)
3 Axillary vein
4 Branch of medial pectoral nerve
5 Branches of lateral pectoral nerve
6 Cephalic vein
7 Clavicle
8 Coracobrachialis
9 Coracoid process and acromial branch of thoracoacromial artery
10 Deltoid
11 First rib
12 Inferior belly of omohyoid (displaced upwards)
13 Intercostobrachial nerve
14 Internal jugular vein
15 Lateral thoracic artery
16 Long thoracic nerve (to serratus anterior)
17 Median nerve
18 Nerve to sternothyroid
19 Pectoral branch of thoracoacromial artery
20 Pectoralis major
21 Pectoralis minor
22 Phrenic nerve overlying scalenus anterior
23 Scalenus medius
24 Short head of biceps
25 Sternohyoid
26 Sternothyroid
27 Subclavian vein
28 Subclavius
29 Subscapularis
30 Suprascapular nerve
31 Tendon of long head of biceps
32 Trapezius
33 Trunks of brachial plexus

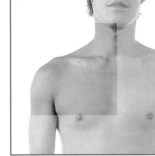

Most of deltoid (10) and pectoralis major (20) have been removed to show the underlying pectoralis minor (21) and its associated vessels and nerves. The clavipectoral fascia which passes between the clavicle (7) and the upper (medial) border of the pectoralis minor (21) has also been removed to show the axillary vein (3) receiving the cephalic vein (6) and continuing as the subclavian vein (27) as it crosses the first rib (11).

## Shoulder arthroscopy

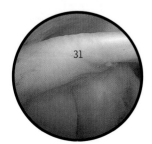

This shows the arthroscopic view of the right shoulder seen from behind. The supraspinatus tendon and the long head of biceps is in pristine condition. The anterior edge of the glenoid labrum shows some wear.

*Klumpke's paralysis, see page 175.*

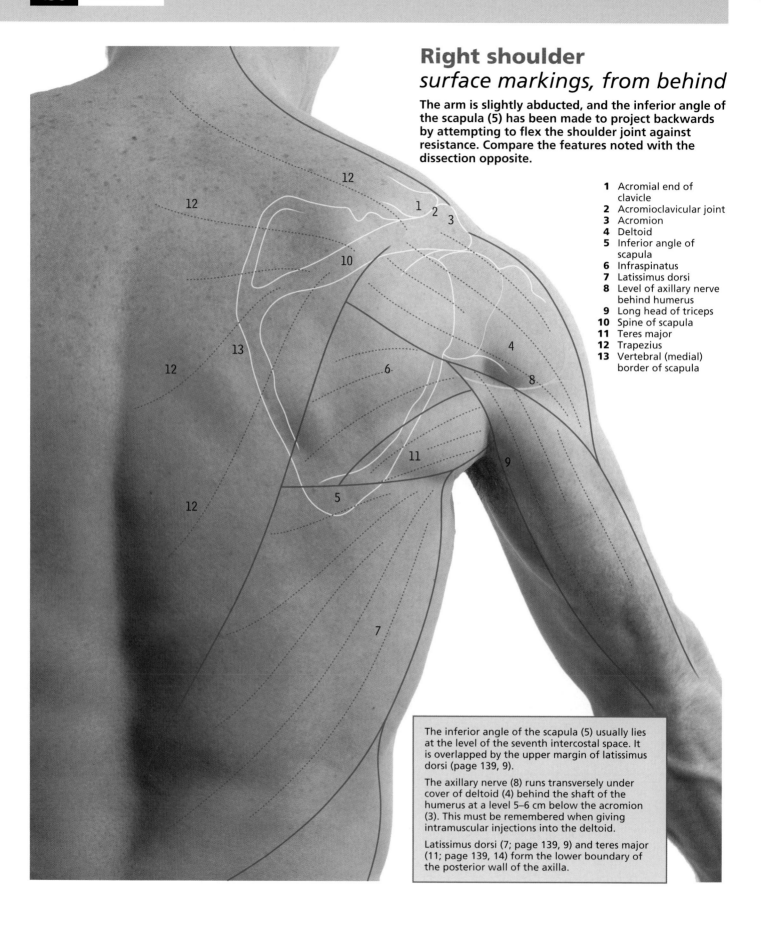

# Right shoulder
## *surface markings, from behind*

The arm is slightly abducted, and the inferior angle of the scapula (5) has been made to project backwards by attempting to flex the shoulder joint against resistance. Compare the features noted with the dissection opposite.

1 Acromial end of clavicle
2 Acromioclavicular joint
3 Acromion
4 Deltoid
5 Inferior angle of scapula
6 Infraspinatus
7 Latissimus dorsi
8 Level of axillary nerve behind humerus
9 Long head of triceps
10 Spine of scapula
11 Teres major
12 Trapezius
13 Vertebral (medial) border of scapula

The inferior angle of the scapula (5) usually lies at the level of the seventh intercostal space. It is overlapped by the upper margin of latissimus dorsi (page 139, 9).

The axillary nerve (8) runs transversely under cover of deltoid (4) behind the shaft of the humerus at a level 5–6 cm below the acromion (3). This must be remembered when giving intramuscular injections into the deltoid.

Latissimus dorsi (7; page 139, 9) and teres major (11; page 139, 14) form the lower boundary of the posterior wall of the axilla.

# Right shoulder *superficial dissection, from behind*

From above and below, trapezius (16) converges on to the spine of the scapula (13). The upper margin of latissimus dorsi (9) overlaps the inferior angle of the scapula and the lowest part of teres major (14). The long head of triceps (10) is seen emerging between teres minor (15) and teres major (14). As at the front, deltoid (5) covers the shoulder joint and upper part of the humerus.

The triangle of auscultation (17) is bounded by the trapezius, latissimus dorsi and the medial border of the scapula; its floor is partly formed by rhomboid major. If the arms are brought forwards, the sixth intercostal space becomes available for auscultation.

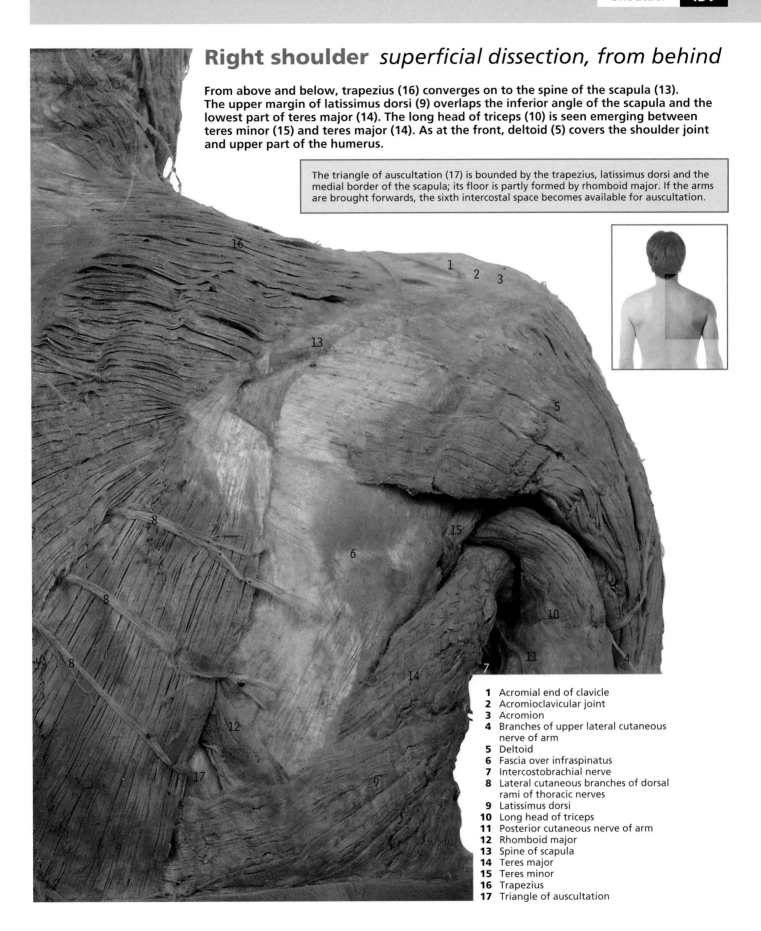

1  Acromial end of clavicle
2  Acromioclavicular joint
3  Acromion
4  Branches of upper lateral cutaneous
   nerve of arm
5  Deltoid
6  Fascia over infraspinatus
7  Intercostobrachial nerve
8  Lateral cutaneous branches of dorsal
   rami of thoracic nerves
9  Latissimus dorsi
10 Long head of triceps
11 Posterior cutaneous nerve of arm
12 Rhomboid major
13 Spine of scapula
14 Teres major
15 Teres minor
16 Trapezius
17 Triangle of auscultation

*Intramuscular injections, see page 175.*

# Right shoulder *from behind*

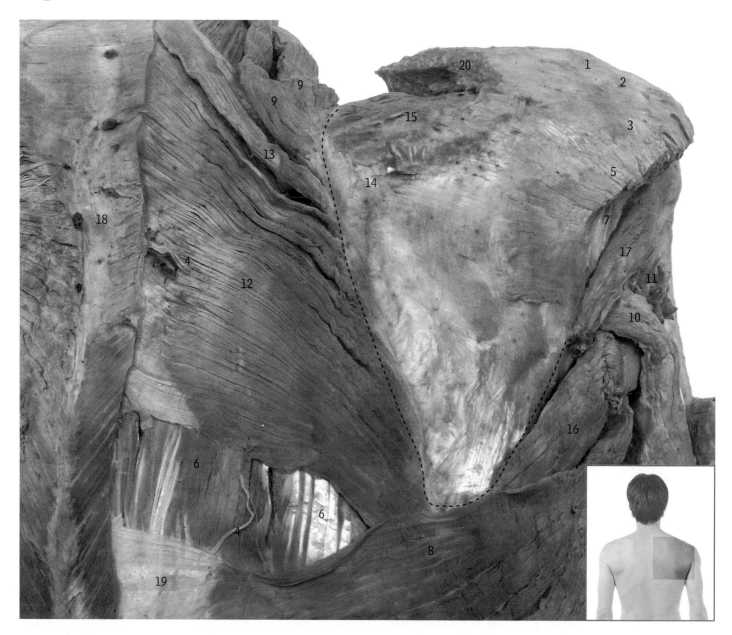

Interrupted line, outline of scapula

**Most of trapezius (20) and deltoid (5) have been removed to show the underlying muscles. The medial cut edge of trapezius remains near the line of the thoracic spines (18). Levator scapulae (9), rhomboid minor (13) and rhomboid major (12) are seen converging on to the vertebral (medial) border of the scapula, and supraspinatus (15) lies above the spine of the scapula (14).**

1 Acromial end of clavicle
2 Acromioclavicular joint
3 Acromion
4 Branch of dorsal ramus of a thoracic nerve
5 Deltoid
6 Erector spinae
7 Infraspinatus
8 Latissimus dorsi
9 Levator scapulae
10 Long head of triceps
11 Posterior circumflex humeral vessels and axillary nerve
12 Rhomboid major
13 Rhomboid minor
14 Spine of scapula
15 Supraspinatus
16 Teres major
17 Teres minor
18 Third thoracic spinous process
19 Thoracic part of thoracolumbar fascia
20 Trapezius

*Shoulder joint injection, see page 175.*

## A Right shoulder *from the right and behind*

The central parts of supraspinatus (13) and infraspinatus (5) have been removed to show the suprascapular nerve (12) which supplies both muscles. The removal of parts of infraspinatus and teres minor (15) displays the anastomosis between the circumflex scapular branch of the subscapular artery (3) and the suprascapular artery (11). Deltoid (4) has been reflected laterally to show the axillary nerve (2) and the posterior circumflex humeral vessels passing backwards through the quadrilateral space (see note below).

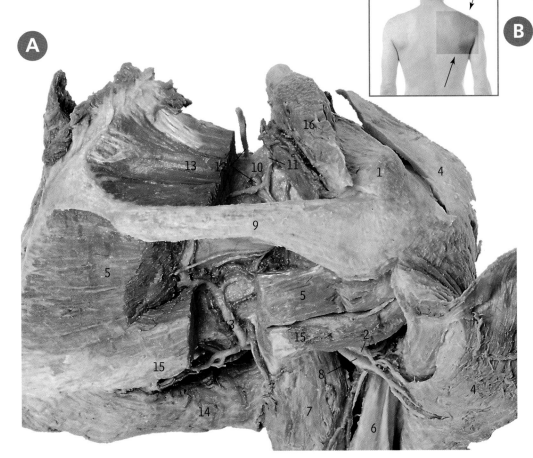

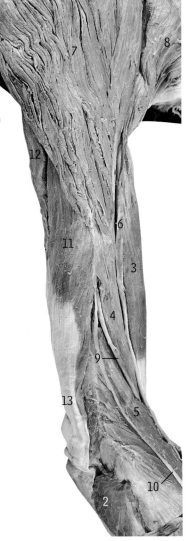

1  Acromioclavicular joint
2  Axillary nerve
3  Circumflex scapular artery
4  Deltoid
5  Infraspinatus
6  Lateral head of triceps
7  Long head of triceps
8  Posterior circumflex humeral artery
9  Spine of scapula
10  Superior transverse scapular (suprascapular) ligament
11  Suprascapular artery
12  Suprascapular nerve
13  Supraspinatus
14  Teres major
15  Teres minor
16  Trapezius

The axillary nerve (A2) and posterior circumflex humeral vessels (A8) pass backwards through the quadrilateral space which (viewed from behind) is bounded by teres minor (A15) above, below by teres major (A14), medially by the long head of triceps (A7), and laterally by the humerus. (Viewed from the front, the upper boundary of the space is subscapularis – see page 146, 23.)

## B Right shoulder and upper arm *from the right*

Deltoid (7) extends over the tip of the shoulder to its attachment halfway down the lateral side of the shaft of the humerus. Biceps (3) is on the front of the arm below pectoralis major (8) and triceps (11 and 12) is at the back.

1  Acromion
2  Anconeus
3  Biceps brachii
4  Brachialis
5  Brachioradialis
6  Cephalic vein
7  Deltoid
8  Pectoralis major
9  Radial nerve
10  Radial nerve, cutaneous branch
11  Triceps, lateral head
12  Triceps, long head
13  Triceps, tendon

*Posterior dislocation of the shoulder, see page 175.*

# Right shoulder joint Ⓐ cross section Ⓑ axial MR image

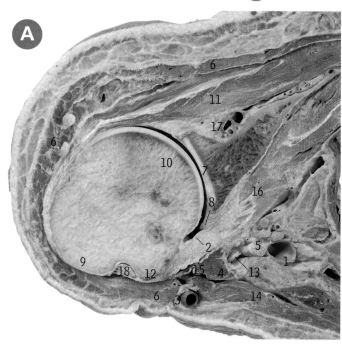

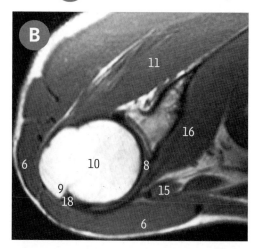

Viewed from below, this cadaveric section shows the articulation of the head of the humerus (10) with the glenoid cavity of the scapula (7). The tendon of the long head of biceps (18) lies in the groove between the greater and lesser tubercles of the humerus (9 and 12). Subscapularis (16) passes immediately in front of the joint, and infraspinatus (11) behind it. Compare the MR image in B with features in A.

| | | | |
|---|---|---|---|
| 1 | Axillary artery | 12 | Lesser tubercle |
| 2 | Capsule | 13 | Musculocutaneous nerve |
| 3 | Cephalic vein | 14 | Pectoralis major |
| 4 | Coracobrachialis | 15 | Short head of biceps |
| 5 | Cords of brachial plexus | 16 | Subscapularis |
| 6 | Deltoid | 17 | Suprascapular nerve and vessels |
| 7 | Glenoid cavity | 18 | Tendon of long head of biceps in intertubercular groove |
| 8 | Glenoid labrum | | |
| 9 | Greater tubercle | | |
| 10 | Head of humerus | | |
| 11 | Infraspinatus | | |

# Right shoulder joint Ⓒ from the front

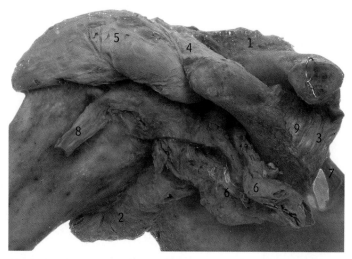

The synovial joint cavity inside the capsule (2) and the subacromial bursa (5) have been injected separately with green resin.

1 Acromioclavicular joint
2 Capsule of shoulder joint
3 Conoid ligament
4 Coracoacromial ligament
5 Subacromial bursa
6 Subscapularis bursa
7 Superior transverse scapular (suprascapular) ligament
8 Tendon of long head of biceps
9 Trapezoid ligament

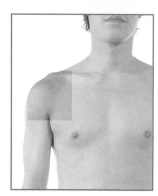

# Ⓓ Shoulder coronal oblique MR arthrogram

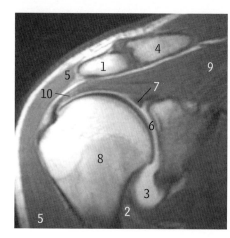

1 Acromion
2 Axillary nerve and circumflex humeral vessels
3 Axillary recess of shoulder joint
4 Clavicle
5 Deltoid
6 Glenoid cavity
7 Glenoid labrum
8 Humerus
9 Supraspinatus muscle
10 Supraspinatus tendon

## E  Shoulder *dissection, coronal section*

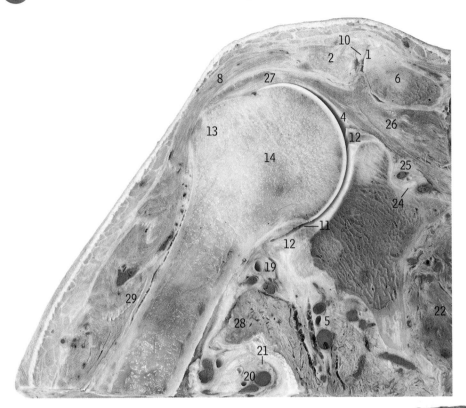

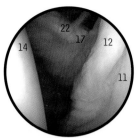

This is the first view of the shoulder on entering the joint from the posterior aspect with an arthroscope. The humerus head is on the left, the subscapularis tendon is in the middle and the glenoid and the surrounding labrum is on the right. The joint is slightly distracted with the aid of traction and also the fluid in the joint used in the arthroscopy.

## G  Right shoulder joint *opened from behind*

In this view, after removing all the posterior part of the capsule, the inner surface of the front of the capsule (4) is seen, with its reinforcing glenohumeral ligaments (15, 17 and 23).

## F  Shoulder *radiograph*
**anteroposterior projection in a 9-year-old child**

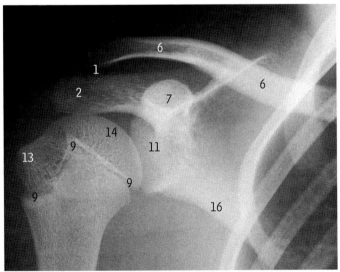

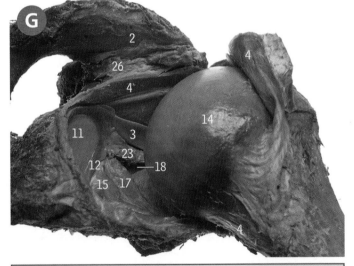

The joint cavity communicates with the subscapularis bursa through an opening (18, 23, 17) between the superior (10) and middle (8) glenohumeral ligaments.

The tendon of the long head of biceps (3, 12) is continuous with the glenoid labrum (4).

| | | | |
|---|---|---|---|
| **1** Acromioclavicular joint | **10** Fibrocartilaginous disc | **18** Opening into subscapularis bursa | **24** Suprascapular nerve |
| **2** Acromion | **11** Glenoid cavity | **19** Posterior circumflex humeral vessels | **25** Suprascapular vessels |
| **3** Biceps, long head | **12** Glenoid labrum | **20** Profunda brachii vessels | **26** Supraspinatus |
| **4** Capsule | **13** Greater tubercle | **21** Radial nerve | **27** Supraspinatus tendon |
| **5** Circumflex scapular vessels | **14** Head of humerus | **22** Subscapularis | **28** Teres major |
| **6** Clavicle | **15** Inferior glenohumeral ligament | **23** Superior glenohumeral ligament | **29** Triceps, lateral head |
| **7** Coracoid process | **16** Lateral border of scapula | | |
| **8** Deltoid | **17** Middle glenohumeral ligament | | |
| **9** Epiphysial line | | | |

*Calcific tendinitis, rotator cuff tears, bicipital tendinitis, painful arc syndrome see pages 174, 175.*

# A Right axilla *anterior wall*

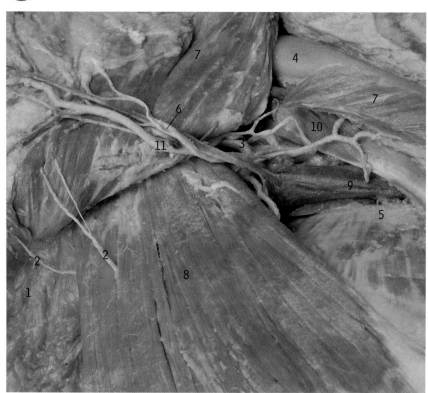

Pectoralis major (7) has been reflected upwards and laterally, and the clavipectoral fascia which passes from subclavius (10) to pectoralis minor (8) has been removed.

1 Axillary sheath
2 Branches of medial pectoral nerve
3 Cephalic vein
4 Clavicle
5 First rib
6 Lateral pectoral nerve
7 Pectoralis major
8 Pectoralis minor
9 Subclavian vein
10 Subclavius
11 Thoracoacromial vessels

---

The clavipectoral fascia (here removed, between subclavius, 10, and pectoralis minor, 8) is pierced by the cephalic vein (3), thoracoacromial vessels (11), lateral pectoral nerve (6) and lymphatics.

The axillary sheath (1) is the downward continuation of the prevertebral fascia of the neck and forms a dense covering for the axillary artery and the surrounding parts of the brachial plexus.

The lateral pectoral nerve (6) is related to the medial (upper) border of pectoralis minor (8). The medial pectoral nerve (2) is related to the lateral (lower) border of pectoralis minor.

---

# B Right axilla and brachial plexus *from the front*

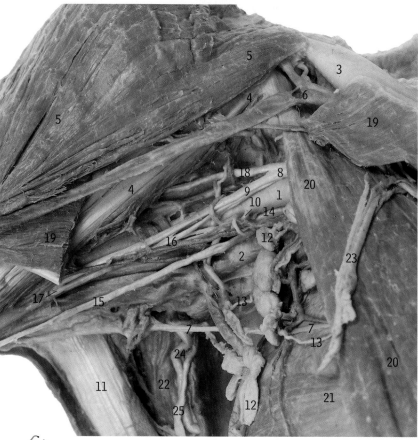

Pectoralis major (19) has been reflected and the clavipectoral fascia removed, together with the axillary sheath (A1) which surrounded the axillary artery and brachial plexus.

1 Axillary artery
2 Axillary vein
3 Clavicle
4 Coracobrachialis
5 Deltoid
6 Entry of cephalic vein into deltoid vein
7 Intercostobrachial nerve
8 Lateral cord of brachial plexus
9 Lateral root of median nerve
10 Lateral thoracic artery
11 Latissimus dorsi
12 Lymph nodes
13 Lymph vessels
14 Medial cord of the brachial plexus
15 Medial cutaneous nerve of arm
16 Medial root of median nerve
17 Median nerve
18 Musculocutaneous nerve
19 Pectoralis major
20 Pectoralis minor
21 Serratus anterior
22 Subscapularis
23 Thoracoacromial vessels and lateral pectoral nerve
24 Thoracodorsal artery
25 Thoracodorsal nerve

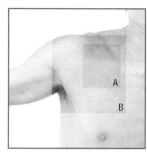

*Axillary-subclavian vein thrombosis, see page 174.*

# Right brachial plexus *from the front*

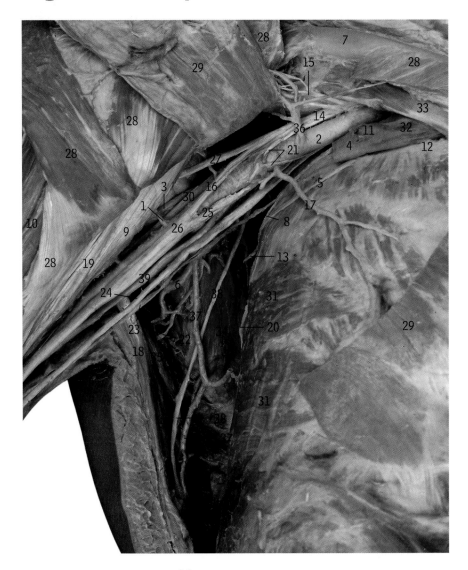

Pectoralis major and minor (28 and 29) have been reflected and the axillary sheath (page 144, A1) removed, together with most of the axillary vein (4) and its tributaries.

1 Anterior circumflex humeral artery
2 Axillary artery
3 Axillary nerve
4 Axillary vein
5 Branch from first thoracic nerve to intercostobrachial nerve
6 Circumflex scapular artery
7 Clavicle
8 Communication between 23 and 13
9 Coracobrachialis and short head of biceps
10 Deltoid
11 Entry of cephalic vein
12 First rib
13 Intercostobrachial nerve (cut end)
14 Lateral cord
15 Lateral pectoral nerve
16 Lateral root of median nerve
17 Lateral thoracic artery
18 Latissimus dorsi
19 Long head of biceps
20 Long thoracic nerve
21 Loop between medial and lateral pectoral nerves
22 Lower subscapular nerve
23 Medial cutaneous nerve of arm
24 Medial cutaneous nerve of forearm
25 Medial root of median nerve
26 Median nerve
27 Musculocutaneous nerve
28 Pectoralis major
29 Pectoralis minor
30 Radial nerve
31 Serratus anterior
32 Subclavian vein
33 Subclavius
34 Subscapularis
35 Teres major
36 Thoracoacromial artery
37 Thoracodorsal artery
38 Thoracodorsal nerve
39 Ulnar nerve

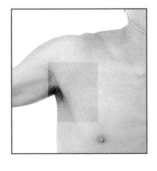

*Erb's paralysis (Erb-Duchenne palsy), winging of the scapula, see pages 175, 176.*

# Right brachial plexus and branches

In this front view of the plexus, all the blood vessels have been removed to show the cords of the plexus and their branches more clearly. Note the 'capital M' pattern formed by the musculocutaneous nerve (18), the lateral root of the median nerve (8), the median nerve itself (17), the medial root of the median nerve (16) and the ulnar nerve (26). In this specimen, the tendon of latissimus dorsi (9) is unusually broad and has become blended with the long head of triceps (10).

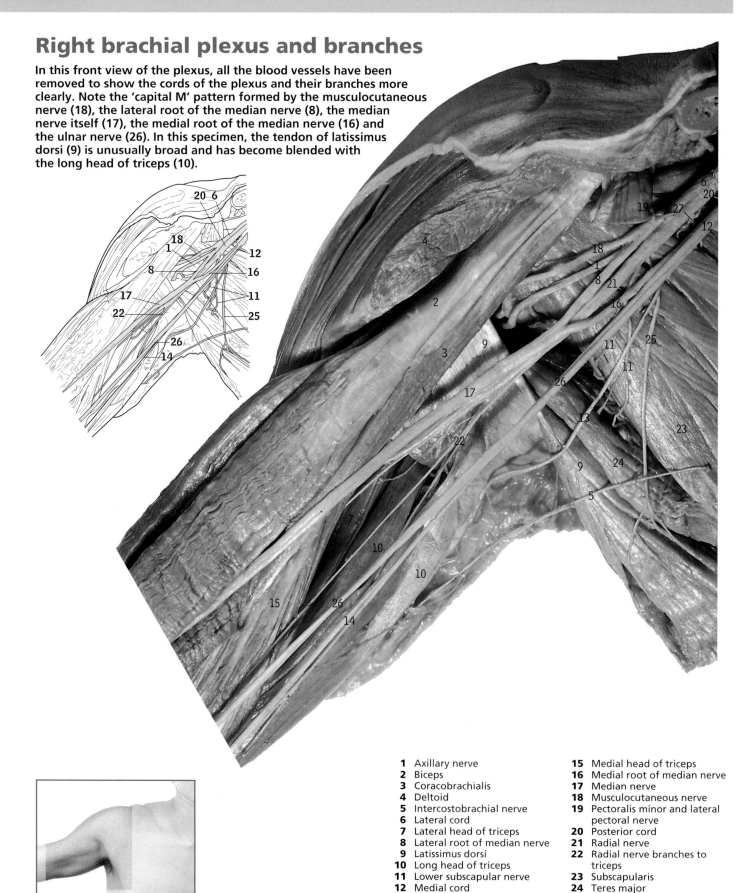

| | |
|---|---|
| **1** Axillary nerve | **15** Medial head of triceps |
| **2** Biceps | **16** Medial root of median nerve |
| **3** Coracobrachialis | **17** Median nerve |
| **4** Deltoid | **18** Musculocutaneous nerve |
| **5** Intercostobrachial nerve | **19** Pectoralis minor and lateral |
| **6** Lateral cord | pectoral nerve |
| **7** Lateral head of triceps | **20** Posterior cord |
| **8** Lateral root of median nerve | **21** Radial nerve |
| **9** Latissimus dorsi | **22** Radial nerve branches to |
| **10** Long head of triceps | triceps |
| **11** Lower subscapular nerve | **23** Subscapularis |
| **12** Medial cord | **24** Teres major |
| **13** Medial cutaneous nerve of arm | **25** Thoracodorsal nerve |
| **14** Medial cutaneous nerve of | **26** Ulnar nerve |
| forearm | **27** Upper subscapular nerves |

*Posterior dislocation of humerus, see page 174.*

# A Right arm *vessels and nerves, from the front*

Biceps (16 and 8) has been turned laterally to show the musculocutaneous nerve (12) emerging from coracobrachialis (6), giving branches to biceps and brachialis (14 and 13) and becoming the lateral cutaneous nerve of the forearm (7) on the lateral side of the biceps tendon (17).

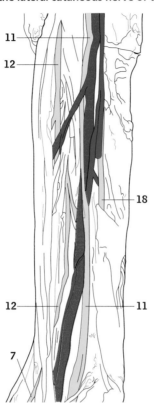

The median nerve (11) gradually crosses over in front of the brachial artery (2) from the lateral to the medial side. The ulnar nerve (18) passes behind the medial intermuscular septum (10), and the end of the basilic vein (1) is seen joining a vena comitans (19) of the brachial artery to form the brachial vein (3).

| | | | |
|---|---|---|---|
| 1 | Basilic vein (cut end) | 11 | Median nerve |
| 2 | Brachial artery | 12 | Musculocutaneous nerve |
| 3 | Brachial vein | 13 | Nerve to brachialis |
| 4 | Brachialis | 14 | Nerve to short head of |
| 5 | Brachioradialis | | biceps |
| 6 | Coracobrachialis | 15 | Pronator teres |
| 7 | Lateral cutaneous nerve | 16 | Short head of biceps |
| | of forearm | 17 | Tendon of biceps |
| 8 | Long head of biceps | 18 | Ulnar nerve |
| 9 | Long head of triceps | 19 | Vena comitans of brachial |
| 10 | Medial intermuscular | | artery |
| | septum | | |

The musculocutaneous nerve (A12) supplies coracobrachialis (A6), biceps (A16 and 8) and brachialis (A4), and at the level where the muscle fibres of biceps become tendinous (A17) it pierces the deep fascia to become the lateral cutaneous nerve of the forearm (A7).

The median nerve does not give off any muscular branches in the arm.

The ulnar nerve (A18) leaves the anterior compartment of the arm by piercing the medial intermuscular septum (A10), and does not give off any muscular branches in the arm.

# B Right arm *cross-section, from below*

Looking from the elbow towards the shoulder, the section is taken through the middle of the arm. The musculocutaneous nerve (9) lies between brachialis (4) and biceps (2), and the median nerve (8) is on the medial side of the brachial artery (3) which has several venae comitantes adjacent (unlabelled). The ulnar nerve (13), with the superior ulnar collateral artery (11) beside it, is behind the median nerve (8) and the basilic vein (1). The radial nerve and the profunda brachii vessels (10) are in the posterior compartment at the lateral side of the humerus (6).

FRONT

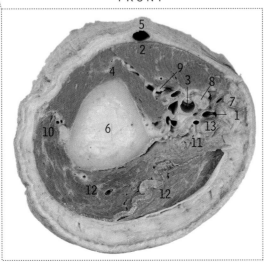

| | |
|---|---|
| 1 | Basilic vein |
| 2 | Biceps |
| 3 | Brachial artery |
| 4 | Brachialis |
| 5 | Cephalic vein |
| 6 | Humerus |
| 7 | Medial cutaneous nerve of forearm |
| 8 | Median nerve |
| 9 | Musculocutaneous nerve |
| 10 | Radial nerve and profunda brachii vessels |
| 11 | Superior ulnar collateral artery |
| 12 | Triceps |
| 13 | Ulnar nerve |

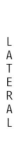

# Right arm *posterior view*

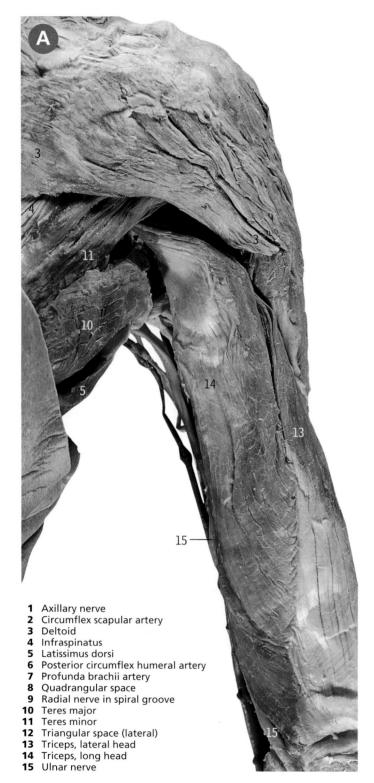

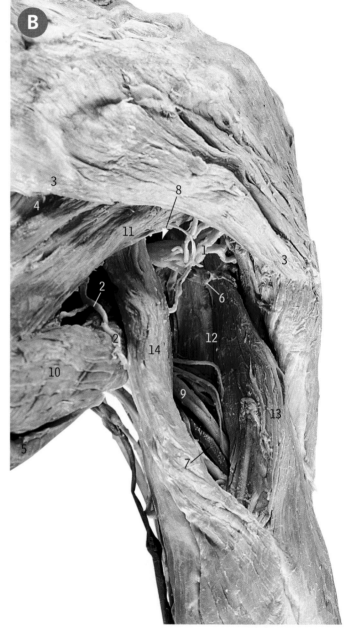

1   Axillary nerve
2   Circumflex scapular artery
3   Deltoid
4   Infraspinatus
5   Latissimus dorsi
6   Posterior circumflex humeral artery
7   Profunda brachii artery
8   Quadrangular space
9   Radial nerve in spiral groove
10   Teres major
11   Teres minor
12   Triangular space (lateral)
13   Triceps, lateral head
14   Triceps, long head
15   Ulnar nerve

**A**   after removal of skin and subcutaneous fat

**B**   after muscle separation to demonstrate spaces and neurovascular bundle

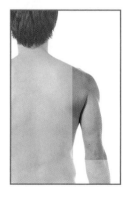

*Radial nerve palsy, see page 175.*

## C Left elbow *surface markings, from behind*

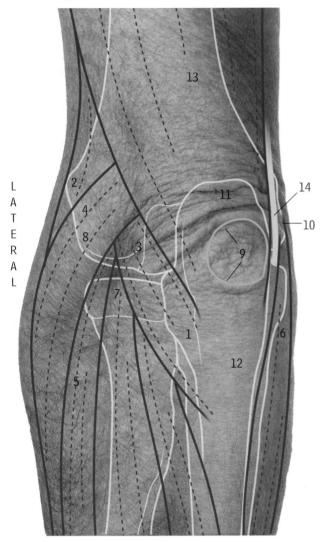

L
A
T
E
R
A
L

## D Right elbow *medial view from behind*

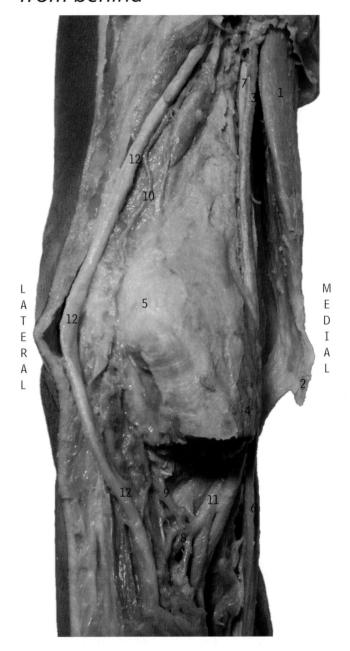

L
A
T
E
R
A
L

M
E
D
I
A
L

With the elbow fully extended, the extensor muscles (5, 4) form a bulge on the lateral side. In the adjacent hollow can be felt the head of the radius (7) and the capitulum of the humerus (3) which indicate the line of the humeroradial part of the elbow joint. The lateral and medial epicondyles of the humerus (8 and 10) are palpable on each side. Wrinkled skin lies at the back of the prominent olecranon of the ulna (11), and in this arm the margin of the olecranon bursa (9) is outlined. The most important structure in this region is the ulnar nerve (14) which is palpable as it lies in contact with the humerus behind the medial epicondyle (10). The posterior border of the ulna (12) is subcutaneous throughout its whole length.

| | | | |
|---|---|---|---|
| **1** | Anconeus | **9** | Margin of olecranon bursa |
| **2** | Brachioradialis | **10** | Medial epicondyle of |
| **3** | Capitulum of humerus | | humerus |
| **4** | Extensor carpi radialis longus | **11** | Olecranon of ulna |
| **5** | Extensor muscles | **12** | Posterior border of ulna |
| **6** | Flexor carpi ulnaris | **13** | Triceps |
| **7** | Head of radius | **14** | Ulnar nerve |
| **8** | Lateral epicondyle of humerus | | |

**1** Biceps muscle
**2** Bicipital aponeurosis
**3** Brachial artery
**4** Common flexor origin
**5** Medial epicondyle
**6** Median artery
**7** Median nerve
**8** Muscular arterial branches to flexors of forearm
**9** Posterior ulnar recurrent artery
**10** Superior ulnar collateral artery
**11** Ulnar artery
**12** Ulnar nerve

**Note: high division and persistent median artery**

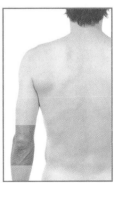

*Olecranon bursitis, triceps tendon reflex, ulnar nerve palsy, see pages 175, 176.*

# Left elbow and radioulnar joint

**A** from the medial side   **B** from the lateral side

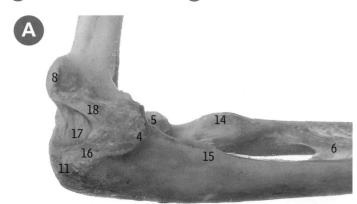

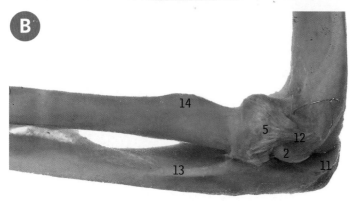

# Right elbow and radioulnar joint

**D** from the medial side   **E** from the lateral side

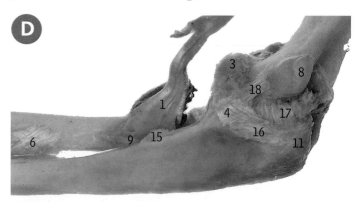

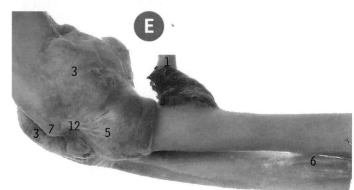

In A and B the forearm is flexed to a right angle. In D and E the forearm is partially flexed, and the synovial cavity within the capsule (3) and the bursa beneath the biceps tendon (1) have been injected with green resin.

# Elbow *radiographs*

**C** lateral projection

**F** AP projection

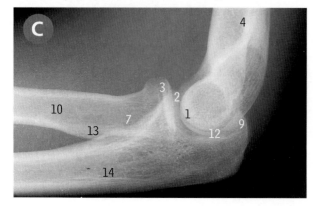

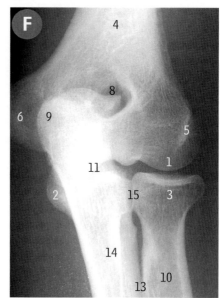

| | | |
|---|---|---|
| **1** | Biceps tendon and underlying bursa | |
| **2** | Capitulum | |
| **3** | Capsule (distended) | |
| **4** | Coronoid process of ulna | |
| **5** | Head and neck of radius covered by annular ligament | |
| **6** | Interosseous membrane | |
| **7** | Lateral epicondyle | |
| **8** | Medial epicondyle | |
| **9** | Oblique cord | |
| **10** | Olecranon fossa | |
| **11** | Olecranon process of ulna | |
| **12** | Radial collateral ligament | |
| **13** | Supinator crest of ulna | |
| **14** | Tuberosity of radius | |
| **15** | Tuberosity of ulna | |
| **16** | Ulnar collateral ligament: oblique band | |
| **17** | Ulnar collateral ligament: posterior band | |
| **18** | Ulnar collateral ligament: upper band | |

**1** Capitulum of humerus
**2** Coronoid process of ulna
**3** Head of radius
**4** Humerus
**5** Lateral epicondyle of humerus
**6** Medial epicondyle of humerus
**7** Neck of radius
**8** Olecranon fossa of humerus
**9** Olecranon process of ulna
**10** Radius
**11** Trochlea of humerus
**12** Trochlear notch of ulna
**13** Tuberosity of radius
**14** Ulna
**15** Radioulnar joint

*Dislocation of the radial head, see page 175.*

# Left elbow joint

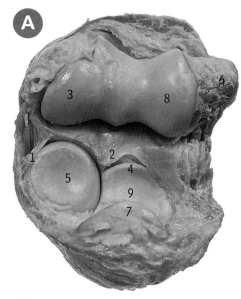

**A**

## A opened from behind

The joint has been 'forced open' from behind: the capitulum (3) and trochlea (8) of the lower end of the humerus are seen from below with the forearm in forced flexion to show the upper ends of the radius and ulna (5 and 9) from above.

1. Annular ligament
2. Anterior part of capsule
3. Capitulum of humerus
4. Coronoid process of ulna
5. Head of radius
6. Medial epicondyle of humerus
7. Olecranon process of ulna
8. Trochlea of humerus
9. Trochlear notch of ulna

# Left elbow

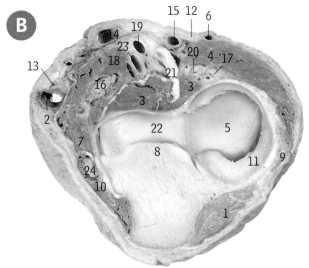

**B**

## D Elbow *coronal section*

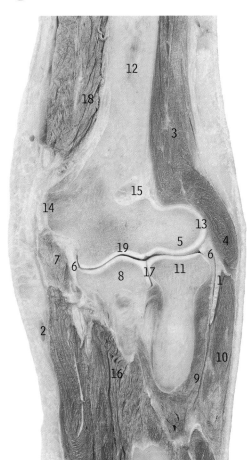

1. Annular ligament
2. Basilic vein
3. Brachialis
4. Brachioradialis
5. Capitulum of humerus
6. Capsule
7. Common flexor origin
8. Coronoid process of ulna
9. Extensor carpi radialis brevis
10. Extensor carpi radialis longus
11. Head of radius
12. Humerus
13. Lateral epicondyle
14. Medial epicondyle
15. Olecranon fossa
16. Pronator teres
17. Radio-ulnar joint, proximal
18. Triceps, medial head
19. Trochlea of humerus

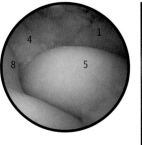

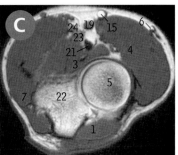

**C**

This is the arthroscopic view of an elbow joint. The view is from the superior aspect showing the orientation and the articulation of the radio-capitellar joint. Just distal to the radial head is the proximal edge of the annular ligament. The radial head is seen articulating with the coronoid process of the ulna.

## B cross-section     C axial MR image

The section is viewed from below, looking towards the shoulder, and is just below the point where the brachial artery has divided into radial and ulnar arteries (19 and 23). The cut has passed immediately below the trochlea (22) and capitulum (5) of the humerus, and has gone through the coronoid process of the ulna (8). The radial nerve (20) and its posterior interosseous branch (17) lie between brachioradialis (4) and brachialis (3). The median nerve (16) is under the main part of pronator teres (18), and the ulnar nerve (24) is passing under flexor carpi ulnaris (10).

1. Anconeus
2. Basilic vein
3. Brachialis
4. Brachioradialis
5. Capitulum of humerus
6. Cephalic vein
7. Common flexor origin
8. Coronoid process of ulna
9. Extensor carpi radialis longus and brevis
10. Flexor carpi ulnaris
11. Fringe of synovial membrane
12. Lateral cutaneous nerve of forearm
13. Medial cutaneous nerve of forearm
14. Median basilic vein
15. Median cephalic vein
16. Median nerve
17. Posterior interosseous nerve
18. Pronator teres
19. Radial artery
20. Radial nerve
21. Tendon of biceps
22. Trochlea of humerus
23. Ulnar artery
24. Ulnar nerve

*Wrist arthroscopy, see page 176.*

# Left cubital fossa Ⓐ surface markings Ⓑ superficial veins

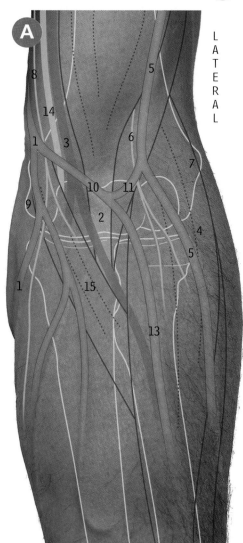

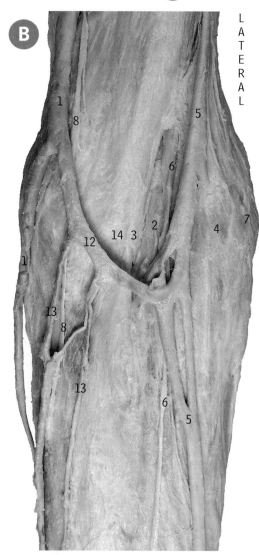

1 Basilic vein
2 Biceps tendon
3 Brachial artery
4 Brachioradialis
5 Cephalic vein
6 Lateral cutaneous nerve of forearm
7 Lateral epicondyle
8 Medial cutaneous nerve of forearm
9 Medial epicondyle
10 Median basilic vein
11 Median cephalic vein
12 Median cubital vein
13 Median forearm vein
14 Median nerve
15 Pronator teres

The superficial veins on the front of the elbow such as the cephalic (5) and basilic (1) and their intercommunicating tributaries are those most commonly used for intravenous injections and obtaining specimens of venous blood. The pattern of veins is typically M-shaped (as in A) or H-shaped (as in B), but there is much variation and it is not always possible or necessary to name every vessel.

The order of the structures in the cubital fossa from lateral to medial is: biceps tendon (2), brachial artery (3) and median nerve (14).

In A there is an M-shaped pattern of superficial veins (see notes). In B the cephalic (5) and basilic (1) veins are joined by a median cubital vein (12) into which drain two small median forearm veins (13). In C (page 153) the deep fascia has been removed but the bicipital aponeurosis (C2) is preserved; it runs downwards and medially from the biceps tendon (B2), crossing the brachial artery (C3) and the median nerve (C9). The musculocutaneous nerve becomes the lateral cutaneous nerve of the forearm (B6, C8) at the lateral border of biceps where the muscle becomes tendinous.

Brachioradialis (A4, B4, C5) forms the lateral boundary and pronator teres (A15, C12) the medial boundary of the cubital fossa. The brachial latex arterial injection in D (page 153) outlines the main arteries (D2, 5 and 7).

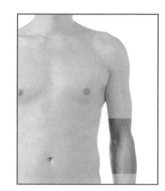

*Auscultation of the brachial pulse, biceps tendon reflex, golfer's elbow, tennis elbow, see pages 174, 175, 176.*

# Left elbow and upper forearm
**C** *from the front* **D** *deeper dissection of nerves and arteries*

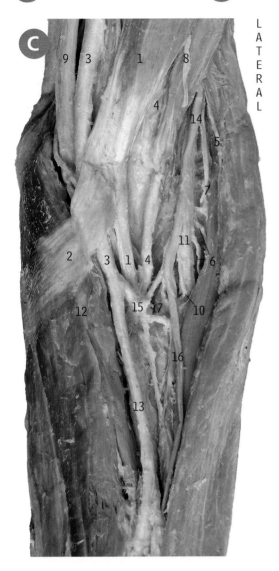

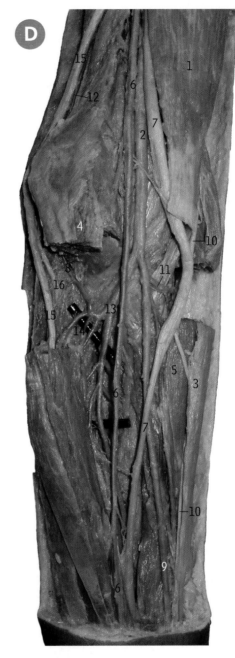

Brachioradialis (5) and extensor carpi radialis longus (7) have been displaced laterally to show the radial nerve (14) giving off branches to those muscles and then dividing into the superficial (cutaneous) branch (16) and the deep (posterior interosseous) branch (11) which enters supinator.

| | | | |
|---|---|---|---|
| **1** | Biceps | **9** | Median nerve |
| **2** | Bicipital aponeurosis | **10** | Nerve to supinator |
| **3** | Brachial artery | **11** | Posterior interosseous nerve |
| **4** | Brachialis | **12** | Pronator teres |
| **5** | Brachioradialis and nerve | **13** | Radial artery |
| **6** | Branches to extensor carpi radialis brevis | **14** | Radial nerve |
| | | **15** | Radial recurrent artery |
| **7** | Extensor carpi radialis longus and nerve | **16** | Superficial branch of radial nerve |
| **8** | Lateral cutaneous nerve of forearm | **17** | Supinator |

| | | | |
|---|---|---|---|
| **1** | Biceps | **11** | Radial recurrent artery |
| **2** | Brachial artery | **12** | Superior ulnar collateral artery |
| **3** | Brachioradialis | | |
| **4** | Common flexor origin | **13** | Ulnar artery |
| **5** | Extensor carpi radialis longus | **14** | Ulnar artery, branches to forearm flexors |
| **6** | Median artery | | |
| **7** | Median nerve, pulled laterally | **15** | Ulnar nerve |
| **8** | Posterior ulnar recurrent artery | **16** | Ulnar nerve, branch to flexor carpi ulnaris |
| **9** | Radial artery | | |
| **10** | Radial nerve, superficial branch | | |

**Note: high division and persistent median artery**

*Arterial puncture, see page 174.*

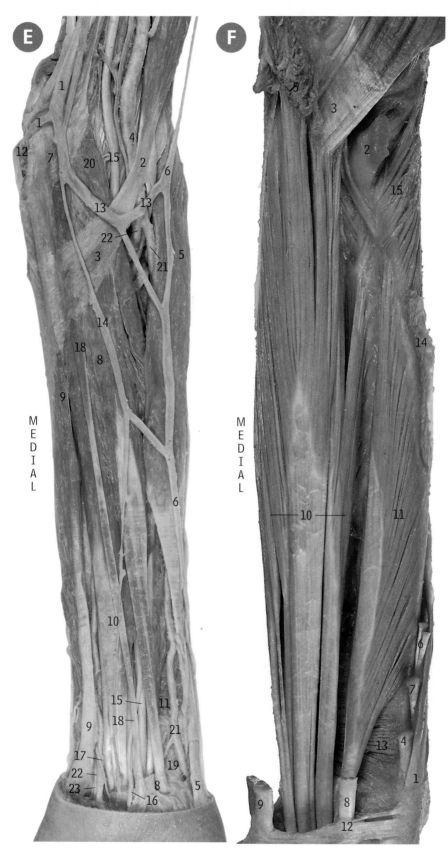

## E Left forearm superficial muscles, from the front

Skin and fascia have been removed, but the larger superficial veins (1, 6 and 13) have been preserved. On the lateral side, the radial artery (21) is largely covered by brachioradialis (5). At the wrist the tendon of flexor carpi radialis (8) has the radial artery (21) on its lateral side; on its medial side is the median nerve (15), slightly overlapped from the medial side by the tendon of palmaris longus (18) (if present; it is absent in 13% of arms).

| | |
|---|---|
| **1** Basilic vein | **13** Median cubital vein |
| **2** Biceps tendon | **14** Median forearm vein |
| **3** Bicipital aponeurosis | **15** Median nerve |
| **4** Brachial artery | **16** Palmar branch of |
| **5** Brachioradialis | median nerve |
| **6** Cephalic vein | **17** Palmar branch of |
| **7** Common flexor | ulnar nerve |
| origin | **18** Palmaris longus |
| **8** Flexor carpi radialis | **19** Pronator quadratus |
| **9** Flexor carpi ulnaris | **20** Pronator teres |
| **10** Flexor digitorum | **21** Radial artery |
| superficialis | **22** Ulnar artery |
| **11** Flexor pollicis longus | **23** Ulnar nerve |
| **12** Medial epicondyle | |

## F Left forearm *deep muscles, from the front*

All vessels and nerves have been removed, together with the superficial muscles, to show the deep flexor group – flexor digitorum profundus (10), flexor pollicis longus (11) and pronator quadratus (13).

**1** Abductor pollicis longus
**2** Biceps
**3** Brachialis
**4** Brachioradialis
**5** Common flexor origin
**6** Extensor carpi radialis brevis
**7** Extensor carpi radialis longus
**8** Flexor carpi radialis
**9** Flexor carpi ulnaris
**10** Flexor digitorum profundus
**11** Flexor pollicis longus
**12** Flexor retinaculum
**13** Pronator quadratus
**14** Pronator teres
**15** Supinator

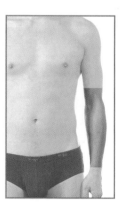

*Venous cutdown, venepuncture of the upper limb, see page 176.*

**A** ## Right cubital fossa and forearm *arteries*

The arteries have been injected, and after removal of most of the superficial muscles, the brachial artery (4) is seen dividing into the radial artery (18) and the ulnar artery (20). The radial artery gives off the radial recurrent (19) which runs upwards in front of supinator, giving branches to the carpal extensor muscles (10 and 9). The ulnar artery gives off the anterior and posterior ulnar recurrent vessels (2 and 15), and its common interosseous branch (8) is seen giving off the anterior interosseous (1) which passes down in front of the interosseous membrane between flexor pollicis longus (13) and flexor digitorum profundus (12).

| | | |
|---|---|---|
| **1** Anterior interosseous artery overlying interosseous membrane | **7** Common flexor origin | **15** Posterior ulnar recurrent artery |
| **2** Anterior ulnar recurrent artery | **8** Common interosseous artery | **16** Pronator quadratus |
| **3** Biceps tendon | **9** Extensor carpi radialis brevis | **17** Pronator teres |
| **4** Brachial artery | **10** Extensor carpi radialis longus | **18** Radial artery |
| **5** Brachialis | **11** Flexor carpi ulnaris | **19** Radial recurrent artery overlying supinator |
| **6** Brachioradialis | **12** Flexor digitorum profundus | **20** Ulnar artery |
| | **13** Flexor pollicis longus | |
| | **14** Medial epicondyle of humerus | |

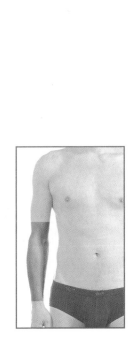

**B** ## Right cubital fossa and forearm *arteries and nerves*

Most of the humeral origins of pronator teres and flexor carpi radialis (from the common flexor origin, 9 and 7) and palmaris longus have been removed to show the median nerve (12) passing superficial to the deep head of pronator teres (18) and then deep to the upper border of the radial head of flexor digitorum superficialis (14).

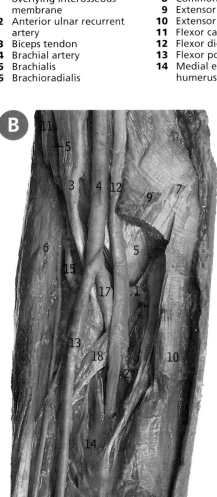

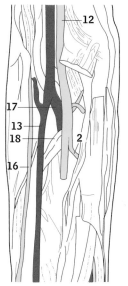

| | |
|---|---|
| **1** A muscular branch of median nerve | |
| **2** Anterior interosseous nerve | |
| **3** Biceps | |
| **4** Brachial artery | |
| **5** Brachialis | |
| **6** Brachioradialis (displaced laterally) | |
| **7** Common flexor origin | |
| **8** Flexor carpi ulnaris (displaced medially) | |
| **9** Humeral head of pronator teres | |
| **10** Humero-ulnar head of flexor digitorum superficialis | |
| **11** Lateral cutaneous nerve of forearm | |
| **12** Median nerve | |
| **13** Radial artery | |
| **14** Radial head of flexor digitorum superficialis | |
| **15** Radial recurrent artery | |
| **16** Superficial terminal branch of radial nerve overlying extensor carpi radialis longus | |
| **17** Ulnar artery | |
| **18** Ulnar head of pronator teres | |
| **19** Ulnar nerve and artery | |

*Anterior interosseous nerve entrapment, Volkmann's contracture, see pages 174, 176.*

## **A** Left elbow

### *from the lateral side*

With the forearm in mid-pronation and seen from the lateral side so that the radius (7) lies in front of the ulna, all muscles have been removed except supinator (8) to show its humeral and ulnar origins (see notes).

1 Annular ligament
2 Capitulum of humerus
3 Interosseous membrane
4 Lateral epicondyle
5 Posterior interosseous nerve
6 Radial collateral ligament
7 Radius
8 Supinator
9 Supinator crest of ulna

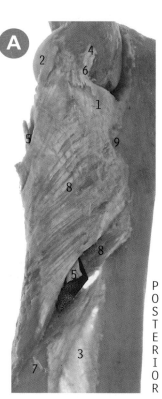

## **B** Left forearm

### *deep muscles, from the lateral side*

1 Abductor pollicis longus
2 Biceps
3 Extensor carpi radialis brevis
4 Extensor carpi radialis longus (double)
5 Extensor indicis
6 Extensor pollicis brevis
7 Extensor pollicis longus
8 Extensor retinaculum
9 Flexor pollicis longus
10 Pronator teres
11 Supinator

## **C** Left forearm

### *posterior interosseous nerve, from behind*

1 Abductor pollicis longus
2 Branch of posterior interosseous artery
3 Extensor carpi radialis brevis
4 Extensor carpi radialis longus
5 Extensor carpi ulnaris
6 Extensor digitorum
7 Extensor indicis
8 Extensor pollicis brevis
9 Extensor pollicis longus
10 Extensor retinaculum
11 Posterior interosseous nerve
12 Supinator

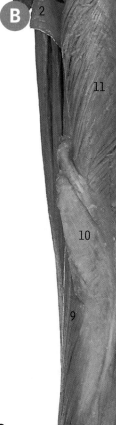

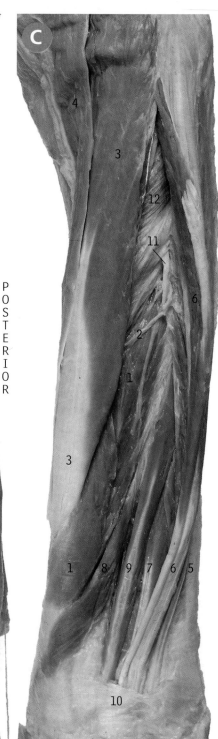

The fibres of the interosseous membrane (A3) pass obliquely downwards from the radius (A7) to the ulna, so transmitting weight from the hand and radius to the ulna.

The supinator muscle (A8) arises from the lateral epicondyle of the humerus (A4), radial collateral ligament (A6), annular ligament (A1), supinator crest of the ulna (A9) and bone in front of the crest (page 127, D10), and an aponeurosis overlying the muscle. From these origins, the fibres wrap themselves round the upper end of the radius above the pronator teres attachment, to be attached to the lateral surface of the radius and extending anteriorly and posteriorly as far as the tuberosity of the radius.

*Posterior interosseous nerve entrapment, see page 175.*

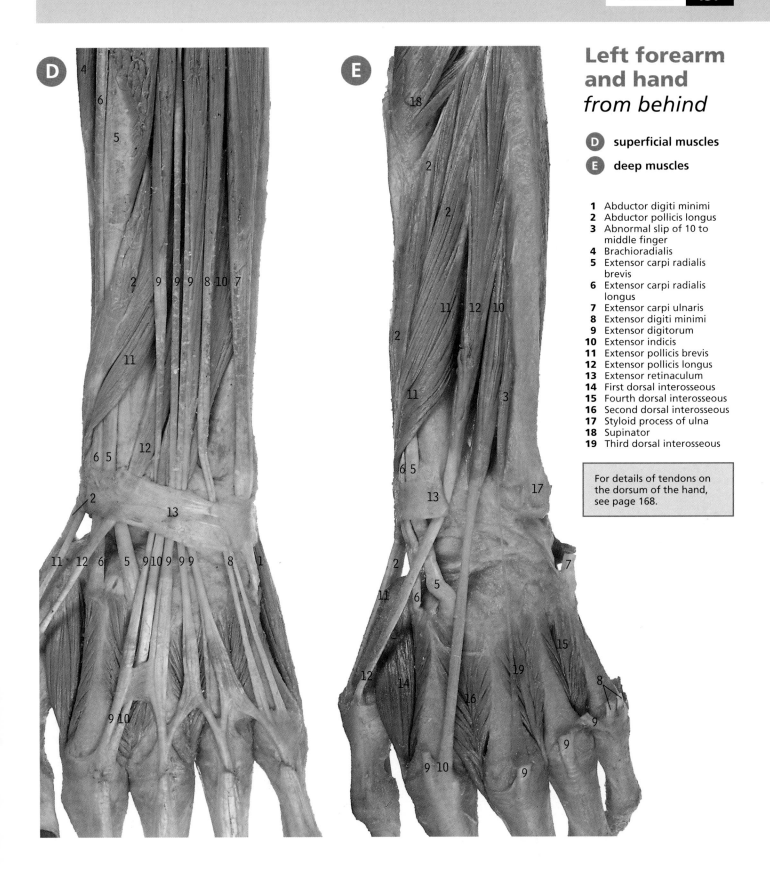

**Left forearm and hand** *from behind*

**D** superficial muscles

**E** deep muscles

1 Abductor digiti minimi
2 Abductor pollicis longus
3 Abnormal slip of 10 to middle finger
4 Brachioradialis
5 Extensor carpi radialis brevis
6 Extensor carpi radialis longus
7 Extensor carpi ulnaris
8 Extensor digiti minimi
9 Extensor digitorum
10 Extensor indicis
11 Extensor pollicis brevis
12 Extensor pollicis longus
13 Extensor retinaculum
14 First dorsal interosseous
15 Fourth dorsal interosseous
16 Second dorsal interosseous
17 Styloid process of ulna
18 Supinator
19 Third dorsal interosseous

For details of tendons on the dorsum of the hand, see page 168.

*De Quervain's disease, wrist drop, see pages 174, 176.*

## A Palm of left hand

1 Abductor digiti minimi
2 Abductor pollicis brevis
3 Adductor pollicis
4 Distal transverse crease
5 Distal wrist crease
6 Flexor carpi radialis
7 Flexor carpi ulnaris
8 Flexor digiti minimi brevis
9 Flexor pollicis brevis
10 Head of metacarpal
11 Hook of hamate
12 Level of deep palmar arch
13 Level of superficial palmar arch
14 Longitudinal crease
15 Median nerve
16 Middle wrist crease
17 Palmaris brevis
18 Palmaris longus
19 Pisiform
20 Proximal transverse crease
21 Proximal wrist crease
22 Radial artery
23 Thenar eminence
24 Ulnar artery and nerve

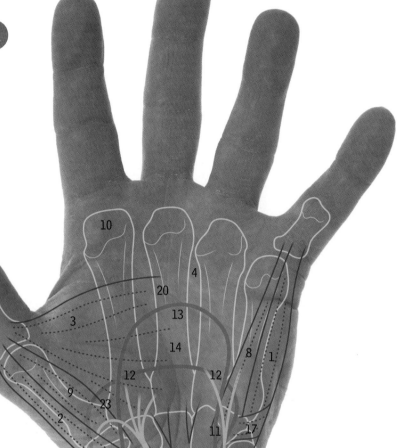

## B Dorsum of left hand

The fingers are extended at the metacarpophalangeal joints, causing the extensor tendons of the fingers (2, 3 and 4) to stand out, and partially flexed at the interphalangeal joints. The thumb is extended at the carpometacarpal joint and partially flexed at the metacarpophalangeal and interphalangeal joints. The lines proximal to the bases of the fingers indicate the ends of the heads of the metacarpals and the level of the metacarpophalangeal joints. The anatomical snuffbox (1) is the hollow between the tendons of abductor pollicis longus and extensor pollicis brevis (5) laterally and extensor pollicis longus (6) medially.

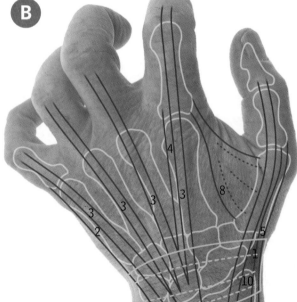

1 Anatomical snuffbox
2 Extensor digiti minimi
3 Extensor digitorum
4 Extensor indicis
5 Extensor pollicis brevis and abductor pollicis longus
6 Extensor pollicis longus
7 Extensor retinaculum
8 First dorsal interosseous
9 Head of ulna
10 Styloid process of radius

# Fingers *movements*

**A** flexion of the metacarpophalangeal joints and flexion of the interphalangeal joints

**B** extension of the metacarpophalangeal joints and flexion of the interphalangeal joints

**C** extension of the metacarpophalangeal and interphalangeal joints

When 'making a fist' with all finger joints flexed (A), the heads of the metacarpals (6) form the knuckles. To extend the metacarpophalangeal joints (B9) requires the activity of the long extensor tendons of the fingers, but to extend the interphalangeal joints (C10 and 5) as well requires the activity of the interossei and lumbricals, pulling on the dorsal extensor expansions (page 170). Only if the metacarpophalangeal joints remain flexed can the long extensors extend the interphalangeal joints.

| | | | |
|---|---|---|---|
| **1** | Base of distal phalanx | **7** | Head of middle phalanx |
| **2** | Base of metacarpal | **8** | Head of proximal phalanx |
| **3** | Base of middle phalanx | **9** | Metacarpophalangeal joint |
| **4** | Base of proximal phalanx | **10** | Proximal interphalangeal joint |
| **5** | Distal interphalangeal joint | | |
| **6** | Head of metacarpal | | |

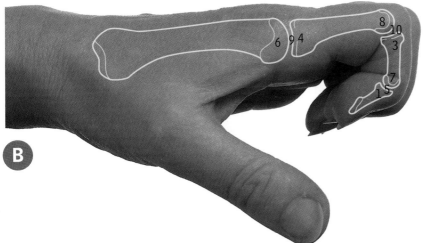

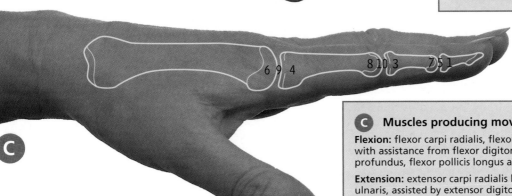

**A** **Muscles producing movements at the metacarpophalangeal joints**

**Flexion:** flexor digitorum profundus, flexor digitorum superficialis, lumbricals, interossei, with flexor digiti minimi brevis for the little finger and flexor pollicis longus, flexor pollicis brevis and the first palmar interosseous for the thumb.

**Extension:** extensor digitorum, extensor indicis (index finger) and extensor digiti minimi (little finger), with extensor pollicis longus and extensor pollicis brevis for the thumb.

**Adduction:** palmar interossei; when flexed, the long flexors assist.

**Abduction:** dorsal interossei and the long extensors, with abductor digiti minimi for the little finger.

**B** **Muscles producing movements at the interphalangeal joints**

**Flexion:** at the proximal joints, flexor digitorum superficialis and flexor digitorum profundus; at the distal joints, flexor digitorum profundus. For the thumb, flexor pollicis longus.

**Extension:** with the metacarpophalangeal joints flexed, extensor digitorum, extensor indicis and extensor digiti minimi; with the metacarpophalangeal joints extended, interossei and lumbricals. For the thumb, extensor pollicis longus.

**C** **Muscles producing movements at the wrist joint**

**Flexion:** flexor carpi radialis, flexor carpi ulnaris, palmaris longus, with assistance from flexor digitorum superficialis, flexor digitorum profundus, flexor pollicis longus and abductor pollicis longus.

**Extension:** extensor carpi radialis longus and brevis, extensor carpi ulnaris, assisted by extensor digitorum, extensor indicis, extensor digiti minimi and extensor pollicis longus.

**Abduction:** flexor carpi radialis, extensor carpi radialis longus and brevis, abductor pollicis longus and extensor pollicis brevis.

**Adduction:** flexor carpi ulnaris, extensor carpi ulnaris.

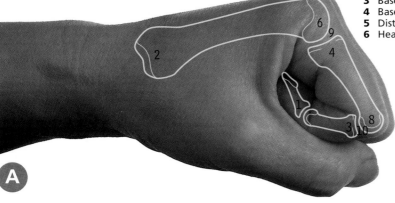

# Thumb *movements*

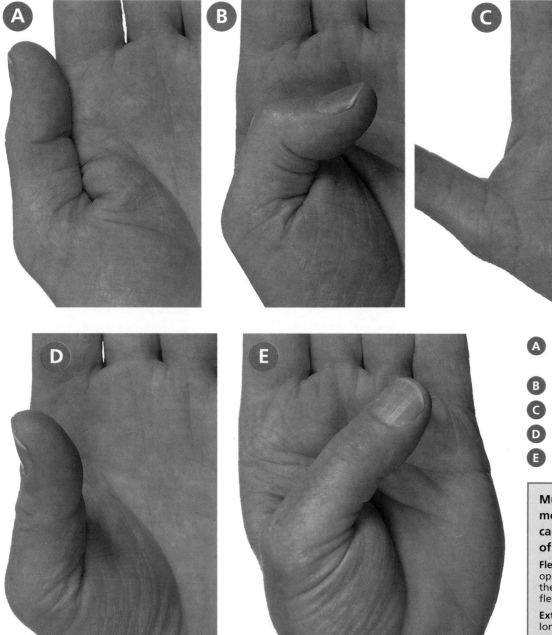

A in the anatomical position

B in flexion

C in extension

D in abduction

E in opposition

---

**Muscles producing movements at the carpometacarpal joint of the thumb**

**Flexion:** flexor pollicis brevis, opponens pollicis, and (when the other thumb joints are flexed) flexor pollicis longus.

**Extension:** abductor pollicis longus, extensor pollicis longus, extensor pollicis brevis.

**Abduction:** abductor pollicis brevis, abductor pollicis longus.

**Adduction:** adductor pollicis.

**Opposition:** opponens pollicis, flexor pollicis brevis, reinforced by adductor pollicis and flexor pollicis longus.

---

With the thumb in the anatomical position (A), the thumb nail is at right angles to the fingers because the first metacarpal is at right angles to the others (page 130). This is a rather artificial position; in the normal position of rest, the thumb makes an angle of about 60° with the plane of the palm (i.e. it is partially abducted). Flexion (B) means bending the thumb across the palm, keeping the phalanges at right angles to the palm. Extension (C) is the opposite movement, away from the palm. In abduction (D) the thumb is lifted forwards from the plane of the palm, and continuation of this movement inevitably leads to opposition (E), with rotation of the first metacarpal, twisting the whole digit so that the pulp of the thumb can be brought towards the palm at the base of the little finger (or more commonly in everyday use, to contact or overlap any of the flexed fingers). Opposition is a combination of abduction with flexion and medial rotation at the carpometacarpal joint; it is not necessarily accompanied by flexion at the other thumb joints.

*Wrist drop, see page 176.*

# Palm of left hand

**A** *palmar aponeurosis*

Removal of the palmar skin reveals the palmar aponeurosis.

**B** *after removal of palmar aponeurosis*

Deeper dissection of the palm reveals the flexor retinaculum, the palmar branches of the median and ulnar nerves and the superficial palmar arch, flanked by the muscles of the thenar and hypothenar eminences.

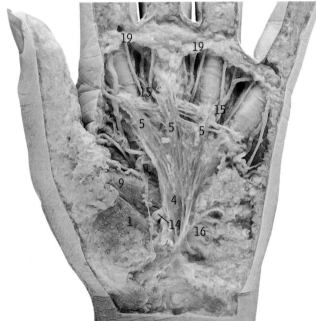

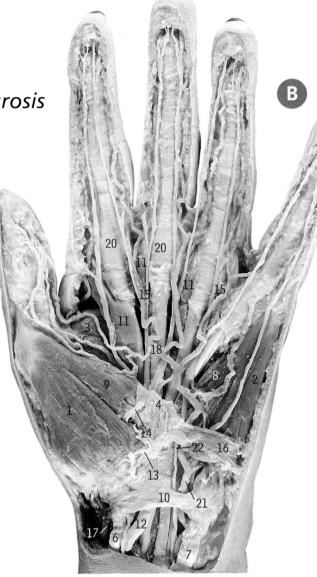

| | | |
|---|---|---|
| **1** Abductor pollicis brevis | **9** Flexor pollicis brevis | **17** Radial artery |
| **2** Abductor digiti minimi | **10** Flexor retinaculum | **18** Superficial palmar arch |
| **3** Adductor pollicis | **11** Lumbrical | **19** Superficial transverse metacarpal ligaments |
| **4** Aponeurosis, central part | **12** Median nerve | **20** Synovial sheaths of flexor tendons |
| **5** Aponeurosis, digital slips | **13** Median nerve, palmar branch | **21** Ulnar artery |
| **6** Flexor carpi radialis | **14** Median nerve, recurrent branch | **22** Ulnar nerve |
| **7** Flexor carpi ulnaris | **15** Palmar digital vessels and nerves | |
| **8** Flexor digiti minimi brevis | **16** Palmaris brevis | |

*Arteriovenous fistula, Dupuytren's contracture, see pages 174, 175.*

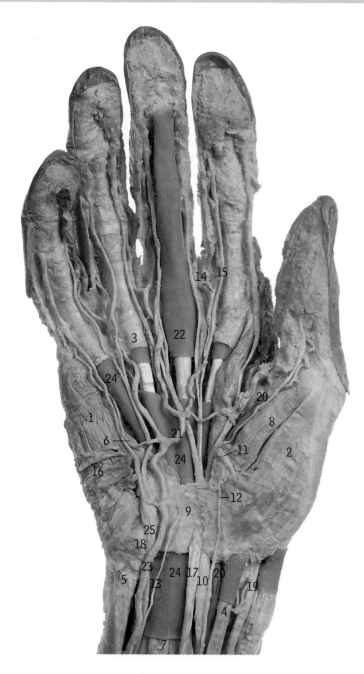

## A Palm of right hand
### with synovial sheaths

The synovial sheaths of the wrist and fingers have been emphasised by blue tissue. On the middle finger, the fibrous flexor sheath has been removed (but retained on the other fingers, as at 3) to show the whole length of the synovial sheath (22). On the index and ring fingers, the synovial sheath projects slightly proximal to the fibrous sheath. The synovial sheath of the little finger is continuous with the sheath surrounding the finger flexor tendons under the flexor retinaculum (the ulnar bursa, 24), and the sheath of flexor pollicis longus is the radial bursa (20), which also continues under the retinaculum (9).

| | |
|---|---|
| **1** Abductor digiti minimi | **13** Palmar branch of ulnar nerve |
| **2** Abductor pollicis brevis | **14** Palmar digital artery |
| **3** Fibrous flexor sheath | **15** Palmar digital nerve |
| **4** Flexor carpi radialis | **16** Palmaris brevis |
| **5** Flexor carpi ulnaris | **17** Palmaris longus |
| **6** Flexor digiti minimi brevis | **18** Pisiform bone |
| **7** Flexor digitorum superficialis | **19** Radial artery |
| **8** Flexor pollicis brevis | **20** Radial bursa and flexor |
| **9** Flexor retinaculum | pollicis longus |
| **10** Median nerve | **21** Superficial palmar arch |
| **11** Muscular (recurrent) branch | **22** Synovial sheath |
| of median nerve | **23** Ulnar artery |
| **12** Palmar branch of median | **24** Ulnar bursa |
| nerve | **25** Ulnar nerve |

In the carpal tunnel (beneath the flexor retinaculum), one synovial sheath envelops the eight tendons of flexor digitorum superficialis and profundus (A24), another envelops the flexor pollicis longus tendon (A20), and flexor carpi radialis (in its own compartment of the flexor retinaculum) has its own sheath also (A4). The synovial sheaths for flexor carpi radialis and flexor pollicis longus extend as far as the tendon insertions.

The sheath of the long finger flexors is continuous with the digital synovial sheath of the little finger, but is *not* continuous with the digital synovial sheaths of the ring, middle or index fingers; these fingers have their own synovial sheaths whose proximal ends project slightly beyond the *fibrous* sheaths within which the digital *synovial* sheaths lie.

The muscular (recurrent) branch (A11) of the median nerve usually supplies abductor pollicis brevis, flexor pollicis brevis and opponens pollicis, but of all the muscles in the body flexor pollicis brevis (A8) is the one most likely to have an anomalous supply: in about one-third of hands by the median nerve, in another third by the ulnar nerve, and in the rest by both the median and ulnar nerves.

## B Right index finger *long tendons, vincula and relations*

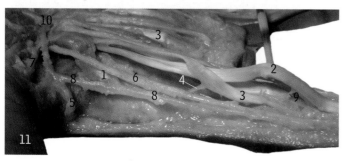

**1** First lumbrical muscle
**2** Flexor digitorum profundus
**3** Flexor digitorum superficialis
**4** Long vinculum of superficialis tendon
**5** Metacarpal arterial branch
**6** Palmar digital nerve
**7** Princeps pollicis artery
**8** Radialis indicis artery
**9** Short vinculum of profundus tendon
**10** Superficial palmar arterial arch
**11** Thumb

*Digital nerve block, see page 174.*

# Left wrist and hand
**A** *palmar surface* **B** *axial MR image*

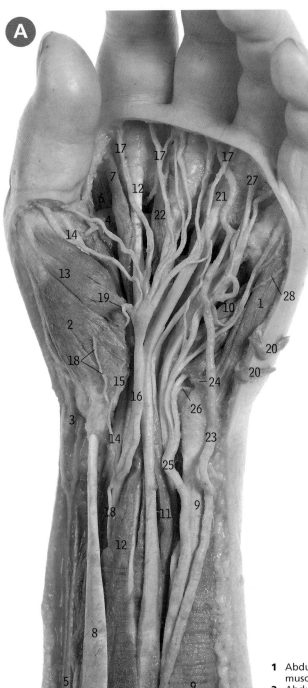

Parts of the fibrous flexor sheaths of the fingers (A21) have also been excised to show the contained tendons of flexor digitorum superficialis (A12) and flexor digitorum profundus (A11). In the palm, the lumbrical muscles (A7 and 22) arise from the profundus tendons. Compare features in the MR image with the dissection.

| | |
|---|---|
| 1 Abductor digiti minimi | 18 Median nerve, palmar cutaneous branch |
| 2 Abductor pollicis brevis | 19 Median nerve, recurrent branch |
| 3 Abductor pollicis longus | 20 Palmaris brevis |
| 4 Adductor pollicis | 21 Remaining parts of fibrous flexor sheath |
| 5 Brachioradialis | 22 Second lumbrical |
| 6 First dorsal interosseous | 23 Ulnar artery |
| 7 First lumbrical | 24 Ulnar artery, deep branch |
| 8 Flexor carpi radialis | 25 Ulnar nerve |
| 9 Flexor carpi ulnaris | 26 Ulnar nerve, deep branch |
| 10 Flexor digiti minimi brevis | 27 Ulnar nerve, digital branch |
| 11 Flexor digitorum profundus | 28 Ulnar nerve, muscular branch |
| 12 Flexor digitorum superficialis | |
| 13 Flexor pollicis brevis | |
| 14 Flexor pollicis longus | |
| 15 Flexor retinaculum cut edge | |
| 16 Median nerve | |
| 17 Median nerve, digital branch | |

The lumbrical muscles have no bony attachments. They arise from the tendons of flexor digitorum profundus (A11) – the first and second (A7 and A22) from the tendons of the index and middle fingers respectively, and the third and fourth from adjacent sides of the middle and ring, and ring and little fingers respectively. Each is attached distally to the radial side of the dorsal digital expansion of each finger (page 170).

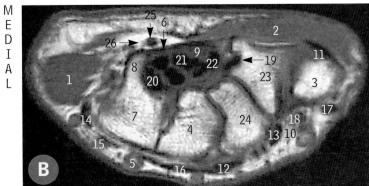

| | |
|---|---|
| 1 Abductor digiti minimi muscle | 14 Tendon of extensor carpi ulnaris muscle |
| 2 Abductor pollicis brevis muscle | 15 Tendon of extensor digiti minimi muscle |
| 3 Base of first metacarpal | 16 Tendon of extensor digitorum muscle |
| 4 Capitate | 17 Tendon of extensor pollicis brevis muscle |
| 5 Dorsal venous arch | 18 Tendon of extensor pollicis longus muscle |
| 6 Flexor retinaculum | 19 Tendon of flexor carpi radialis muscle |
| 7 Hamate | 20 Tendon of flexor digitorum profundus muscle |
| 8 Hook of hamate | 21 Tendon of flexor digitorum superficialis muscle |
| 9 Median nerve | 22 Tendon of flexor pollicis longus muscle |
| 10 Radial artery | 23 Trapezium |
| 11 Tendon of abductor pollicis longus muscle | 24 Trapezoid |
| 12 Tendon of extensor carpi radialis brevis muscle | 25 Ulnar artery |
| 13 Tendon of extensor carpi radialis longus muscle | 26 Ulnar nerve |

*Carpal tunnel syndrome, median nerve palsy, see pages 174, 175.*

# Superficial palmar arch

**(A)** *incomplete in the left hand*

**(B)** *complete in the right hand*

In two-thirds of hands, the superficial palmar arch is not complete (as in A29). In the other third, it is usually completed by the superficial palmar branch of the radial artery (B30).

In the palm the superficial arterial arch (29) and its branches (as at 1) lie superficial to the common palmar digital nerves (22 and 7), but on the fingers the palmar digital nerves (as at 3) lie superficial (anterior) to the palmar digital arteries (as at 2).

**1** A common palmar digital artery
**2** A palmar digital artery
**3** A palmar digital nerve
**4** Abductor digiti minimi
**5** Abductor pollicis brevis
**6** Abductor pollicis longus
**7** Common palmar digital branch of ulnar nerve
**8** Common origin of 28 and 26
**9** Deep branch of ulnar artery
**10** Deep branch of ulnar nerve
**11** Deep palmar arch
**12** First lumbrical
**13** Flexor carpi radialis
**14** Flexor carpi ulnaris and pisiform
**15** Flexor digitorum profundus
**16** Flexor digitorum superficialis
**17** Flexor pollicis brevis
**18** Flexor pollicis longus
**19** Flexor retinaculum
**20** Fourth lumbrical
**21** Median nerve
**22** Median nerve dividing into common palmar digital branches
**23** Muscular (recurrent) branch of median nerve
**24** Opponens digiti minimi
**25** Palmaris brevis
**26** Princeps pollicis artery
**27** Radial artery
**28** Radialis indicis artery
**29** Superficial palmar arch
**30** Superficial palmar branch of radial artery
**31** Ulnar artery
**32** Ulnar nerve

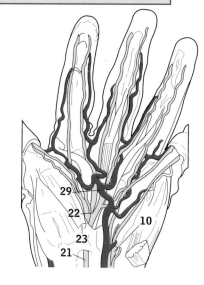

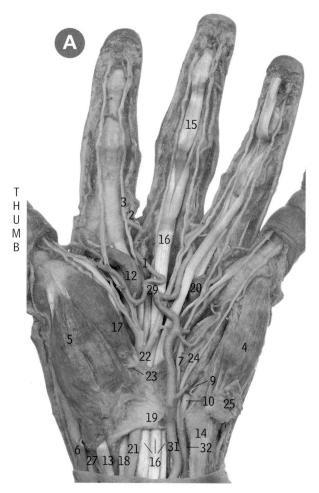

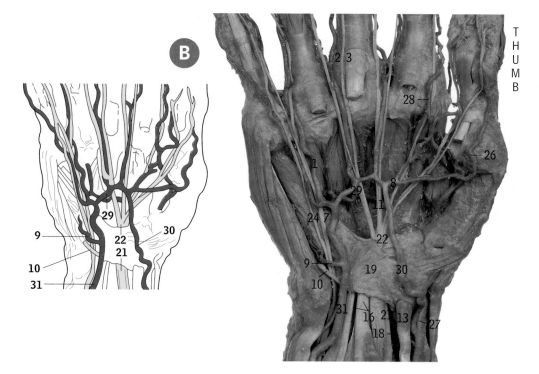

*Arterial puncture at the wrist, see page 174.*

# Palm of right hand

**C** *deep palmar arch*   **D** *arteriogram of palmar arteries*

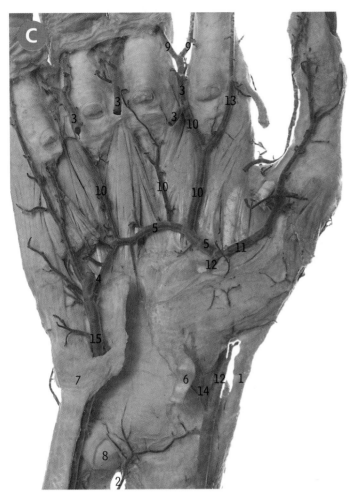

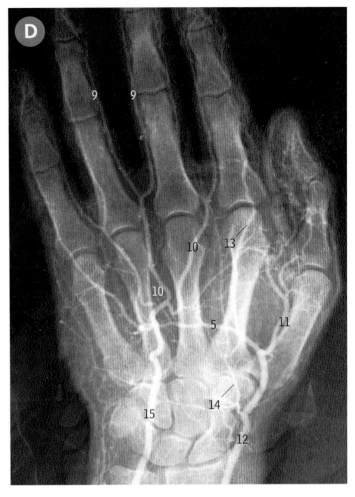

Most muscles and tendons have been removed and the arteries have been distended by injection. The deep palmar arch (5) is seen giving off the palmar metacarpal arteries (10) which join the common palmar digital arteries (3) from the superficial arch. Compare C with the vessels in the arteriogram.

1  Abductor pollicis longus
2  Branch of anterior interosseous artery to anterior carpal arch
3  Common palmar digital arteries (from superficial arch)
4  Deep branch of ulnar artery
5  Deep palmar arch
6  Flexor carpi radialis
7  Flexor carpi ulnaris and pisiform
8  Head of ulna
9  Palmar digital arteries
10  Palmar metacarpal arteries
11  Princeps pollicis artery
12  Radial artery
13  Radialis indicis artery (anomalous origin)
14  Superficial palmar branch of radial artery
15  Ulnar artery

 *Trigger finger, see page 176.*

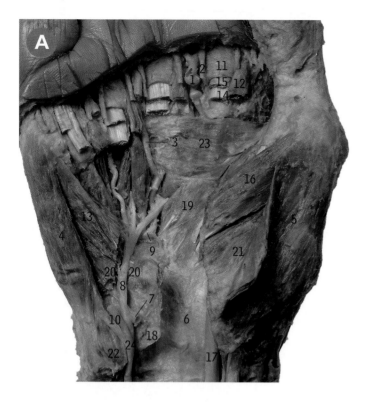

## A Palm of right hand
## *deep branch of the ulnar nerve*

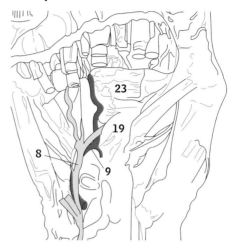

The long flexor tendons (15 and 14) and lumbricals (12) have been cut off near the heads of the metacarpals, and parts of the hypothenar muscles removed to show the deep branches of the ulnar nerve and artery (8 and 7) running into the palm and curling laterally to pass between the transverse and oblique heads of adductor pollicis (23 and 19).

| | |
|---|---|
| **1** A common palmar digital artery | **13** Flexor digiti minimi brevis |
| **2** A palmar digital nerve | **14** Flexor digitorum profundus |
| **3** A palmar metacarpal artery | **15** Flexor digitorum superficialis |
| **4** Abductor digiti minimi | **16** Flexor pollicis brevis |
| **5** Abductor pollicis brevis | **17** Flexor pollicis longus |
| **6** Carpal tunnel | **18** Flexor retinaculum (cut edge) |
| **7** Deep branch of ulnar artery | **19** Oblique head of adductor pollicis |
| **8** Deep branch of ulnar nerve | **20** Opponens digiti minimi |
| **9** Deep palmar arch | **21** Opponens pollicis |
| **10** Digital branches of ulnar nerve | **22** Pisiform |
| **11** Fibrous flexor sheath | **23** Transverse head of adductor pollicis |
| **12** First lumbrical | **24** Ulnar nerve |

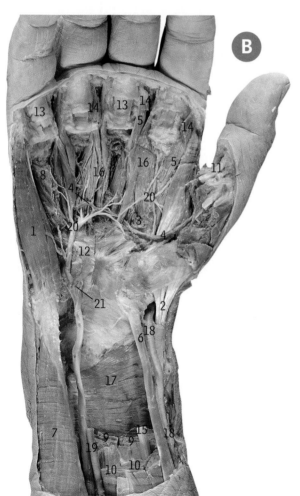

## B Palm of right hand

## *deep dissection*

Deep to the adductor pollicis and the flexor tendons lie the pronator quadratus proximally and the extensive deep palmar branches of the ulnar nerve and deep palmar arch distally.

| | |
|---|---|
| **1** Abductor digiti minimi | **12** Flexor retinaculum – cut |
| **2** Abductor pollicis longus | **13** Flexor tendon sheaths |
| **3** Adductor pollicis – cut | **14** Lumbrical – cut |
| **4** Deep palmar arch | **15** Median nerve – cut |
| **5** Dorsal interossei | **16** Palmar interossei |
| **6** Flexor carpi radialis | **17** Pronator quadratus |
| **7** Flexor carpi ulnaris | **18** Radial artery |
| **8** Flexor digiti minimi – cut | **19** Ulnar artery – cut |
| **9** Flexor digitorum profundus – cut | **20** Ulnar nerve, deep branches to intrinsic hand muscles |
| **10** Flexor digitorum superficialis – cut | **21** Ulnar nerve, superficial branch (cut at wrist) |
| **11** Flexor pollicis longus | |

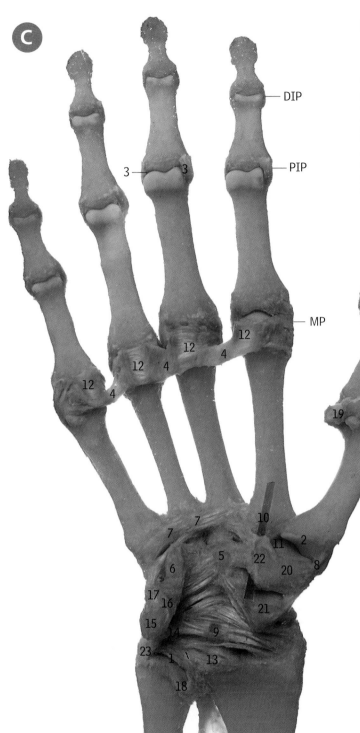

**C** DIP

3 — 3

PIP

MP

12

12

12 4

12 4 4

12

4

19

19

10

7 7

11 2

5 22

6 20 8

17 16

15 21

23 14 9

1 13

18

**DIP** distal interphalangeal joint
**PIP** proximal interphalangeal joint
**MP** metacarpophalangeal joint

## **C** Palm of right hand

### *ligaments and joints*

The capsule of the carpometacarpal joint of the thumb (between the base of the first metacarpal and the trapezium) has been removed, to show the saddle-shaped joint surfaces, which allow the unique movement of opposition of the thumb to occur. The palmar and lateral ligaments (11 and 8) of the joint remain intact. The capsule of the distal radio-ulnar joint has also been removed to show the articular disc, but the wrist joint, the ulnar part of which lies distal to the disc, has not been opened.

1   Articular disc of distal radio-ulnar joint
2   Base of first metacarpal
3   Collateral ligament of interphalangeal joint
4   Deep transverse metacarpal ligament
5   Head of capitate
6   Hook of hamate
7   Interosseous metacarpal ligament
8   Lateral ligament of carpometacarpal joint of thumb
9   Lunate
10  Marker in groove on trapezium for flexor carpi radialis tendon
11  Palmar ligament of carpometacarpal joint of thumb
12  Palmar ligament of metacarpophalangeal joint with groove for flexor tendon
13  Palmar radiocarpal ligament
14  Palmar ulnocarpal ligament
15  Pisiform
16  Pisohamate ligament
17  Pisometacarpal ligament
18  Sacciform recess of capsule of distal radio-ulnar joint
19  Sesamoid bones of flexor pollicis brevis tendons (with adductor pollicis on ulnar side)
20  Trapezium
21  Tubercle of scaphoid
22  Tubercle of trapezium
23  Ulnar collateral ligament of wrist joint

---

The collateral ligaments of the metacarpophalangeal and interphalangeal joints (D2, C3) pass obliquely forwards from the posterior part of the side of the head of the proximal bone to the anterior part of the side of the base of the distal bone.

Opposition of the thumb is a combination of flexion and abduction with medial rotation of the first metacarpal (page 160). The saddle-shape of the joint between the base of the first metacarpal and the trapezium, together with the way that the capsule and its reinforcing ligaments are attached to the bones, ensures that when flexor pollicis brevis and opponens pollicis contract they produce the necessary metacarpal rotation.

The articular disc (1) holds the lower ends of the radius and ulna together, and separates the distal radio-ulnar joint from the wrist joint, so that the cavities of these joints are not continuous (unlike those of the elbow and proximal radio-ulnar joints, which have one continuous cavity – page 150).

---

## **D** Right index finger

### *metacarpophalangeal (MP) joint, from the radial side*

Part of the capsule has been removed to define the collateral ligament (2).

**D**

1 2 4

3

1   Base of proximal phalanx
2   Collateral ligament
3   Fibrous flexor sheath
4   Head of second metacarpal

*Game-keeper's thumb, see page 175.*

# Dorsum of left hand

**A** *Radial side view of 'Anatomical snuff box'*

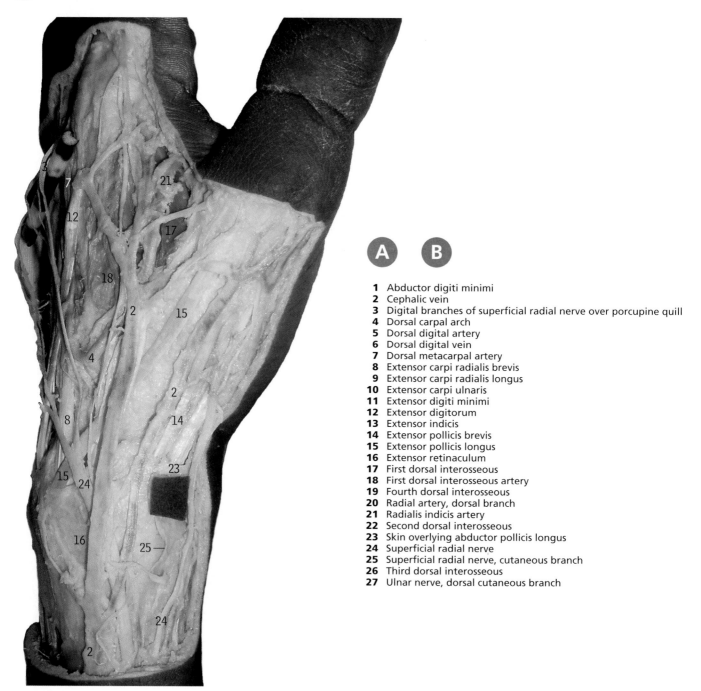

**A** **B**

1 Abductor digiti minimi
2 Cephalic vein
3 Digital branches of superficial radial nerve over porcupine quill
4 Dorsal carpal arch
5 Dorsal digital artery
6 Dorsal digital vein
7 Dorsal metacarpal artery
8 Extensor carpi radialis brevis
9 Extensor carpi radialis longus
10 Extensor carpi ulnaris
11 Extensor digiti minimi
12 Extensor digitorum
13 Extensor indicis
14 Extensor pollicis brevis
15 Extensor pollicis longus
16 Extensor retinaculum
17 First dorsal interosseous
18 First dorsal interosseous artery
19 Fourth dorsal interosseous
20 Radial artery, dorsal branch
21 Radialis indicis artery
22 Second dorsal interosseous
23 Skin overlying abductor pollicis longus
24 Superficial radial nerve
25 Superficial radial nerve, cutaneous branch
26 Third dorsal interosseous
27 Ulnar nerve, dorsal cutaneous branch

*Mallet finger, see page 175.*

## B Dorsum of left hand

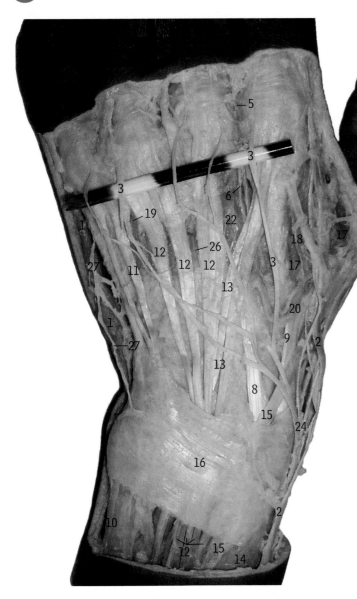

## C Dorsum of right wrist and hand
### synovial sheaths

Fascia and cutaneous branches of the ulnar nerve have been removed; the extensor reticulum (13) and the radial nerve (2) have been preserved and the synovial sheaths have been emphasised by blue tissue. From the radial to the ulnar side, the six compartments of the extensor retinaculum contain the tendons of: (a) abductor pollicis longus and extensor pollicis brevis (1 and 11); (b) extensor carpi radialis longus and brevis (6 and 5); (c) extensor pollicis longus (12); (d) extensor digitorum and extensor indicis (9 and 10); (e) extensor digiti minimi (8); (f) extensor carpi ulnaris (7).

C

1   Abductor pollicis longus
2   Branches of radial nerve
3   Cephalic vein
4   Common sheath for 5 and 6
5   Extensor carpi radialis brevis
6   Extensor carpi radialis longus
7   Extensor carpi ulnaris
8   Extensor digiti minimi
9   Extensor digitorum
10  Extensor indicis
11  Extensor pollicis brevis
12  Extensor pollicis longus
13  Extensor retinaculum

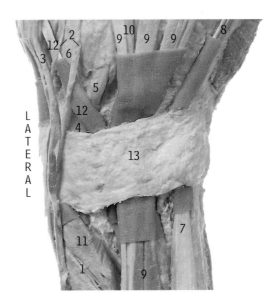

*Wrist ganglion, see page 176.*

## A Dorsum of right hand *arteries*

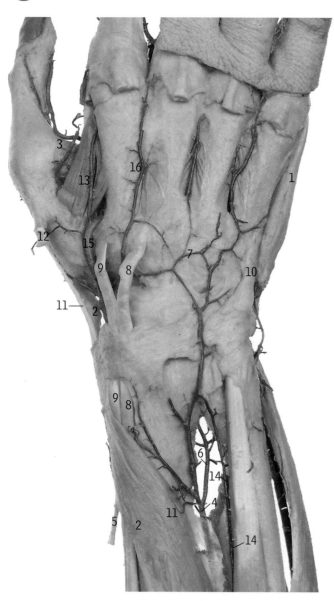

The arteries have been injected and the long finger tendons removed to display the dorsal carpal arch (7) and dorsal metacarpal arteries (as at 13 and 16). Above the wrist pronator quadratus has been removed to show the branch (6) of the anterior interosseous artery (4), which continues towards the palm; the anterior interosseous itself passes to the dorsal surface to join the posterior interosseous artery (14).

## B Left ring finger *extensor expansion (dorsal digital expansion)*

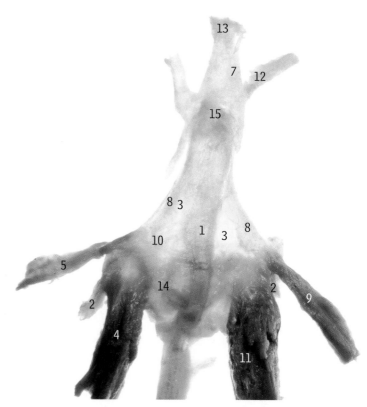

| | | | |
|---|---|---|---|
| **1** | Abductor digiti minimi | **9** | Extensor carpi radialis longus |
| **2** | Abductor pollicis longus | **10** | Extensor carpi ulnaris |
| **3** | Adductor pollicis and branch of princeps pollicis artery | **11** | Extensor pollicis brevis |
| | | **12** | Extensor pollicis longus |
| **4** | Anterior interosseous artery | **13** | First dorsal interosseous and first dorsal metacarpal artery |
| **5** | Brachioradialis | **14** | Posterior interosseous artery |
| **6** | Branch of anterior interosseous artery to anterior carpal arch | **15** | Radial artery |
| | | **16** | Second dorsal interosseous and second dorsal metacarpal artery |
| **7** | Dorsal carpal arch | | |
| **8** | Extensor carpi radialis brevis | | |

| | | | |
|---|---|---|---|
| **1** | Common extensor tendon | **8** | Lateral tendon "wing tendon" |
| **2** | Deep transverse metacarpal ligament | **9** | Lumbrical muscle |
| **3** | Dorsal digital expansion | **10** | Oblique interosseous fibres |
| **4** | Dorsal interosseous muscle | **11** | Palmar interosseous muscle |
| **5** | Dorsal interosseous muscle, phalangeal attachment | **12** | Retinacular ligament, transverse band |
| | | **13** | Terminal conjoint extensor tendon |
| **6** | Extensor digitorum tendon | **14** | Transverse ligament |
| **7** | Lateral conjoined extensor tendon | **15** | Triangular ligament |

Three tendons pass to different levels of the thumb: abductor pollicis longus (A2) to the base of the first metacarpal, extensor pollicis brevis (A11) to the base of the proximal phalanx, and extensor pollicis longus (A12) to the base of the distal phalanx.

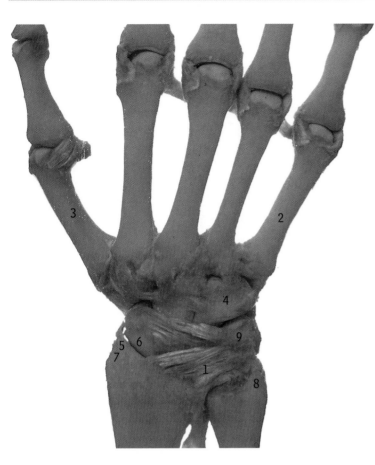

# A Dorsum of right hand
## ligaments and joints

Most joint capsules have been removed, including the radial parts of the wrist joint capsule, thus showing the articulation between the scaphoid (6) and the lower end of the radius (7).

1 Dorsal radiocarpal ligament
2 Fifth metacarpal
3 First metacarpal
4 Hamate
5 Radial collateral ligament of wrist joint
6 Scaphoid
7 Styloid process of radius
8 Styloid process of ulna
9 Triquetral

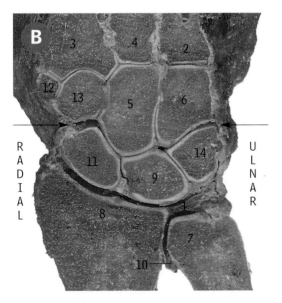

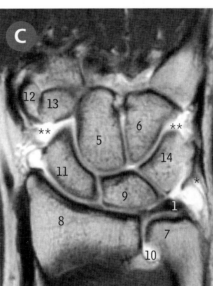

# Right wrist
## coronal section

**B** dissection

**C** coronal MR arthrogram

1 Articular disc (triangular fibrocartilage)
2 Base of fourth metacarpal
3 Base of second metacarpal
4 Base of third metacarpal
5 Capitate
6 Hamate
7 Head of ulna
8 Lower end of radius
9 Lunate
10 Sacciform recess of distal radio-ulnar joint
11 Scaphoid
12 Trapezium
13 Trapezoid
14 Triquetral

\* Normal vascular penetration of triangular fibrocartilage peripherally
\*\* Contrast in midcarpal joint indicates abnormal communication between radiocarpal and midcarpal joints

Viewed from the dorsal surface, the section has passed through the wrist near this surface, and the first and fifth metacarpals have not been included in the cut. The arrows between the two rows of carpal bones indicate the line of the midcarpal joint. Compare the MR image with the section.

*Dislocation of the lunate, avascular necrosis of the scaphoid, see pages 174, 175.*

# Right midcarpal and wrist joints

**A** *midcarpal joint, opened up in forced flexion*

**B** *wrist joint, opened up in forced extension*

BACK OF RIGHT THUMB EDGE

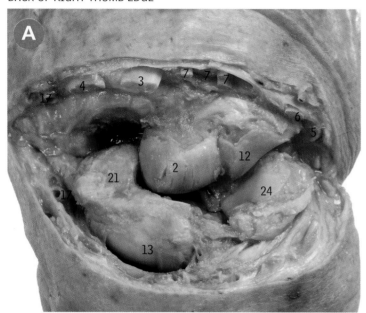

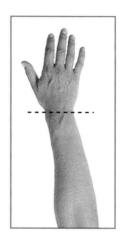

| | |
|---|---|
| **1** | Articular disc |
| **2** | Capitate |
| **3** | Extensor carpi radialis brevis |
| **4** | Extensor carpi radialis longus |
| **5** | Extensor carpi ulnaris |
| **6** | Extensor digiti minimi |
| **7** | Extensor digitorum |
| **8** | Flexor carpi radialis tendon |
| **9** | Flexor carpi ulnaris tendon |
| **10** | Flexor digitorum profundus tendon |
| **11** | Flexor digitorum superficialis tendon |
| **12** | Hamate |
| **13** | Lunate |
| **14** | Median nerve |
| **15** | Palmar arch vein |
| **16** | Palmaris longus tendon |
| **17** | Radial artery |
| **18** | Radial artery, palmar arch branch |
| **19** | Radial surface for lunate |
| **20** | Radial surface for scaphoid |
| **21** | Scaphoid |
| **22** | Styloid process of radius |
| **23** | Styloid process of ulna |
| **24** | Triquetral |
| **25** | Ulnar artery |

FRONT OF RIGHT THUMB EDGE

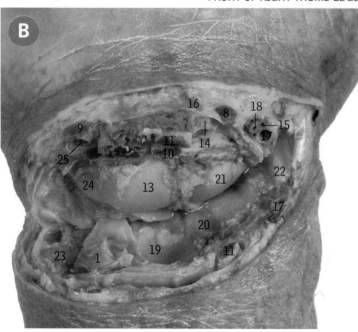

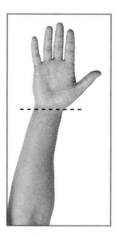

Both joints have been opened up (far beyond the normal range of movement) in order to demonstrate the bones of the joint surfaces. The wrist joint in B has been forced open in flexion, since flexion takes place mostly at this joint, and the midcarpal joint in A has been forced open in extension, since extension takes place mostly at this joint. The proximal (wrist joint) surfaces of the scaphoid (21), lunate (13) and triquetral (24) are seen in B, and their distal (midcarpal joint) surfaces in A.

# Wrist and hand *radiographs*

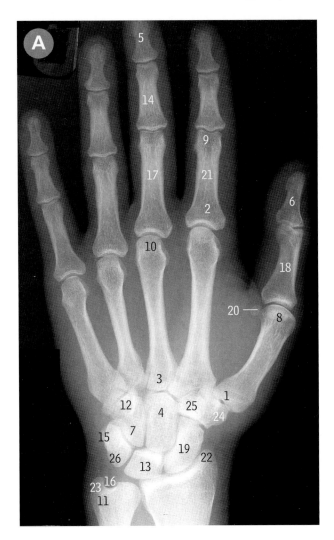

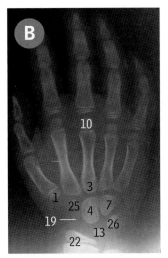

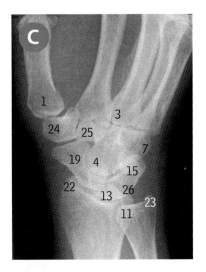

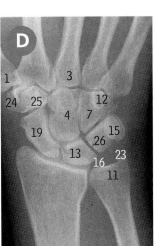

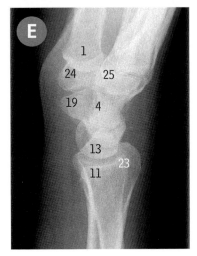

Ⓐ dorsopalmar projection

Ⓑ of a 4-year-old child

Ⓒ oblique projection

Ⓓ posteroanterior projection

Ⓔ lateral projection

The epiphysis at the lower end of the radius appears on a radiograph at 2 years and in the ulna at 6 years. The first carpal bone to appear is the capitate at 1 year.

**Compare the epiphyses of the metacarpals and phalanges seen in B with the bony specimens in J and K on page 133.**

1  Base of first metacarpal
2  Base of phalanx
3  Base of third metacarpal
4  Capitate
5  Distal phalanx of middle finger
6  Distal phalanx of thumb
7  Hamate
8  Head of first metacarpal
9  Head of phalanx
10  Head of third metacarpal
11  Head of ulna
12  Hook of hamate
13  Lunate
14  Middle phalanx of middle finger
15  Pisiform
16  Position of articular disc (triangular fibrocartilage) of distal radio-ulnar joint
17  Proximal phalanx of middle finger
18  Proximal phalanx of thumb
19  Scaphoid
20  Sesamoid bone in flexor pollicis brevis
21  Shaft of phalanx
22  Styloid process at lower end of radius
23  Styloid process of ulna
24  Trapezium
25  Trapezoid
26  Triquetral

# Upper limb

Clinical thumbnails, see DVD Upper limb for details and further clinical images

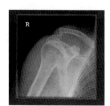
Acromioclavicular separation

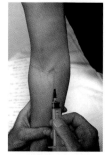
Anterior interosseous nerve entrapment

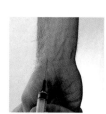
Arterial puncture at the elbow

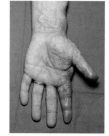
Arterial puncture at the wrist

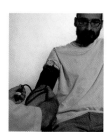
Arteriovenous fistula

Auscultation of the brachial pulse

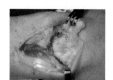
Avascular necrosis of the scaphoid

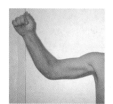
Axillary-subclavian vein thrombosis

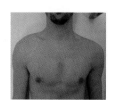
Biceps tendon reflex

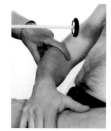
Bicipital tendinitis and rupture

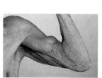
Calcific tendinitis

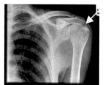
Carpal tunnel syndrome

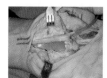

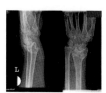
Colles' fracture

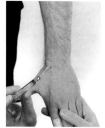
de Quervain's disease

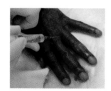
Digital nerve block

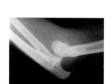
Dislocation of the elbow

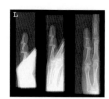
Dislocation of the finger

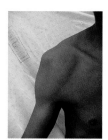
Dislocation of humerus

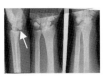
Dislocation of the lunate

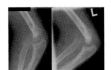
Dislocation of the radial head

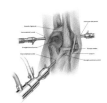
Dupuytren's contracture

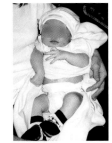
Elbow arthroscopy

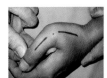
Erb's palsy

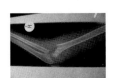

Gamekeeper's thumb

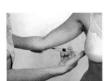
Golfer's elbow – injection

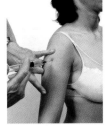
Intramuscular injection – deltoid

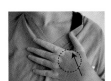
Klumpke's paralysis

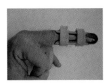
Mallet finger

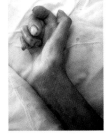
Median nerve palsy

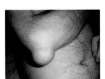
Olecranon bursitis

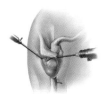
Painful arc syndrome/ rotator cuff tear

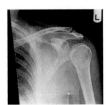
Posterior dislocation of the shoulder

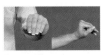
Posterior interosseous nerve entrapment

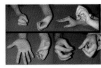
Radial nerve palsy

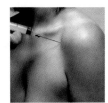
Shoulder joint injection

Supracondylar fracture of the humerus

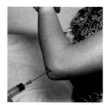

Tennis elbow

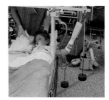

Traction of forearm fractures

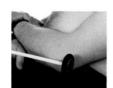

Triceps tendon reflex

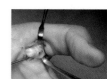

Trigger finger

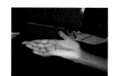

Ulnar nerve palsy

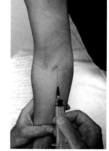

Venepuncture

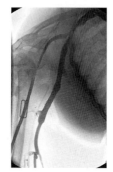

Venous cutdown

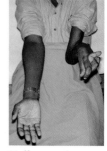

Volkmann's contracture

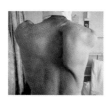

Winging of the scapula

Wrist arthroscopy

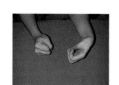

Wrist drop

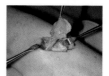

Wrist ganglion

# Thorax

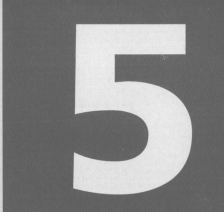

**Thorax** **A** *surface anatomy, from the front*

**B** *axial skeleton, from behind*

**C** *axial skeleton, from the front
(skull, vertebral column and thoracic cage)*

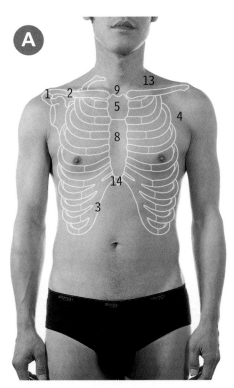

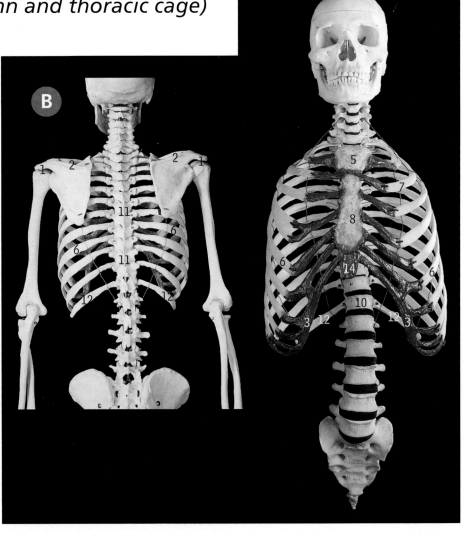

1 Acromion
2 Clavicle
3 Costal margin
4 Deltopectoral groove
5 Manubrium
6 Rib
7 Second rib
8 Sternal body
9 Suprasternal notch
10 Thoracic vertebra, body
11 Thoracic vertebra, spine
12 Twelfth rib
13 Trapezius
14 Xiphisternum

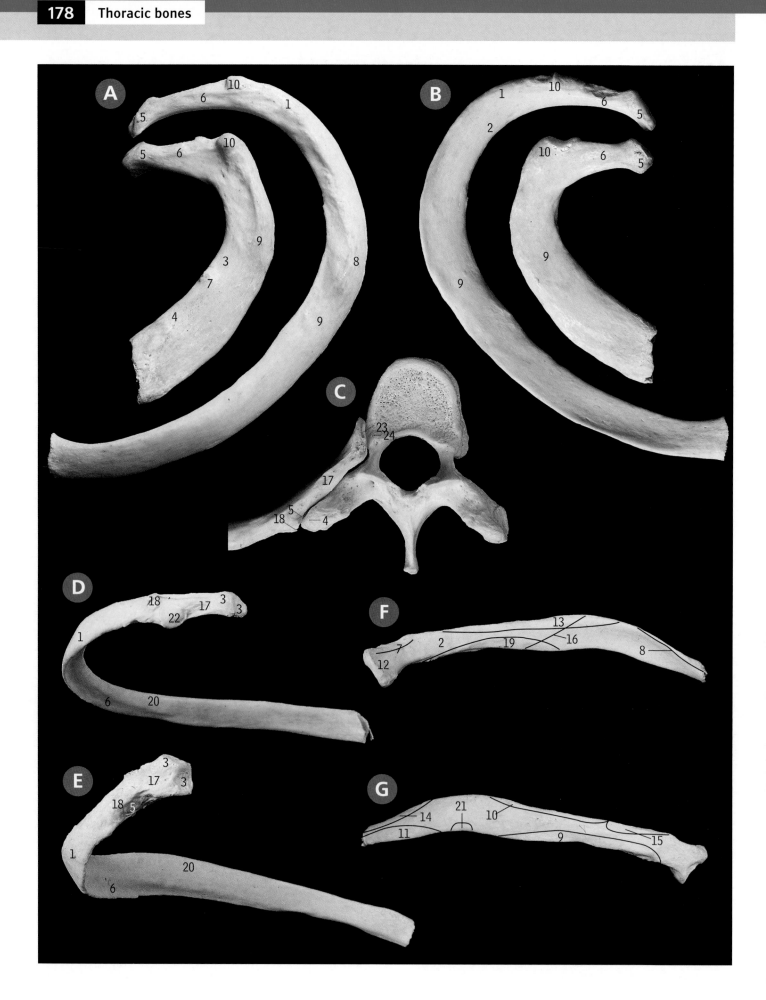

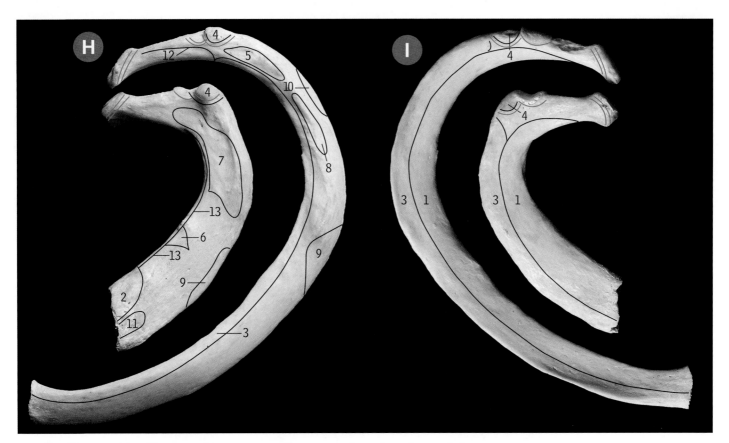

## Left first rib (inner) and second rib (outer)

**A** from above

**B** from below

1  Angle
2  Costal groove
3  Groove for subclavian artery and first thoracic nerve
4  Groove for subclavian vein
5  Head
6  Neck
7  Scalene tubercle
8  Serratus anterior tuberosity
9  Shaft
10  Tubercle

The atypical ribs are the first, second, tenth, eleventh and twelfth.

The **first rib** has a head with one facet (A5), a prominent tubercle (A10), no angle and no costal groove. The shaft has superior and inferior surfaces.

The **second rib** has a head with two facets (B5), an angle (B1) near the tubercle (B10), a broad costal groove (B2) posteriorly, and an external surface facing upwards and outwards with the inner surface facing correspondingly downwards and inwards.

The **twelfth rib** has a head with one facet (F12) but there is no tubercle, no angle and no costal groove. The shaft tapers at its end (the ends of all other ribs widen slightly).

## Ribs and relationships

**C** a typical rib and vertebra articulated, from above

**D** the left fifth rib from behind (a typical upper rib)

**E** the left seventh rib from behind (a typical lower rib)

**F** the left twelfth rib from the front, with attachments

**G** the left twelfth rib from behind, with attachments

1  Angle of rib
2  Area covered by pleura
3  Articular facet of head
4  Articular facet of transverse process
5  Articular part of tubercle
6  Costal groove
7  Costotransverse ligament
8  Diaphragm
9  Erector spinae
10  External intercostal
11  External oblique
12  Head
13  Internal intercostal
14  Latissimus dorsi
15  Levator costae
16  Line of pleural reflexion
17  Neck of rib
18  Non-articular part of tubercle
19  Quadratus lumborum
20  Shaft of rib
21  Serratus posterior inferior
22  Tubercle
23  Upper costal facet of head of rib
24  Upper costal facet of vertebral body

## Left first rib (inner) and second rib (outer), attachments

 **H** from above          **I** from below

Blue lines, epiphysial lines; green lines, capsule attachments of costovertebral joints

1  Area covered by pleura
2  Costoclavicular ligament
3  Intercostal muscles and membranes
4  Lateral costotransverse ligament
5  Levator costae
6  Scalenus anterior
7  Scalenus medius
8  Scalenus posterior
9  Serratus anterior
10  Serratus posterior superior
11  Subclavius
12  Superior costotransverse ligament
13  Suprapleural membrane

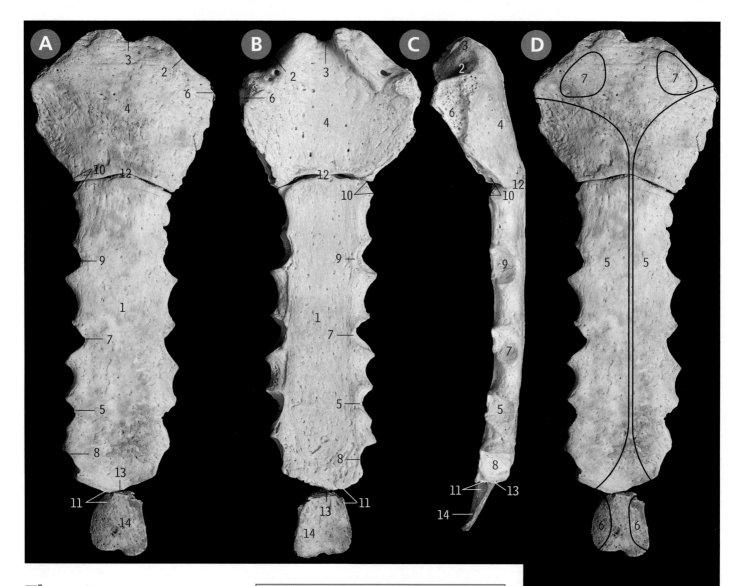

# The sternum

**A** from the front

**B** from behind

**C** from the right

**1** Body
**2** Clavicular notch
**3** Jugular notch
**4** Manubrium
**5** Notch for fifth costal cartilage
**6** Notch for first costal cartilage
**7** Notch for fourth costal cartilage
**8** Notch for sixth costal cartilage
**9** Notch for third costal cartilage
**10** Notches for second costal cartilage
**11** Notches for seventh costal cartilage
**12** Sternal angle and manubriosternal joint
**13** Xiphisternal joint
**14** Xiphoid process

The sternum consists of the manubrium (4), body (1) and xiphoid process (14).

The body of the sternum (1) is formed by the fusion of four sternebrae, the sites of the fusion sometimes being indicated by three slight transverse ridges.

The manubrium (4) and body (1) are bony but the xiphoid process (14), which varies considerably in size and shape, is cartilaginous although it frequently shows some degree of ossification.

The manubriosternal and xiphisternal joints (12 and 13) are both symphyses, the surfaces being covered by hyaline cartilage and united by a fibrocartilaginous disc.

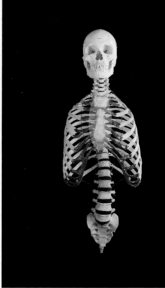

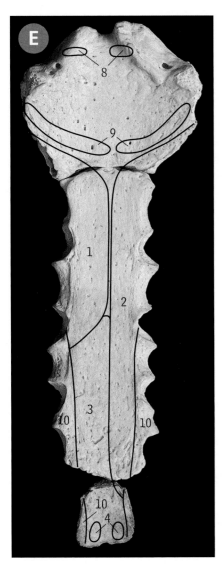

## The sternum attachments

**D** from the front

**E** from behind

1 Area covered by left pleura
2 Area covered by right pleura
3 Area in contact with pericardium
4 Diaphragm
5 Pectoralis major
6 Rectus abdominis
7 Sternocleidomastoid
8 Sternohyoid
9 Sternothyroid
10 Transversus thoracis

> The two pleural sacs are in contact from the levels of the second to fourth costal cartilages (E2 and 1).

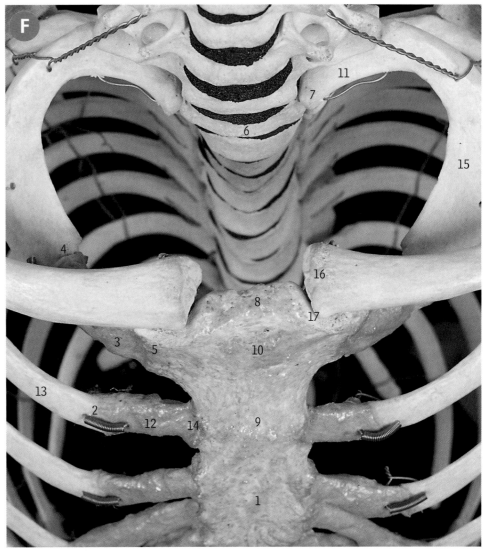

## **F** Thoracic inlet *in an articulated skeleton, from above and in front*

The thoracic inlet or outlet (upper aperture of the thorax) is approximately the same size and shape as the outline of the kidney, and is bounded by the first thoracic vertebra (6), first ribs (15), and costal cartilages (3) and the upper border of the manubrium of the sternum (jugular notch, 8). It does not lie in a horizontal plane but slopes downwards and forwards.

The second costal cartilage (12) joins the manubrium and body of the sternum (10 and 1) at the level of the manubriosternal joint (9). This is an important landmark, since the joint line is palpable as a ridge at the slight angle between the manubrium and body, and the second costal cartilage and rib can be identified lateral to it. Other ribs can be identified by counting down from the second.

1 Body of sternum
2 Costochondral joint
3 First costal cartilage
4 First costochondral joint
5 First sternocostal joint
6 First thoracic vertebra
7 Head of first rib
8 Jugular notch
9 Manubriosternal joint (angle of Louis)
10 Manubrium of sternum
11 Neck of first rib
12 Second costal cartilage
13 Second rib
14 Second sternocostal joint
15 Shaft of first rib
16 Sternal end of clavicle
17 Sternoclavicular joint

*Flail chest, see page 219.*

# Heart, left pleura and lung *surface markings, in the female*

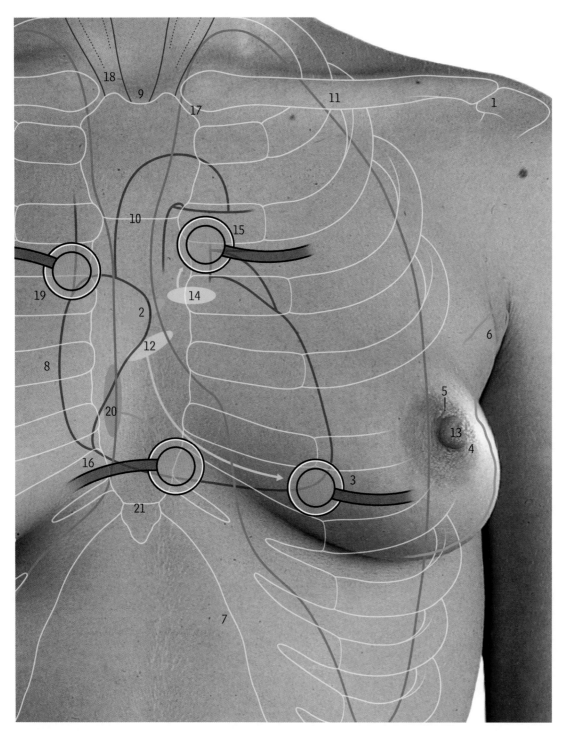

**Brown line, heart; pink line, pleura; green line, axillary tail of breast**

**The positions of the four heart valves are indicated by coloured ellipses, and the sites where the sounds of the corresponding valves are best heard with the stethoscope are shown.**

The manubriosternal joint (10) is palpable and a guide to identifying the second costal cartilage (15) which joins the sternum at this level (see page 181, F9, 14 and 12).

The pleura and lung extend into the neck for 2.5 cm above the medial third of the clavicle.

In the midclavicular line the lower limit of the *pleura* reaches the eighth costal cartilage, in the midaxillary line it reaches the tenth rib, and at the lateral border of the erector spinae muscle it crosses the twelfth rib. The lower border of the *lung* is about two ribs higher than the pleural reflection.

Behind the sternum, the pleural sacs are adjacent to one another in the midline from the level of the second to fourth costal cartilages, but then diverge owing to the mass of the heart on the left.

| | | | |
|---|---|---|---|
| **1** Acromioclavicular joint | **7** Costal margin (at eighth costal cartilage) | **12** Mitral valve | **18** Sternocleidomastoid |
| **2** Aortic valve | **8** Fourth costal cartilage | **13** Nipple of breast | **19** Third costal cartilage |
| **3** Apex of heart | **9** Jugular notch | **14** Pulmonary valve | **20** Tricuspid valve |
| **4** Areola of breast | **10** Manubriosternal joint | **15** Second costal cartilage | **21** Xiphisternal joint |
| **5** Areolar glands of breast | **11** Midpoint of clavicle | **16** Sixth costal cartilage | |
| **6** Axillary tail of breast | | **17** Sternoclavicular joint | |

*Auscultation of heart sounds, see page 219.*

# Female breast *mammary gland*

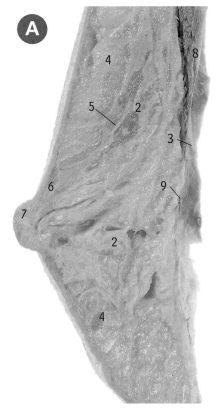

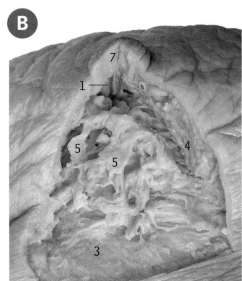

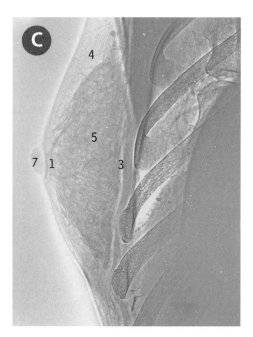

**A** median parasagittal section

**B** dissection of lower part, from the front and below

**C** xeromammogram (obsolete test)

1 Ampulla of lactiferous duct
2 Condensed glandular tissue
3 Fascia over pectoralis major
4 Fat
5 Fibrous septum
6 Lactiferous duct
7 Nipple
8 Pectoralis major
9 Retromammary space

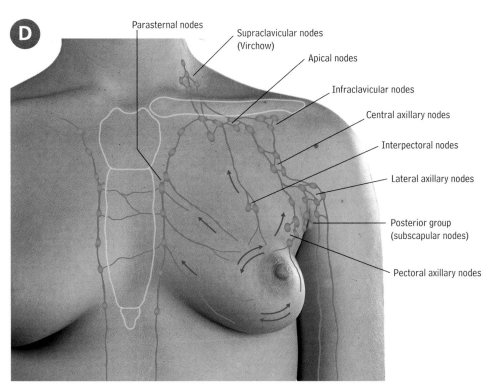

Parasternal nodes
Supraclavicular nodes (Virchow)
Apical nodes
Infraclavicular nodes
Central axillary nodes
Interpectoral nodes
Lateral axillary nodes
Posterior group (subscapular nodes)
Pectoral axillary nodes

## D Breast *lymph drainage*

There is a diffuse network of anastomosing lymphatic channels within the breast, including the overlying skin, and *lymph in any part may travel to any other part*. Larger channels drain most of the lymph to axillary nodes, but some from the medial part pass through the thoracic wall near the sternum to parasternal nodes adjacent to the internal thoracic vessels. These are the commonest and initial sites for cancerous spread, but other nodes may be involved (especially in the later spread of disease); these include infraclavicular and supraclavicular (deep cervical) nodes, nodes in the mediastinum, and nodes in the abdomen (via the diaphragm and rectus sheath). Spread to the opposite breast may also occur.

*Breast examination, carcinoma of the breast, mastectomy, orange-peel skin, see pages 219, 220.*

## A Right side of the thorax *from behind with the arm abducted*

With the arm fully abducted, the medial (vertebral) border of the scapula (5) comes to lie at an angle of about 60° to the vertical, and indicates approximately the line of the oblique fissure of the lung (interrupted line).

1 Deltoid
2 Fifth intercostal space
3 Inferior angle of scapula
4 Latissimus dorsi
5 Medial border of scapula
6 Spine of scapula
7 Spinous process of third thoracic vertebra
8 Teres major
9 Trapezius

> The line of the oblique fissure of the lung runs from the level of the spine of the third thoracic vertebra (7) to the sixth costal cartilage at the lateral border of the sternum (see B). With the arm fully abducted, the vertebral border of the scapula (5) is a good guide to the direction of this fissure.

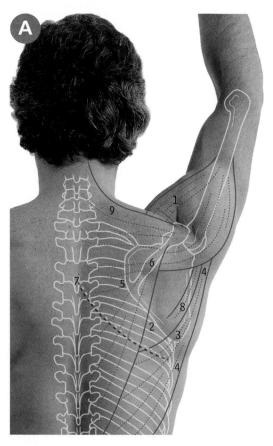

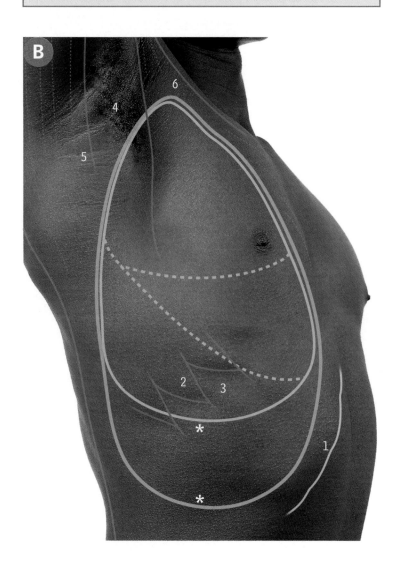

## B Right side of the thorax *surface markings, from the right, with the arm abducted*

The purple line indicates the extent of the pleura, and the solid orange line the lower limit of the lung; note the gap between the two at the lower part of the thorax, indicating the costodiaphragmatic recess of pleura, which does not contain any lung. The transverse and oblique fissures of the lung are represented by the interrupted orange lines.

1 Costal margin
2 Digitations of serratus anterior
3 External oblique
4 Floor of axilla
5 Latissimus dorsi
6 Pectoralis major

> The transverse fissure of the right lung is represented by a line drawn horizontally backwards from the fourth costal cartilage until it meets the line of the oblique fissure (described in A) running forwards to the sixth costal cartilage. The triangle so outlined indicates the middle lobe of the lung, with the superior lobe above it and the inferior lobe below and behind it. It is the area covered by the right breast.
>
> On the left side, where the lung has only two lobes, superior and inferior, there is no transverse fissure; the surface marking for the oblique fissure is similar to that on the right.
>
> * The asterisks represent the places where the lower edges of the lung and pleura cross the eighth and tenth ribs, respectively in the mid-axillary line.

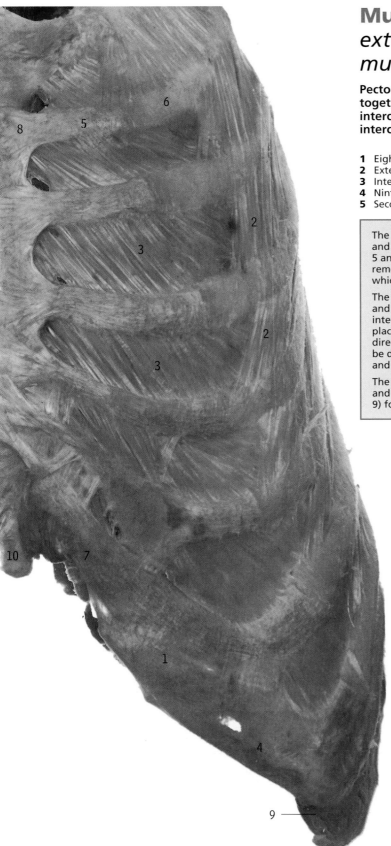

## Muscles of the thorax *left external and internal intercostal muscles, from the front*

**Pectoral and abdominal muscles have been removed, together with all vessels and nerves and the anterior intercostal membranes, to show the external and internal intercostal muscles (as at 2 and 3).**

| | | | |
|---|---|---|---|
| **1** | Eighth costal cartilage | **6** | Second rib |
| **2** | External intercostal | **7** | Seventh costal cartilage |
| **3** | Internal intercostal | **8** | Sternal angle (of Louis) |
| **4** | Ninth costal cartilage | **9** | Tenth costal cartilage |
| **5** | Second costal cartilage | **10** | Xiphoid process |

The fibres of the **external intercostal muscles** (2) run downwards and medially, and near the costochondral junctions (as between 5 and 6) give place to the anterior intercostal membrane (here removed); these are thin sheets of connective tissue through which the underlying internal intercostal muscles (3) can be seen.

The fibres of the **internal intercostal muscles** (3) run downwards and laterally. At the front, they are covered by the anterior intercostal membranes, and at the back of the thorax they give place to the posterior intercostal membranes. The different directions of the muscle fibres enable the two muscle groups to be distinguished – down and medially for the externals (2), down and laterally for the internals (3).

The seventh costal cartilage (7) is the lowest to join the sternum and together with the eighth, ninth and tenth cartilages (1, 4 and 9) forms the costal margin.

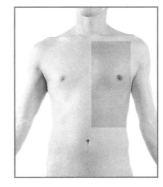

*Flail chest, see page 219.*

# Muscles of the thorax *right intercostal muscles*

**A** from the outside

**B** from the inside

1. Eighth rib
2. External intercostal
3. Fifth intercostal nerve
4. Fifth posterior intercostal artery
5. Fifth posterior intercostal vein
6. Fifth rib
7. Fourth rib
8. Innermost intercostal
9. Internal intercostal
10. Pleura
11. Seventh rib
12. Sixth intercostal nerve
13. Sixth rib

> The **internal intercostal muscles** are continuous posteriorly with the posterior intercostal membranes which are covered up by the medial ends of the external intercostals (as at 2).

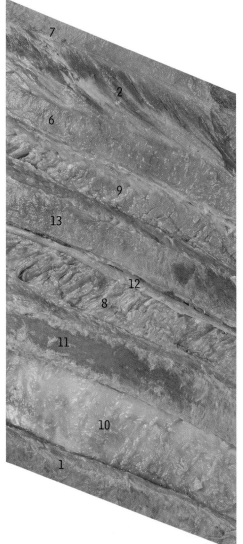

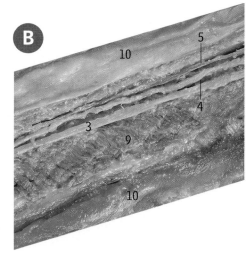

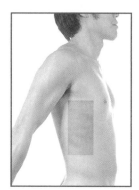

In A, each intercostal space has been dissected to a different depth, showing from above downwards an external intercostal muscle (2), internal intercostal (9), innermost intercostal (8) and pleura (10). The main intercostal vessels and nerve lie between the internal and innermost muscles; the nerve (12) is seen in the sixth interspace immediately below the sixth rib (13) and lying on the outer surface of the innermost intercostal (8), but the artery and vein are under cover of the costal groove. The vessels as well as the nerve are seen in the fifth intercostal space when this is dissected from the inside of the thorax, as in B; here the pleura and innermost intercostal muscle have been removed, and the vessels (5 and 4) and fifth intercostal nerve (3) lie against the inner surface of the internal intercostal (9).

*Intercostal nerve block, see page 219.*

# Muscles of the thorax

**A** *right transversus thoracis, from behind (inside view)*

**B** *left lower subcostal and innermost intercostal muscles*

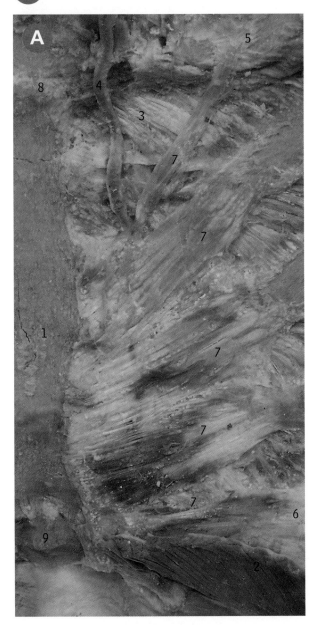

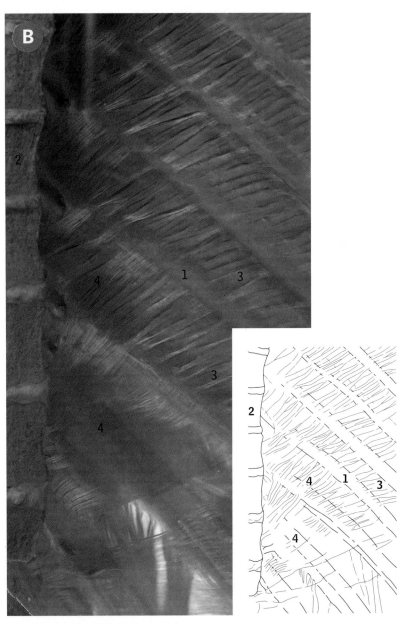

This view of the internal surface of the thoracic wall shows the posterior surface of the right half of the sternum and adjacent wall, with the pleura removed. The internal thoracic artery (4) is seen passing deep to the slips of transversus thoracis (7, previously called sternocostalis).

| | | | |
|---|---|---|---|
| **1** | Body of sternum | **6** | Sixth rib |
| **2** | Diaphragm | **7** | Slips of transversus |
| **3** | Internal intercostal | | thoracis muscle |
| **4** | Internal thoracic artery | **8** | Sternal angle |
| **5** | Second rib | **9** | Xiphoid process |

**Transversus thoracis** (A7) is in the same plane as the **innermost intercostal muscles** at the lateral side of the thoracic wall (B3) and the subcostal muscles on the posterior part (B4).

The **subcostal muscles** (B4) span more than one rib. They and the innermost intercostals (B3, intercostales intimi) are often poorly developed or absent in the upper part of the thorax.

This view of the lower left hemithorax is seen from the right and in front, with vertebral bodies (as at 2) sectioned and the pleura, vessels and nerves removed, and shows part of the innermost layer of thoracic wall muscles (3 and 4).

| | | | |
|---|---|---|---|
| **1** | Eighth rib | **3** | Innermost |
| **2** | Eighth thoracic | | intercostal |
| | vertebra | **4** | Subcostal |

# Lungs, pericardium and pleura *from the front*

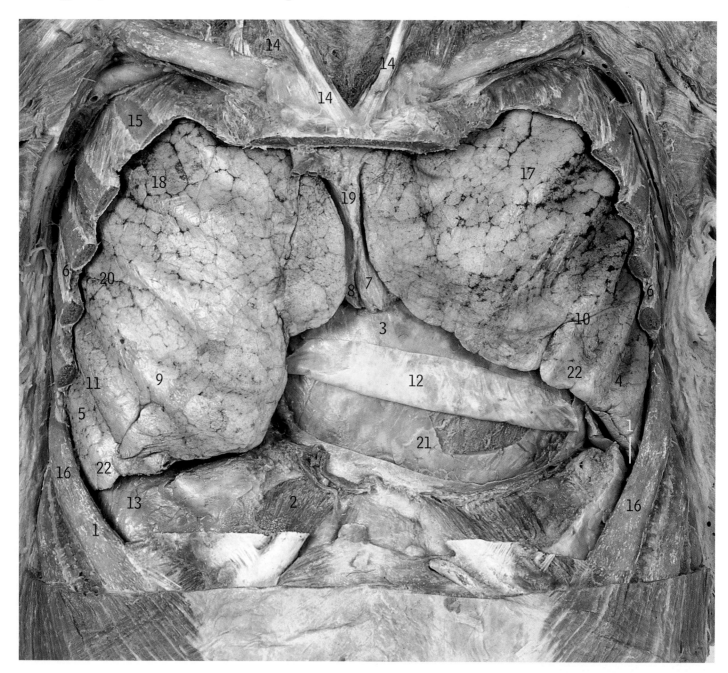

| | | |
|---|---|---|
| **1** Costodiaphragmatic recess | **9** Middle lobe of right lung | **17** Superior lobe of left lung |
| **2** Diaphragm | **10** Oblique fissure of left lung | **18** Superior lobe of right lung |
| **3** Fibrous pericardium | **11** Oblique fissure of right lung | **19** Thymic remnants, see page 359 |
| **4** Inferior lobe of left lung | **12** Parietal pericardium | **20** Transverse fissure of right lung |
| **5** Inferior lobe of right lung | **13** Parietal diaphragmatic pleura | **21** Visceral pericardium overlying myocardium |
| **6** Intercostal muscles | **14** Sternocleidomastoid | **22** Visceral pleura |
| **7** Line of anterior reflection of left pleura | **15** Second rib | |
| **8** Line of anterior reflection of right pleura | **16** Seventh rib | |

*Cardio-pulmonary resuscitation (CPR), thymus, see pages 219, 220.*

# Heart and pericardium

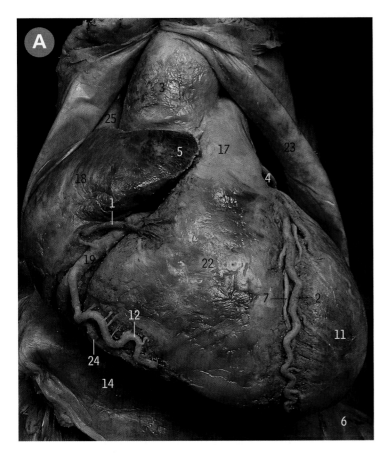

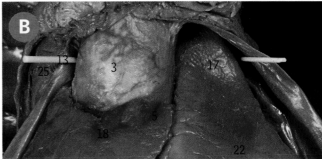

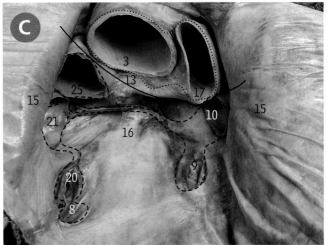

**A** from the front

**B** with marker in the transverse sinus

**C** oblique sinus after removal of the heart

| | |
|---|---|
| **1** Anterior cardiac vein | **15** Pericardium turned laterally over lung |
| **2** Anterior interventricular branch of left coronary artery | **16** Posterior wall of pericardial cavity and oblique sinus |
| **3** Ascending aorta | **17** Pulmonary trunk |
| **4** Auricle of left atrium | **18** Right atrium |
| **5** Auricle of right atrium | **19** Right coronary artery |
| **6** Diaphragm | **20** Right inferior pulmonary vein |
| **7** Great cardiac vein | **21** Right superior pulmonary vein |
| **8** Inferior vena cava | **22** Right ventricle |
| **9** Left inferior pulmonary vein | **23** Serous pericardium overlying fibrous pericardium (turned laterally) |
| **10** Left superior pulmonary vein | **24** Small cardiac vein |
| **11** Left ventricle | **25** Superior vena cava |
| **12** Marginal branch of right coronary artery | |
| **13** Marker in transverse sinus | |
| **14** Pericardium fused with central tendon of diaphragm | |

The **right border of the heart** is formed by the right atrium (A18).

The **left border** is formed mostly by the left ventricle (A11) with at the top the uppermost part (infundibulum) of the right ventricle (A22) and the tip of the left auricle (A4).

The **inferior border** is formed by the right ventricle (A22) with a small part of the left ventricle at the apex.

In A, the pericardium has been incised and turned back (23) to display the anterior surface of the heart. The pulmonary trunk (17) leaves the right ventricle (22) in front and to the left of the ascending aorta (3), which is overlapped by the auricle (5) of the right atrium (18). The superior vena cava (25) is to the right of the aorta and still largely covered by pericardium. The anterior interventricular branch (2) of the left coronary artery and the great cardiac vein (7) lie in the interventricular groove between the right and left ventricles (22 and 11), and the right coronary artery (19) is in the atrioventricular groove between the right ventricle (22) and right atrium (18). In B, only the upper part of another heart is shown, with a marker in the transverse sinus, the space behind the aorta (3) and pulmonary trunk (17). In C, the heart has been removed from the pericardium, leaving the orifices of the great vessels. The dotted line indicates the attachment of the single sleeve of serous pericardium surrounding the aorta (3) and pulmonary trunk (17). The interrupted line indicates the attachment of another more complicated but still single sleeve of serous pericardium surrounding all the other six great vessels (the four pulmonary veins, 10, 9, 20 and 21, and the superior and inferior venae cavae, 25 and 8). The narrow interval between the two sleeves is the transverse sinus; the solid line in C indicates the path of the marker in B. The area of the pericardium (16) between the pulmonary veins and limited above by the reflection of the serious pericardium on to the back of the heart is the oblique sinus.

 *Cardiac tamponade, pericardial effusion, see pages 219, 220.*

# Heart *with blood vessels injected* Ⓐ *from the front* Ⓑ *from behind*

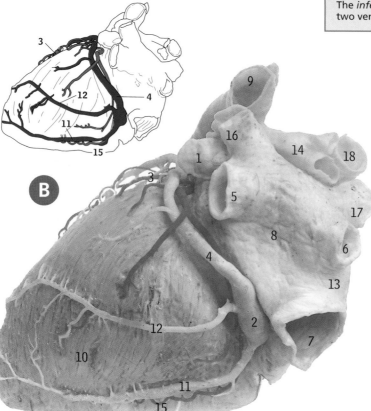

The coronary arteries have been injected with red latex and the cardiac veins with grey latex. The pulmonary trunk (8) passes upwards from the infundibulum (5) of the right ventricle (11), and at its commencement it is just in front and to the left of the ascending aorta (3).

1 Anterior interventricular branch of left coronary artery and great cardiac vein in interventricular groove
2 Apex
3 Ascending aorta
4 Auricle of right atrium (displaced laterally)
5 Infundibulum of right ventricle
6 Left ventricle
7 Marginal branch of right coronary artery
8 Pulmonary trunk
9 Right atrium
10 Right coronary artery in anterior atrioventricular groove
11 Right ventricle
12 Superior vena cava

The *sternocostal* surface of the heart is the *anterior* surface (as seen in A on page 189 and A here) formed mainly by the right ventricle (A11, D7), with parts of the left ventricle (A6) and right atrium (A9 and D10).

The *apex* of the heart (A2) is formed by the left ventricle.

The *base* of the heart is the *posterior* surface, formed mainly by the left atrium (B8) with a small part of the right atrium (B13).

The *inferior* surface is the *diaphragmatic* surface, formed by the two ventricles (mainly the left) (B10 and B15).

1 Auricle of left atrium
2 Coronary sinus in posterior atrioventricular groove
3 Great cardiac vein and anterior interventricular branch of left coronary artery
4 Great cardiac vein and circumflex branch of left coronary artery
5 Inferior left pulmonary vein
6 Inferior right pulmonary vein
7 Inferior vena cava
8 Left atrium
9 Left pulmonary artery
10 Left ventricle
11 Middle cardiac vein and posterior interventricular branch of right coronary artery in posterior interventricular groove
12 Posterior vein of left ventricle
13 Right atrium
14 Right pulmonary artery
15 Right ventricle
16 Superior left pulmonary vein
17 Superior right pulmonary vein
18 Superior vena cava

*Coronary artery bypass, myocardial infarction, see pages 219, 220.*

## C Right atrium *from the front and right*

The anterior wall has been incised near its left margin and reflected to the right, showing on its internal surface the vertical crista terminalis (2) and horizontal pectinate muscles (7). The fossa ovalis (3) is on the interatrial septum, and the opening of the coronary sinus (6) is to the left of the inferior vena caval opening (4).

| | |
|---|---|
| 1 Auricle | 8 Position of |
| 2 Crista terminalis | atrioventricular node |
| 3 Fossa ovalis | 9 Position of intervenous |
| 4 Inferior vena cava | tubercle |
| 5 Limbus | 10 Superior vena cava |
| 6 Opening of coronary | 11 Tricuspid valve |
| sinus | 12 Valve of coronary sinus |
| 7 Pectinate muscles | 13 Valve of inferior vena cava |

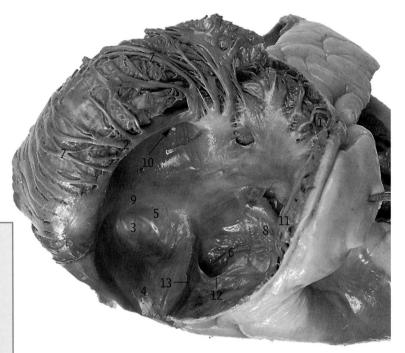

The fossa ovalis (3) forms part of the interatrial septum, and is part of the embryonic primary septum.

The limbus (5), which forms the margin of the fossa ovalis (3), represents the lower margin of the embryonic secondary septum. Before the primary and secondary septa fuse (at birth), the gap between them forms the foramen ovale.

The sinuatrial node (SA node, not illustrated) is embedded in the anterior wall of the atrium at the upper end of the crista terminalis, just below the opening of the superior vena cava.

The atrioventricular node (AV node, 8) is embedded in the interatrial septum, just above and to the left of the opening of the coronary sinus (6).

## D Right ventricle *from the front*

| | |
|---|---|
| 1 | Anterior cusp of tricuspid valve |
| 2 | Anterior papillary muscle |
| 3 | Ascending aorta |
| 4 | Auricle of right atrium |
| 5 | Chordae tendineae |
| 6 | Inferior vena cava |
| 7 | Infundibulum of right ventricle |
| 8 | Posterior papillary muscle |
| 9 | Pulmonary trunk |
| 10 | Right atrium |
| 11 | Septomarginal trabeculum |
| 12 | Superior vena cava |
| 13 | Trabeculae on interventricular septum |

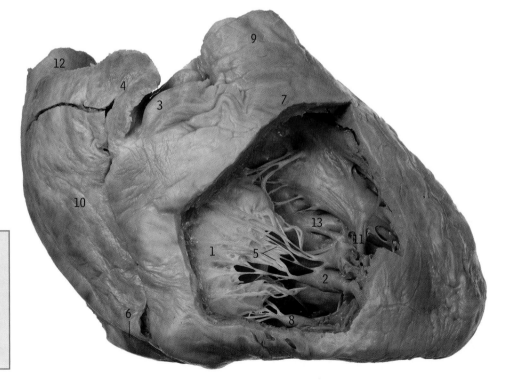

The septomarginal trabeculum (11), which conducts part of the right limb of the atrioventricular bundle from the interventricular septum (13) to the anterior papillary muscle (2), was formerly known as the moderator band.

The chordae tendineae (5) connect the cusps of the tricuspid valve to the papillary muscles.

*Cardiac pacemaker, left ventricular enlargement, see page 219.*

## A Left ventricle *from the left and below*

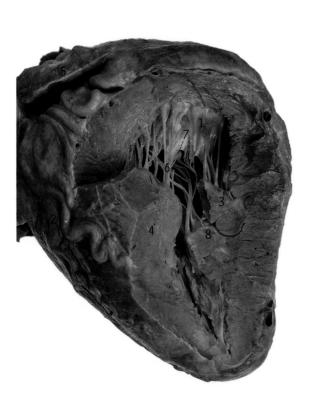

## B Heart *coronal section of the ventricles*

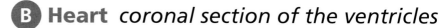
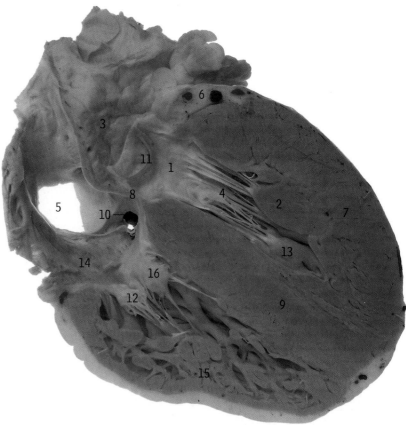

The ventricle has been opened by removing much of the left, anterior and posterior walls, and is viewed from below, looking upwards to the under-surface of the cusps of the mitral valve (1 and 7) which are anchored to the anterior and posterior papillary muscles (3 and 8) by chordae tendineae (6). The posterior cusp (7) is largely hidden by the anterior cusp (1) in this view.

1　Anterior cusp of mitral valve
2　Anterior interventricular branch
　　of left coronary artery
3　Anterior papillary muscle
4　Anterior ventricular wall
5　Auricle of left atrium
6　Chordae tendineae
7　Posterior cusp of mitral valve
8　Posterior papillary muscle

The heart has been cut in two in the coronal plane, and this is the posterior section seen from the front, looking towards the back of both ventricles. The section has passed immediately in front of the anterior cusp of the mitral valve (1) and the posterior cusp of the aortic valve (11).

The cusps of the aortic and pulmonary valves are here given their official names but some English texts use slightly different alternatives, as follows:

| | Official | English |
|---|---|---|
| **Aortic** | Right | Anterior |
| | Left | Left posterior |
| | Posterior | Right posterior |
| **Pulmonary** | Left | Posterior |
| | Anterior | Left anterior |
| | Right | Right anterior |

1　Anterior cusp of mitral valve
2　Anterior papillary muscle
3　Ascending aorta
4　Chordae tendineae
5　Inferior vena cava
6　Left coronary artery branches
　　and great cardiac vein
7　Left ventricular wall
8　Membranous part of
　　interventricular septum
9　Muscular part of interventricular
　　septum
10　Opening of coronary sinus
11　Posterior cusp of aortic valve
12　Posterior cusp of tricuspid valve
13　Posterior papillary muscle
14　Right atrium
15　Right ventricular wall
16　Septal cusp of tricuspid valve

*Mitral valve disease, see page 219.*

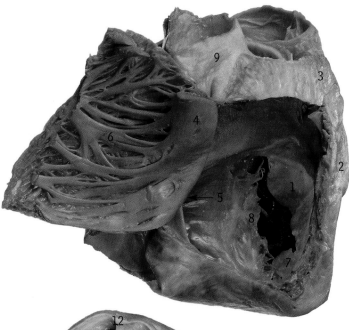

## C Tricuspid valve *from the right atrium*

The atrium has been opened by incising the anterior wall (2) and turning the flap outwards so that the atrial surface of the atrioventricular orifice is seen, guarded by the three cusps of the tricuspid valve – anterior (1), posterior (7) and septal (8).

1 Anterior cusp of tricuspid valve
2 Anterior wall of right atrium
3 Auricle of right atrium
4 Crista terminalis
5 Interatrial septum
6 Pectinate muscles
7 Posterior cusp of tricuspid valve
8 Septal cusp of tricuspid valve
9 Superior vena cava

> The posterior cusp (7) of the tricuspid valve is the smallest.

## D Pulmonary, aortic and mitral valves *from above*

The pulmonary trunk (12) and ascending aorta (3) have been cut off immediately above the three cusps of the pulmonary and aortic valves (7, 2 and 15, and 14, 10 and 6). The upper part of the left atrium (5) has been removed to show the upper surface of the mitral valve cusps (11 and 1).

1 Anterior cusp of mitral valve
2 Anterior cusp of pulmonary valve
3 Ascending aorta
4 Auricle of right atrium
5 Left atrium
6 Left cusp of aortic valve
7 Left cusp of pulmonary valve
8 Marker in ostium of right coronary artery
9 Ostium of left coronary artery
10 Posterior cusp of aortic valve
11 Posterior cusp of mitral valve
12 Pulmonary trunk
13 Right atrium
14 Right cusp of aortic valve
15 Right cusp of pulmonary valve
16 Superior vena cava

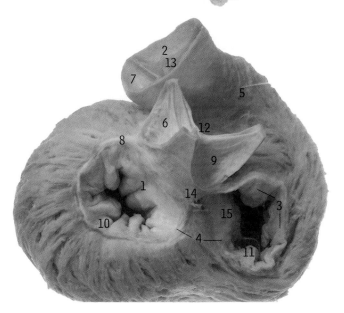

## E Heart *fibrous framework*

The heart is seen from the right and behind after removing both atria, looking down on to the fibrous rings (4) that surround the mitral and tricuspid orifices and form the attachments for the bases of the valve cusps. The cusps of the pulmonary valve (7, 2 and 13) are seen at the top of the infundibulum of the right ventricle (5), and the aortic valve cusps (12, 9 and 6) have been dissected out from the beginning of the ascending aorta.

1 Anterior cusp of mitral valve
2 Anterior cusp of pulmonary valve
3 Anterior cusp of tricuspid valve
4 Fibrous ring
5 Infundibulum of right ventricle
6 Left cusp of aortic valve
7 Left cusp of pulmonary valve
8 Left fibrous trigone
9 Posterior cusp of aortic valve
10 Posterior cusp of mitral valve
11 Posterior cusp of tricuspid valve
12 Right cusp of aortic valve
13 Right cusp of pulmonary valve
14 Right fibrous trigone
15 Septal cusp of tricuspid valve

# Coronary arteries

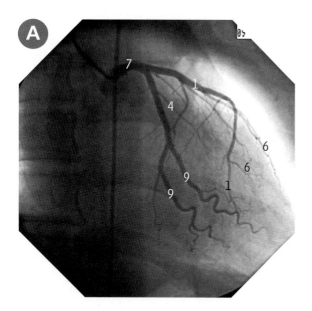

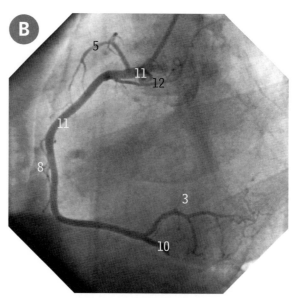

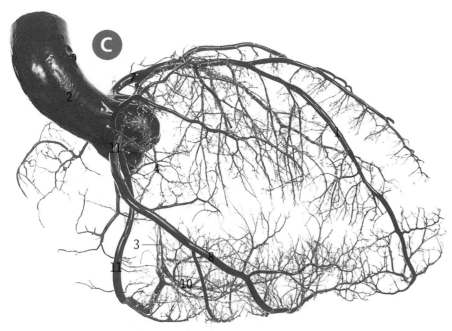

**A**  left coronary arteriogram, right anterior oblique projection

**B**  right coronary arteriogram, left anterior oblique projection

**C**  cast of the coronary arteries, from the front

> The interventricular branches are often called by clinicians the descending branches (anterior interventricular, left anterior descending; posterior interventricular, posterior descending).

**1** Anterior interventricular branch of left coronary artery
**2** Ascending aorta
**3** Atrioventricular nodal artery
**4** Circumflex branch of left coronary artery
**5** Conus artery
**6** Diagonal artery
**7** Left coronary artery
**8** Marginal branch of right coronary artery
**9** Obtuse marginal artery
**10** Posterior interventricular branch of right coronary artery
**11** Right coronary artery
**12** Sinuatrial nodal artery

*Angina pectoris, coronary angiography, see page 219.*

# **D** Coronary arteries *3D CT reconstruction*

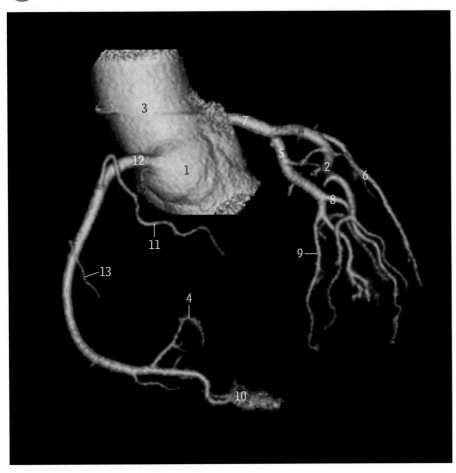

1 Anterior aortic sinus
2 Anterior interventricular, descending branch, left coronary artery (LAD)
3 Aorta, ascending
4 Atrioventricular nodal artery
5 Circumflex branch, left coronary artery
6 Diagonal artery
7 Left coronary artery
8 Marginal artery, left coronary artery
9 Obtuse marginal branch, left coronary artery
10 Posterior interventricular branch, right coronary artery
11 Right conal artery
12 Right coronary artery
13 Right ventricular branch, right coronary artery

# **E** Cast of the heart and great vessels *from below and behind*

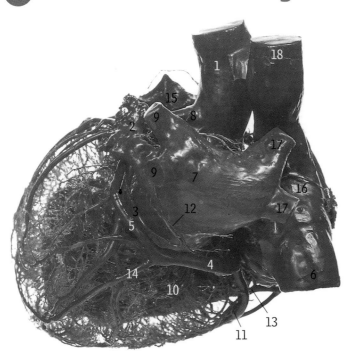

This cast shows the coronary sinus (4) in the atrioventricular groove, and various tributaries (see notes).

1 Ascending aorta
2 Auricle of left atrium
3 Circumflex branch of left coronary artery
4 Coronary sinus
5 Great cardiac vein
6 Inferior vena cava
7 Left atrium
8 Left coronary artery
9 Left pulmonary veins
10 Left ventricle
11 Middle cardiac vein
12 Oblique vein of left atrium
13 Posterior interventricular branch of right coronary artery
14 Posterior vein of left ventricle
15 Pulmonary trunk
16 Right atrium
17 Right pulmonary veins
18 Superior vena cava

The base of the heart is its posterior surface, formed largely by the left atrium (E7). Note that the base is not the part of the heart which joins the superior vena cava, aorta and pulmonary trunk; this part has no special name.

The very small oblique vein of the left atrium (E12) marks the point where the great cardiac vein (E5) becomes the coronary sinus (E4), but in E, the junction is unusually far to the right so that the posterior vein of the left ventricle (E14) joins the great cardiac vein (E5) instead of the coronary sinus itself.

The coronary sinus (E4), which receives most of the venous blood from the heart, lies in the posterior part of the atrioventricular groove between the left atrium and left ventricle and opens into the right atrium.

The coronary sinus normally receives as tributaries the great cardiac vein (E5), middle cardiac vein (E11), and the small cardiac vein, the posterior vein of the left ventricle (E14) and the oblique vein of the left atrium (E12).

# A Right lung root and mediastinal pleura

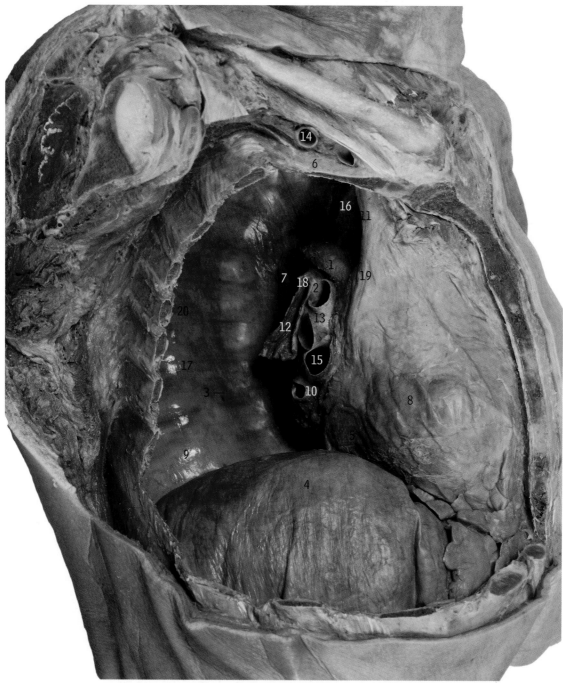

This is the view of the right side of the mediastinum after removing the lung but with the parietal pleura still intact.

1 Azygos vein
2 Branch of right pulmonary artery to superior lobe
3 Branches of sympathetic trunk to greater splanchnic nerve
4 Diaphragm
5 Inferior vena cava
6 Neck of first rib
7 Oesophagus
8 Pericardium over right atrium
9 Pleura, costal
10 Right inferior pulmonary vein
11 Right phrenic nerve
12 Right principal bronchus
13 Right pulmonary artery
14 Right subclavian artery
15 Right superior pulmonary vein
16 Right vagus nerve
17 Sixth right posterior intercostal vessels under parietal pleura
18 Superior lobe bronchus
19 Superior vena cava
20 Sympathetic trunk and ganglion

# B Right lung root and mediastinum

In a similar specimen to A, most of the pleura has been removed to display the underlying structures. The azygos vein (1) arches over the structures forming the lung root to enter the superior vena cava (24). The highest structures in the lung root are the artery (2) and bronchus (14) to the superior lobe of the lung. The right superior pulmonary vein (18) is in front of the right pulmonary artery, with the right inferior pulmonary vein (12) the lowest structure in the root. Above the arch of the azygos vein the trachea (28), with the right vagus nerve (19) in contact with it, lies in front of the oesophagus (8). Part of the first rib has been cut away to show the structures lying in front of its neck (5), the sympathetic trunk (27), supreme intercostal vein (22), superior intercostal artery (20) and the ventral ramus of the first thoracic nerve. The right recurrent laryngeal nerve hooks underneath the right subclavian artery (16). The right phrenic nerve (13) runs down over the superior vena cava (24) and the pericardium overlying the right atrium (9), and pierces the diaphragm (4) beside the inferior vena cava. Contributions from the sympathetic trunk (3) pass over the sides of vertebral bodies superficial to posterior intercostal arteries and veins (as at 20 and 21) to form the greater splanchnic nerve. The lower part of the oesophagus (8) behind the lung root and heart has the azygos vein (1) on its right side.

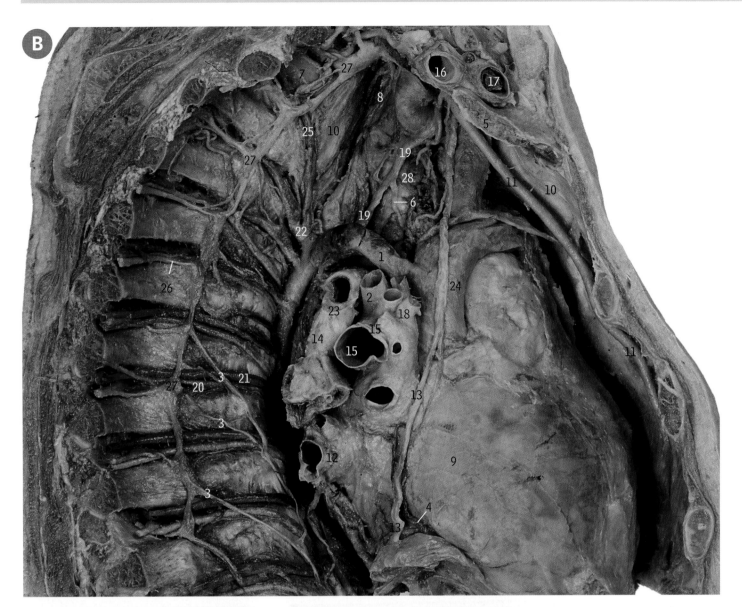

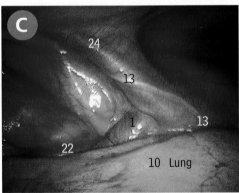

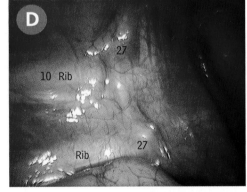

**C  D**

# Thoracoscopies

| | | | |
|---|---|---|---|
| **1** Azygos vein (arch) | **7** Neck of first rib | **16** Right subclavian artery | **22** Superior intercostal vein |
| **2** Branch of right pulmonary artery to superior lobe | **8** Oesophagus | **17** Right subclavian vein (NB: thrombus) | **23** Superior lobe bronchus |
| **3** Branches of sympathetic trunk to greater splanchnic nerve | **9** Pericardium over right atrium | **18** Right superior pulmonary vein | **24** Superior vena cava |
| | **10** Pleura | **19** Right vagus nerve | **25** Supreme intercostal vein |
| **4** Diaphragm | **11** Right internal thoracic artery | **20** Sixth right posterior intercostal artery | **26** Sympathetic rami communicantes |
| **5** First rib (sectioned) | **12** Right inferior pulmonary vein | **21** Sixth right posterior intercostal vein | **27** Sympathetic trunk and ganglion |
| **6** Inferior cardiac branches of vagus nerve | **13** Right phrenic nerve | | **28** Trachea |
| | **14** Right principal bronchus | | |
| | **15** Right pulmonary artery | | |

*Pleural effusion, transthoracic sympathectomy, see page 220.*

# Left lung root and mediastinal pleura

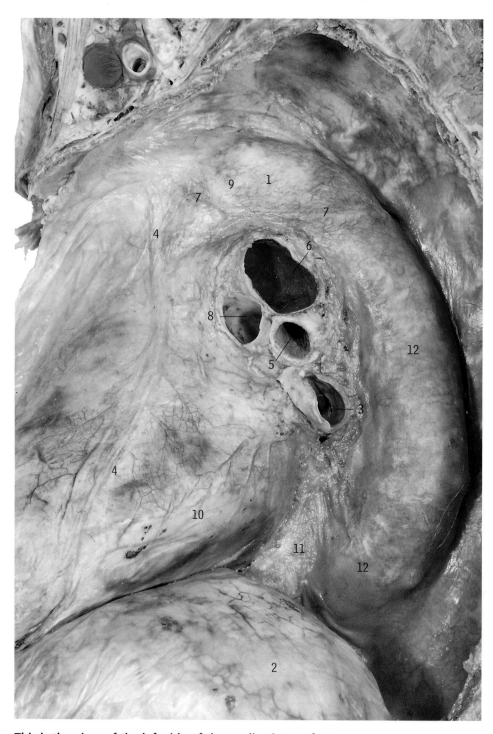

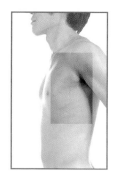

1 Arch of aorta
2 Diaphragm
3 Left inferior pulmonary vein
4 Left phrenic nerve and
   pericardiophrenic vessels
5 Left principal bronchus
6 Left pulmonary artery
7 Left superior intercostal vein
8 Left superior pulmonary vein
9 Left vagus nerve
10 Mediastinal pleura and pericardium
   overlying left ventricle
11 Oesophagus
12 Thoracic aorta

On the left side above the diaphragm, the lower end of the oesophagus lies in a triangle bounded by the diaphragm below (2), the heart in front (10) and the descending aorta behind (12).

This is the view of the left side of the mediastinum after removing the lung but with the parietal pleura still intact. Compare the features seen here with those in the dissection opposite (a different specimen), from which the pleura has been removed.

Pneumothorax, thoracic aortic aneurysm, see pages 219, 220.

# Left lung root and mediastinum

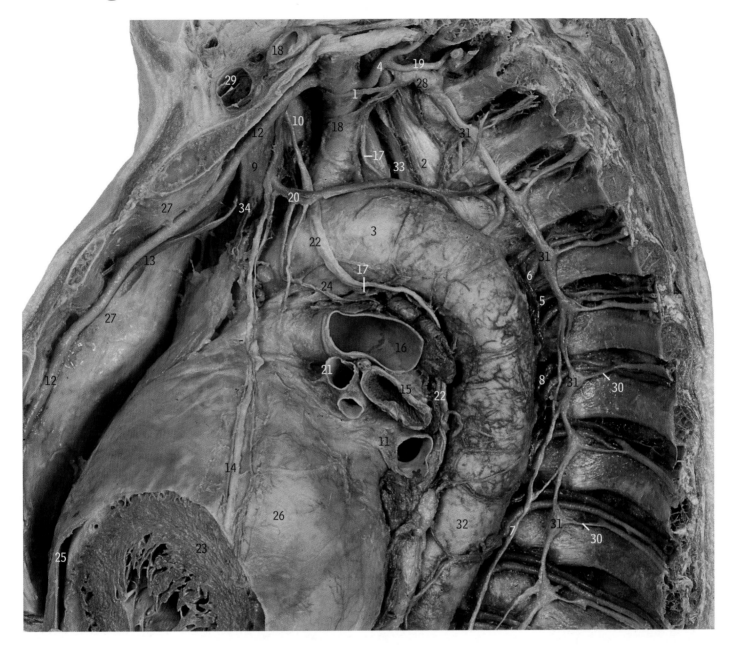

1 Ansa subclavia
2 Anterior longitudinal ligament
3 Arch of aorta
4 Costocervical trunk
5 Fifth left posterior intercostal vein
6 Fourth left posterior intercostal artery
7 Greater splanchnic nerve
8 Hemi-azygos vein
9 Left brachiocephalic vein
10 Left common carotid artery
11 Left inferior pulmonary vein
12 Left internal thoracic artery
13 Left internal thoracic vein
14 Left phrenic nerve and pericardiophrenic vessels
15 Left principal bronchus
16 Left pulmonary artery
17 Left recurrent laryngeal nerve
18 Left subclavian artery
19 Left superior intercostal artery
20 Left superior intercostal vein
21 Left superior pulmonary vein
22 Left vagus nerve
23 Left ventricle (NB thick-walled cavity)
24 Ligamentum arteriosum
25 Pericardial cavity (space)
26 Pericardium overlying left ventricle
27 Pleura (cut edge)
28 Stellate ganglion
29 Subclavian vein
30 Sympathetic rami communicantes
31 Sympathetic trunk and ganglion
32 Thoracic aorta
33 Thoracic duct (page 213, 25)
34 Thymic veins (page 359)

*Coarctation of the aorta, see page 219.*

# Axial CT images *with contrast*

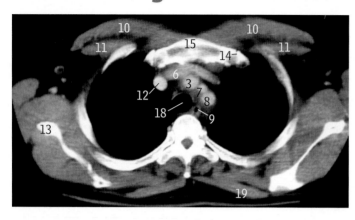

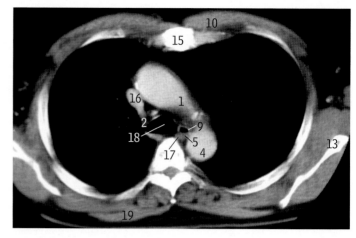

**A** Level of T2

| | | | |
|---|---|---|---|
| **1** | Arch aorta | **6** | Left brachiocephalic vein |
| **2** | Azygos vein | **7** | Left common |
| **3** | Brachiocephalic trunk | | carotid artery |
| | (artery) | **8** | Left subclavian artery |
| **4** | Descending aorta | **9** | Oesophagus |
| **5** | Hemi-azygos vein | **10** | Pectoralis major |

**B** Level of T4

| | | | |
|---|---|---|---|
| **11** | Pectoralis minor | **17** | Thoracic duct |
| **12** | Right brachiocephalic vein | **18** | Trachea |
| **13** | Scapula | **19** | Trapezius |
| **14** | Sternoclavicular joint | | |
| **15** | Sternum | | |
| **16** | Superior vena cava | | |

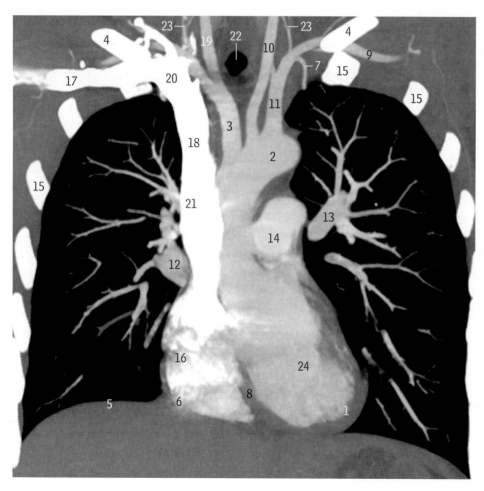

**C** **Thorax** *coronal 64 slice CT reconstruction – venous phase of the cardiac cycle*

**1** Apex of heart
**2** Arch of aorta
**3** Brachiocephalic trunk
**4** Clavicle
**5** Dome of diaphragm, right
**6** Inferior vena cava
**7** Internal thoracic artery
**8** Interventricular septum
**9** Left axillary artery
**10** Left common carotid artery
**11** Left subclavian artery
**12** Pulmonary artery, right
**13** Pulmonary artery, upper lobe branch
**14** Pulmonary trunk
**15** Ribs
**16** Right atrium
**17** Right axillary vein
**18** Right brachiocephalic vein
**19** Right common carotid artery
**20** Right subclavian vein
**21** Superior vena cava
**22** Trachea
**23** Vertebral artery
**24** Ventricle, left

*Phrenic nerve palsy, see page 220.*

# Cast of the lower trachea and bronchi
**Ⓐ** *vertical from the front* **Ⓑ** *oblique from the left*

The principal and lobar bronchi are labelled with letters; the segmental bronchi are labelled with their conventional numbers. In the side view in B, the cast has been tilted to avoid overlap, and the right side is more anterior than the left.

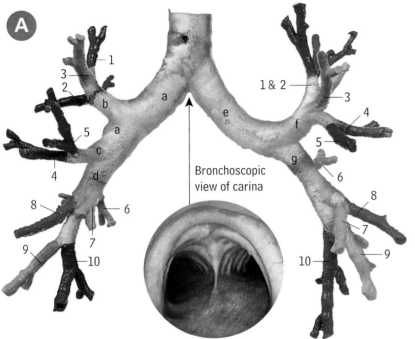

Bronchoscopic view of carina

| Right lung | Left lung |
|---|---|
| **Lobar bronchi** ||
| a Principal | e Principal |
| b Superior lobe | f Superior lobe |
| c Middle lobe | g Inferior lobe |
| d Inferior lobe | |

**Segmental bronchi**

| Superior lobe | Superior lobe |
|---|---|
| **1** Apical | **1 & 2** Apicoposterior |
| **2** Posterior | **3** Anterior |
| **3** Anterior | **4** Superior lingular |
| | **5** Inferior lingular |

| Middle lobe |
|---|
| **4** Lateral |
| **5** Medial |

| Inferior lobe | Inferior lobe |
|---|---|
| **6** Apical (superior) | **6** Apical (superior) |
| **7** Medial basal | **7** Medial basal |
| **8** Anterior basal | **8** Anterior basal |
| **9** Lateral basal | **9** Lateral basal |
| **10** Posterior basal | **10** Posterior basal |

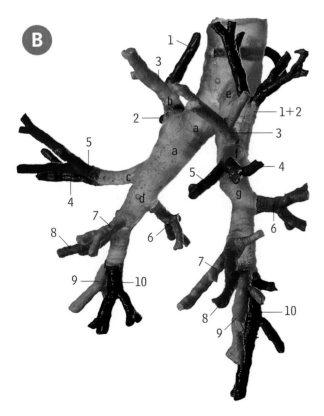

The trachea divides into right and left principal bronchi (a and e).

The right principal bronchus (a) is shorter, wider and more vertical than the left (e).

The left principal bronchus (e) is longer and narrower and lies more transversely than the right. Foreign bodies are therefore more likely to enter the right principal bronchus than the left.

The right principal bronchus (a) gives off a superior lobe bronchus (b) and then enters the hilum of the right lung before dividing into middle and inferior lobe bronchi (c and d).

The left principal bronchus (e) enters the hilum of the lung before dividing into superior and inferior lobe bronchi (f and g).

The branches of the lobar bronchi are called segmental bronchi and each supplies a segment of lung tissue - bronchopulmonary segment. The segmental bronchi and the bronchopulmonary segments have similar names, and the ten segments of each lung are officially numbered (as here and page 202) as well as being named.

The segmental bronchi of the left and right lungs are essentially similar except that the apical and posterior bronchi of the superior lobe of the left lung arise from a common stem, thus called the apicoposterior bronchus and labelled here as 1 and 2; also there is no middle lobe of the left lung, and so the corresponding segments bear similar numbers; and the medial basal bronchus (7) of the left lung usually arises in common with the anterior basal (8).

The apical (superior) bronchus of the inferior lobe (6) of both lungs is the first or highest bronchus to arise from the posterior surface of the bronchial tree, as illustrated in B. When lying on the back fluid may therefore gravitate into this bronchus.

# Cast of the bronchial tree

The bronchi and bronchopulmonary segments have been coloured and labelled with their conventional numbers.

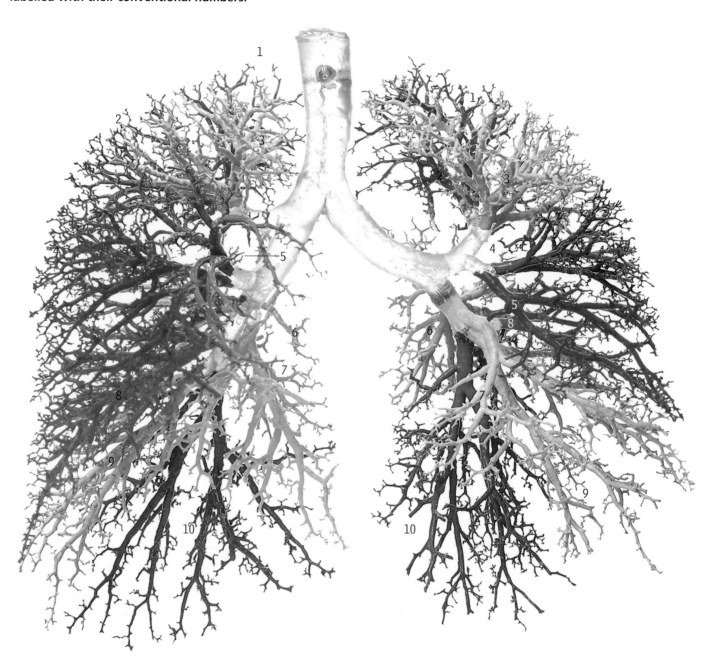

**Right lung**

**Superior lobe**
1 Apical
2 Posterior
3 Anterior

**Middle lobe**
4 Lateral
5 Medial

**Inferior lobe**
6 Apical (superior)
7 Medial basal
8 Anterior basal
9 Lateral basal
10 Posterior basal

**Left lung**

**Superior lobe**
1 Apical
2 Posterior
3 Anterior
4 Superior lingular
5 Inferior lingular

**Inferior lobe**
6 Apical (superior)
7 Medial basal (cardiac)
8 Anterior basal
9 Lateral basal
10 Posterior basal

*Bronchoscopy, see page 219.*

# Bronchopulmonary segments of the right lung

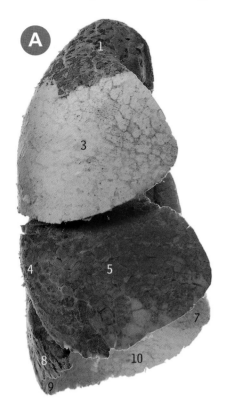

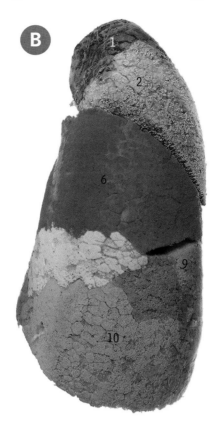

**A** from the front

**B** from behind

**Superior lobe**
1 Apical
2 Posterior
3 Anterior

**Middle lobe**
4 Lateral
5 Medial

**Inferior lobe**
6 Apical (superior)
7 Medial basal
8 Anterior basal
9 Lateral basal
10 Posterior basal

A subapical (subsuperior) segmental bronchus and bronchopulmonary segment are present in over 50% of lungs; in this specimen, this additional segment is shown in white.

The posterior basal segment (10) is coloured with two different shades of yellow ochre.

# Bronchopulmonary segments of the left lung

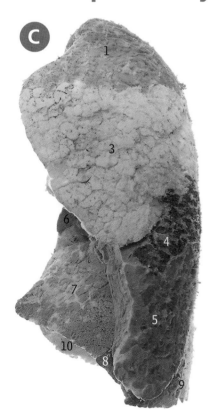

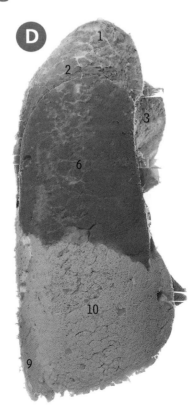

**C** from the front

**D** from behind

**Superior lobe**
1 Apical
2 Posterior
3 Anterior
4 Superior lingular
5 Inferior lingular

**Inferior lobe**
6 Apical (superior)
7 Medial basal (cardiac)
8 Anterior basal
9 Lateral basal
10 Posterior basal

The apical and posterior segments (1 and 2) are both coloured green, having been filled from the common apicoposterior bronchus (see page 201).

**A** **Bronchopulmonary segments of the right lung** *from the lateral side*

**B** **Right bronchogram**

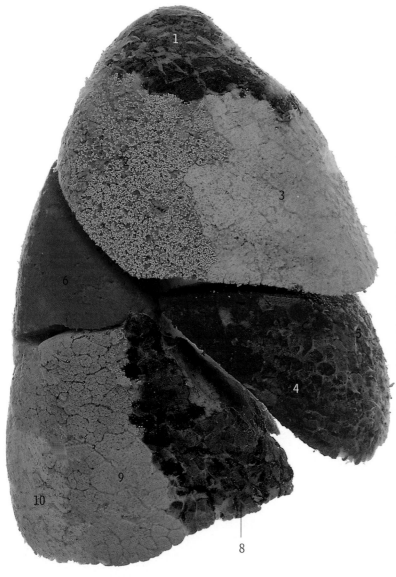

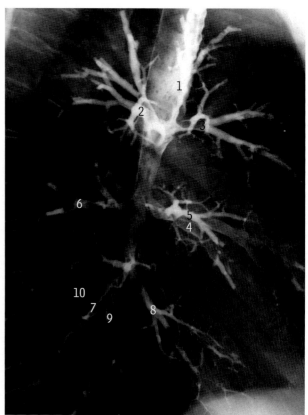

**Superior lobe**
1 Apical
2 Posterior
3 Anterior

**Middle lobe**
4 Lateral
5 Medial

**Inferior lobe**
6 Apical (superior)
7 Medial basal
8 Anterior basal
9 Lateral basal
10 Posterior basal

The medial basal segment (7) is not seen in the view in A.

The posterior basal segment in A (10) is coloured with two different shades of green.

*Empyema, see page 219.*

## C Bronchopulmonary segments of the left lung *from the lateral side*

## D Left bronchogram

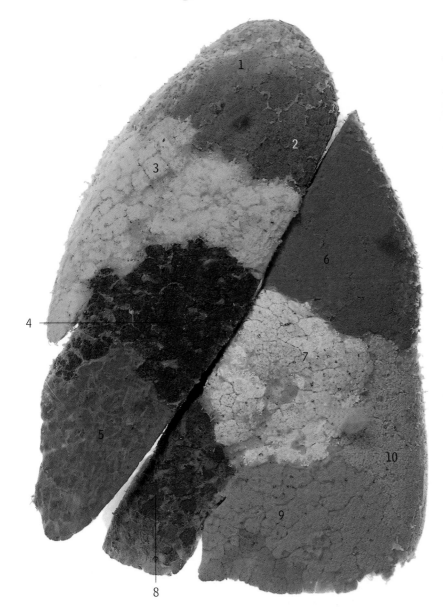

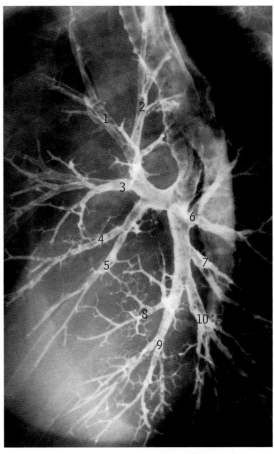

**Superior lobe**
1 Apical
2 Posterior
3 Anterior
4 Superior lingular
5 Inferior lingular

**Inferior lobe**
6 Apical (superior)
7 Medial basal (cardiac)
8 Anterior basal
9 Lateral basal
10 Posterior basal

The apical and posterior segments (1 and 2) are both coloured green, having been filled from the common apicoposterior bronchus (see page 201).

## A  Cast of the bronchial tree and pulmonary vessels *from the front*

## B  Lung roots and bronchial arteries *right side from above*

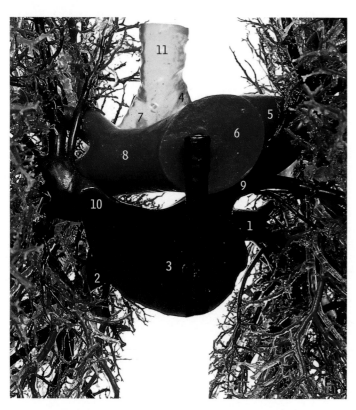

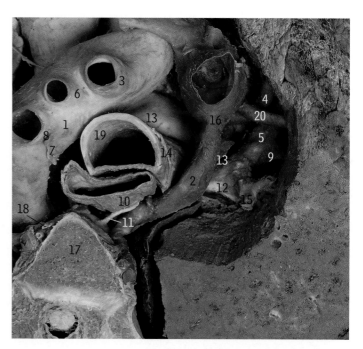

The pulmonary trunk (6) divides into the left and right pulmonary arteries (5 and 8), and these vessels have been injected with red resin. The four pulmonary veins (9, 1, 2 and 10) which drain into the left atrium (3) have been filled with blue resin. Note that in the living body the pulmonary veins are filled with oxygenated blood from the lungs and would normally be represented by a red colour; similarly the pulmonary arteries contain deoxygenated blood and should be represented by a blue colour.

1  Inferior left pulmonary vein
2  Inferior right pulmonary vein
3  Left atrium
4  Left principal bronchus
5  Left pulmonary artery
6  Pulmonary trunk
7  Right principal bronchus
8  Right pulmonary artery
9  Superior left pulmonary vein
10  Superior right pulmonary vein
11  Trachea

The thorax has been sectioned transversely at the level of the third thoracic vertebra (17), just above the arch of the aorta (1) whose three larger branches have been removed (8, 6 and 3), and lung tissue at the hilum has been dissected away from above. The oesophagus (10) and trachea (19) have been tilted forwards to show one of the bronchial arteries (11).

1  Arch of aorta
2  Azygos vein
3  Brachiocephalic trunk
4  Inferior lobe artery
5  Inferior lobe bronchus
6  Left common carotid artery
7  Left recurrent laryngeal nerve
8  Left subclavian artery
9  Middle lobe bronchus
10  Oesophagus
11  Right bronchial artery
12  Right principal bronchus
13  Right pulmonary artery
14  Right vagus nerve
15  Superior lobe bronchus
16  Superior vena cava
17  Third thoracic vertebra
18  Thoracic duct
19  Trachea
20  Tributary of inferior pulmonary vein

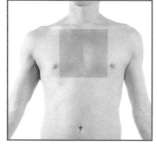

*Carcinoma of the oesophagus, pulmonary embolism, see pages 219, 220.*

# C Cast of the pulmonary arteries and bronchi *from the front*
# D Pulmonary arteriogram

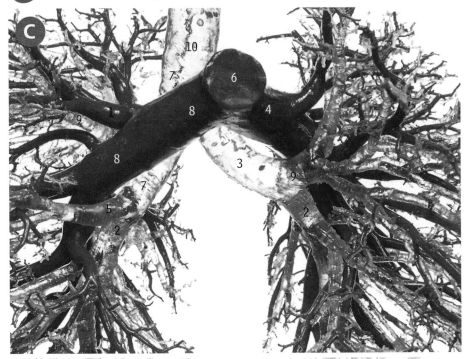

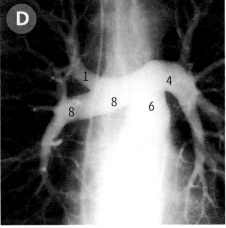

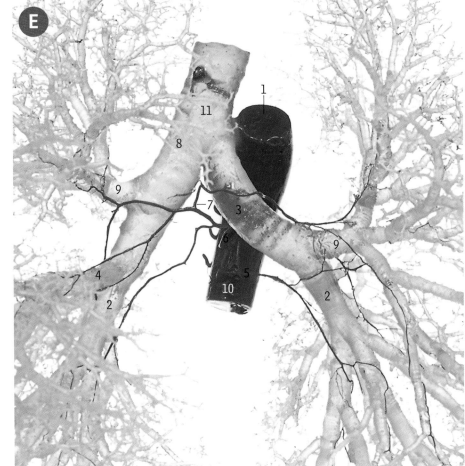

The upper part of the pulmonary trunk (6) is seen end-on after cutting off the lower part, and the bifurcation of the trunk into the left (4) and right (8) pulmonary arteries is in front of the beginning of the left main bronchus (3). In the living body, these pulmonary vessels contain deoxygenated blood and would normally be represented by a blue colour, but here they have been filled with red resin. Compare the vessels in the cast with those in the arteriogram D.

**1** Branch of right pulmonary artery to superior lobe
**2** Inferior lobe bronchus
**3** Left principal bronchus
**4** Left pulmonary artery
**5** Middle lobe bronchus
**6** Pulmonary trunk
**7** Right principal bronchus
**8** Right pulmonary artery
**9** Superior lobe bronchus
**10** Trachea

# E Cast of the bronchi and bronchial arteries *from the front*

Part of the aorta (1 and 10) has been injected with red resin to fill the bronchial arteries. These vessels normally run behind the bronchi and their branches but in this specimen, they are in front.

**1** Arch of aorta
**2** Inferior lobe bronchus
**3** Left principal bronchus
**4** Middle lobe bronchus
**5** Origin of lower left bronchial artery
**6** Origin of right bronchial artery
**7** Origin of upper left bronchial artery
**8** Right principal bronchus
**9** Superior lobe bronchus
**10** Thoracic aorta
**11** Trachea

## Ⓐ Right lung *medial surface*     Ⓑ Left lung *medial surface*

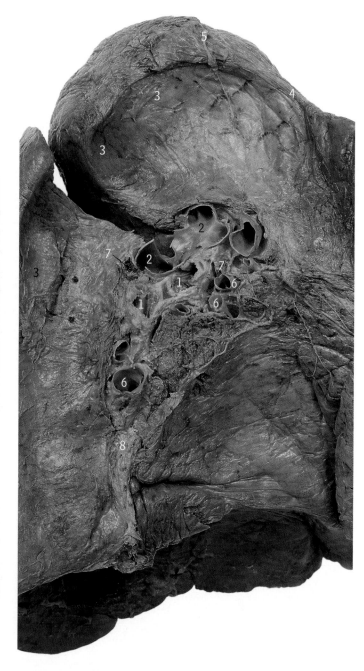

In the hardened dissecting room specimen, adjacent structures make impressions on the medial surface of the lung. The most prominent feature on the right side is the groove for the azygos vein (3), above and behind the structures of the lung root (9, 2 and 1).

1  Branches of right principal bronchus
2  Branches of right pulmonary artery
3  Groove for azygos vein
4  Groove for first rib
5  Groove for subclavian artery
6  Groove for subclavian vein
7  Groove for superior vena cava
8  Oesophageal and tracheal area
9  Right pulmonary veins
10  Transverse fissure

The upper end of the medial surface of the right lung lies against the oesophagus and trachea (A8) with only the pleura intervening, but on the left, the subclavian artery (B5) (and the left common carotid in front of it) keep the lung further away from these structures.

Compare with the right lung in A, and note the large size of the impression made by the aorta on the left lung (B3), in contrast to the smaller azygos groove on the right (A3).

1  Branches of left principal bronchus
2  Branches of left pulmonary artery
3  Groove for aorta
4  Groove for first rib
5  Groove for left subclavian artery
6  Left pulmonary veins
7  Lymph node, containing carbon
8  Pulmonary ligament

*Carcinoma of the lung, mesothelioma, tuberculosis, see pages 219, 220.*

# Lower neck and upper thorax *surface markings*

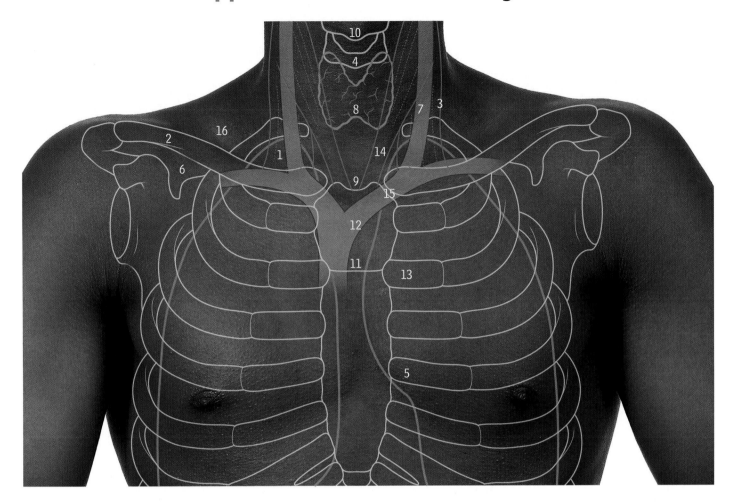

The pink line indicates the extent of the pleura and lung on each side; the apices of the pleura and lung (1) rise into the neck for about 3 cm above the medial third of the clavicle. The lower end of the internal jugular vein (7) lies behind the interval between the sternal (14) and clavicular (3) heads of sternocleidomastoid. Behind the sternoclavicular joint (15) the internal jugular and subclavian veins unite to form the brachiocephalic vein. The trachea (8) is felt in the midline above the jugular notch (9), and the arch of the cricoid cartilage (4) is 4–5 cm above the notch. The manubriosternal joint is at the level of the second costal cartilage (13) and opposite the lower border of the body of the fourth thoracic vertebra, and the horizontal plane through these points indicates the junction between the superior and inferior parts of the mediastinum. The left brachiocephalic vein passes behind the upper half of the manubrium to unite with the right brachiocephalic at the lower border of the right first costal cartilage (to form the superior vena cava). The midpoint of the manubrium (12) marks the highest level of the arch of the aorta and the origin of the brachiocephalic trunk. Compare many of the features mentioned here with the structures in the dissection on page 210.

1 Apex of pleura and lung
2 Clavicle
3 Clavicular head of sternocleidomastoid
4 Cricoid cartilage
5 Fourth costal cartilage
6 Infraclavicular fossa
7 Internal jugular vein
8 Isthmus of thyroid gland overlying trachea
9 Jugular notch (suprasternal)
10 Laryngeal prominence of the thyroid cartilage
11 Manubriosternal joint
12 Midpoint of manubrium of sternum
13 Second costal cartilage
14 Sternal head of sternocleidomastoid
15 Sternoclavicular joint
16 Supraclavicular fossa

# Thoracic inlet and mediastinum *from the front*

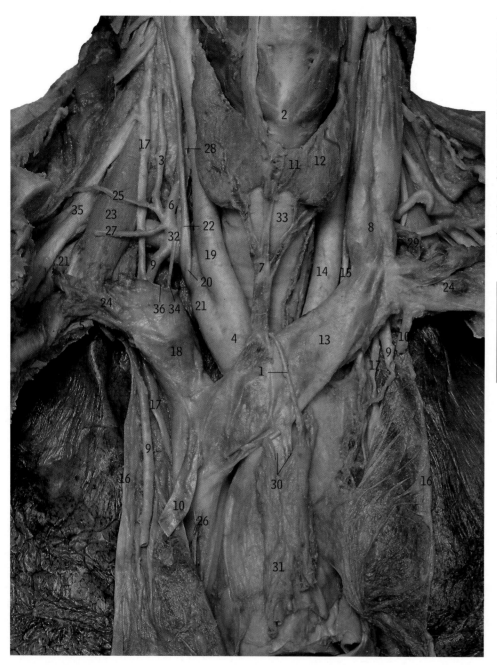

The anterior thoracic wall and the medial ends of the clavicles have been removed, but part of the parietal pleura (16) remains over the medial part of each lung. The right internal jugular vein has also been removed, displaying the thyrocervical trunk (32) and the origin of the internal thoracic artery (9). Inferior thyroid veins (7) run down over the trachea (33) to enter the left brachiocephalic vein (13). The thymus (31) has been dissected out from mediastinal fat; thymic veins (30) enter the left brachiocephalic vein, and an unusual thymic artery (1) arises from the brachiocephalic trunk (4).

The remains of the thymus (31) are in front of the pericardium, but in the child, where the thymus is much larger (see page 188), it may extend upwards in front of the great vessels as high as the lower part of the thyroid gland (12).

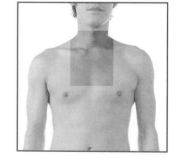

| | | |
|---|---|---|
| **1** A thymic artery | **13** Left brachiocephalic vein | **25** Superficial cervical artery |
| **2** Arch of cricoid cartilage | **14** Left common carotid artery | **26** Superior vena cava |
| **3** Ascending cervical artery | **15** Left vagus nerve | **27** Suprascapular artery |
| **4** Brachiocephalic trunk | **16** Parietal pleura (cut edge) over lung | **28** Sympathetic trunk |
| **5** First rib cut edge | **17** Phrenic nerve | **29** Thoracic duct |
| **6** Inferior thyroid artery | **18** Right brachiocephalic vein | **30** Thymic veins |
| **7** Inferior thyroid veins | **19** Right common carotid artery | **31** Thymus |
| **8** Internal jugular vein | **20** Right recurrent laryngeal nerve | **32** Thyrocervical trunk |
| **9** Internal thoracic artery | **21** Right subclavian artery | **33** Trachea |
| **10** Internal thoracic vein | **22** Right vagus nerve | **34** Unusual cervical tributary of 18 |
| **11** Isthmus of thyroid gland | **23** Scalenus anterior | **35** Upper trunk of brachial plexus |
| **12** Lateral lobe of thyroid gland | **24** Subclavian vein | **36** Vertebral vein |

*Pancoast's tumour, thoracic outlet syndromes, see page 220.*

# Thoracic inlet and superior mediastinum
## *axilla and root of neck*

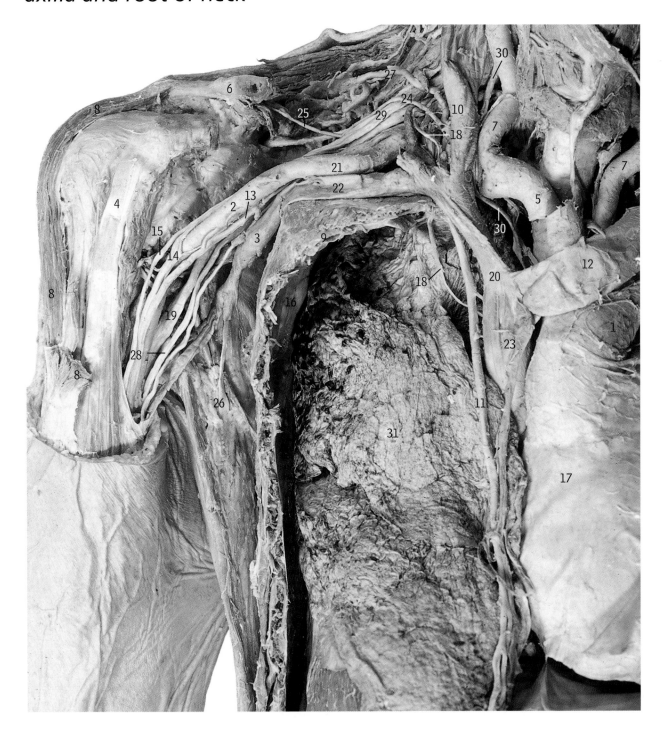

| | | | |
|---|---|---|---|
| **1** Aortic arch | **10** Internal jugular vein | **18** Phrenic nerve | **27** Transverse cervical artery |
| **2** Axillary artery | **11** Internal thoracic artery | **19** Radial nerve | **28** Ulnar nerve |
| **3** Axillary vein | **12** Left brachiocephalic vein | **20** Right brachiocephalic vein | **29** Upper trunk, brachial plexus |
| **4** Biceps, short head | **13** Medial cord, brachial plexus | **21** Subclavian artery | **30** Vagus nerve |
| **5** Brachiocephalic trunk | **14** Median nerve | **22** Subclavian vein | **31** Visceral pleura covering lung |
| **6** Clavicle (cut and removed) | **15** Musculocutaneous nerve | **23** Superior vena cava | |
| **7** Common carotid artery | **16** Parietal pleural covering of | **24** Suprascapular artery | |
| **8** Deltoid | chest wall | **25** Suprascapular nerve | |
| **9** First rib | **17** Pericardium, fibrous layer | **26** Thoracodorsal vein | |

# Thoracic inlet *right upper ribs, from below*

ANTERIOR

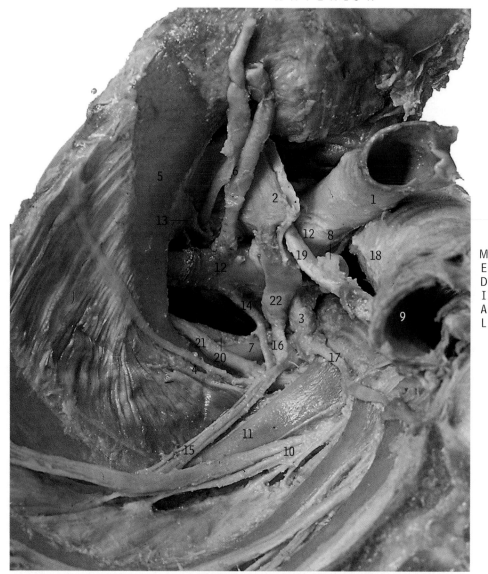

1  Brachiocephalic trunk
2  Brachiocephalic vein
3  Cervicothoracic (stellate) ganglion
4  First intercostal nerve
5  First rib
6  Internal thoracic vessels
7  Neck of first rib
8  Recurrent laryngeal nerve
9  Right principal bronchus
10  Second intercostal nerve
11  Second rib
12  Subclavian artery
13  Subclavian vein
14  Superior intercostal artery
15  Superior intercostal vein
16  Supreme intercostal vein (unusually large)
17  Sympathetic trunk
18  Trachea
19  Vagus nerve
20  Ventral ramus of eighth cervical nerve
21  Ventral ramus of first thoracic nerve
22  Vertebral vein

MEDIAL

The neck of the first rib (7) is crossed in order from medial to lateral by the sympathetic trunk (17), supreme intercostal vein (16), superior intercostal artery (14) and the ventral ramus of the first thoracic nerve (21).

This is the view looking upwards into the right side of the thoracic inlet – the region occupied by the cervical pleura, here removed. The under-surface of most of the first rib (5) is seen from below, with the subclavian artery (12) passing over the top of it after giving off the internal thoracic branch (6) which runs towards the top of the picture (to the anterior thoracic wall), and the costocervical trunk whose superior intercostal branch (14) runs down over the neck of the first rib (7). The vertebral vein (22) has come down from the neck and is labelled on its posterior surface before entering the brachiocephalic vein (2, labelled at its opened cut edge). The vertebral vein receives an unusually large supreme intercostal vein (16). On its medial side is the sympathetic trunk (17) with the cervicothoracic ganglion (3). The neck of the first rib (7) has the ventral ramus of the first thoracic nerve (21) below it.

*Catheterisation of subclavian vein, thoracic outlet syndromes, see pages 219, 220.*

# Posterior mediastinum *from the right hand side of the chest*

1 Ascending aorta
2 Azygos arch
3 Azygos venous system
4 Carinal node
5 Cysterna chyli
6 Descending thoracic aorta
7 Diaphragm, cut edge, light from abdomen inferiorly
8 Diaphragm, right crus
9 Diaphragmatic visceral peritoneum
10 Greater splanchnic nerve
11 Intercostal vein
12 Intercostal artery
13 Intercostal nerve
14 Intestinal lymphatic trunk
15 Lumbar lymphatic trunk, left
16 Lumbar lymphatic trunk, right
17 Oesophagus, displaced anteriorly by marker
18 Phrenic nerve, right
19 Pulmonary vein, left
20 Right lower lobe bronchus
21 Superior vena cava
22 Sympathetic ganglion
23 Sympathetic trunk
24 Thoracic duct
25 Thoracic duct, crossover
26 Vagus nerve, anterior oesophageal plexus

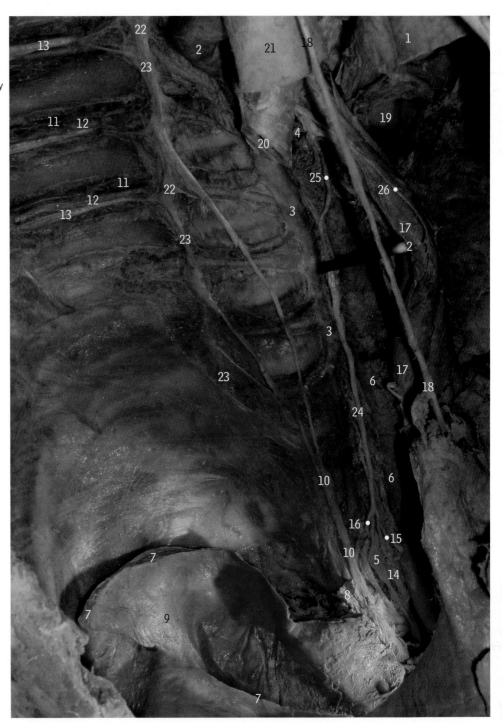

## (A) Oesophagus *lower thoracic part, from the front*

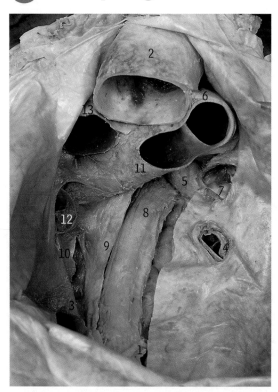

The heart has been removed from the pericardial cavity by transecting the great vessels, the pulmonary trunk being cut at the point where it divides into the two pulmonary arteries (11 and 6). Part of the pericardium (9) at the back has been removed to reveal the oesophagus (8). It is seen below the left principal bronchus (5) and is being crossed by the beginning of the right pulmonary artery (11).

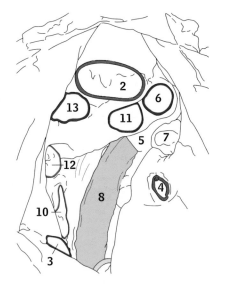

1  Anterior vagal trunk
2  Ascending aorta
3  Inferior vena cava
4  Left inferior pulmonary vein
5  Left principal bronchus
6  Left pulmonary artery
7  Left superior pulmonary vein
8  Oesophagus
9  Pericardium (cut edge)
10  Right inferior pulmonary vein
11  Right pulmonary artery
12  Right superior pulmonary vein
13  Superior vena cava

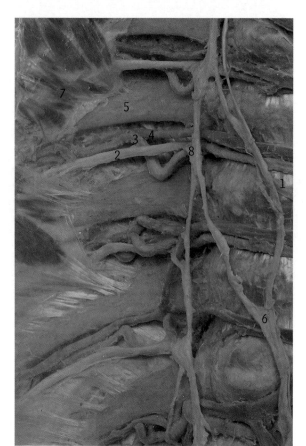

## (B) Intercostal spaces *posterior internal view*

This dissection shows the medial ends of some intercostal spaces of the right side, viewed from the front and slightly from the right. The pleura has been removed, revealing subcostal muscles (7) laterally, the nerves and vessels (4, 3 and 2) in the intercostal spaces, and the sympathetic trunk (8) and greater splanchnic nerve (6) on the sides of the vertebral bodies (as at 1).

1  Body of ninth thoracic vertebra
2  Eighth intercostal nerve
3  Eighth posterior intercostal artery
4  Eighth posterior intercostal vein

5  Eighth rib
6  Greater splanchnic nerve
7  Subcostal muscle
8  Sympathetic trunk and ganglia

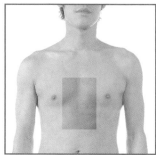

*Intercostal drainage, see page 219.*

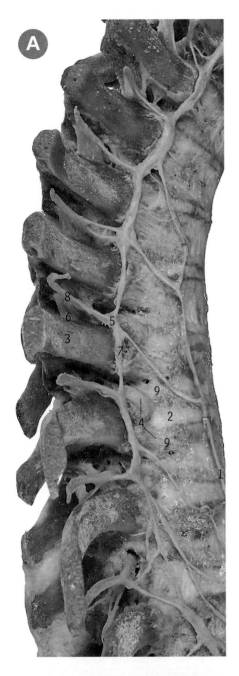

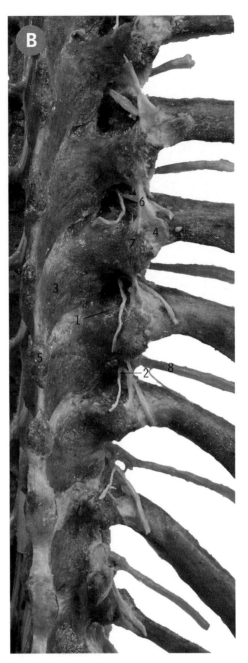

## A Joints of the heads of the ribs *from the right*

In this part of the right mid-thoracic region, the ribs have been cut short beyond their tubercles, and the joints that the two facets of the head of a rib make with the facets on the sides of adjacent vertebral bodies and the intervening disc are shown, as at 4, 9 and 2, where the radiate ligament (4) covers the capsule of these small synovial joints.

1  Greater splanchnic nerve
2  Intervertebral disc
3  Neck of rib
4  Radiate ligament of joint of head of rib
5  Rami communicantes
6  Superior costotransverse ligament
7  Sympathetic trunk
8  Ventral ramus of spinal nerve
9  Vertebral body

## B Costotrans-verse joints *from behind*

In this view of the right half of the thoracic vertebral column from behind, costotransverse joints between the transverse processes of vertebrae and the tubercles of ribs are covered by the lateral costotransverse ligaments (as at 4). The dorsal rami of spinal nerves (2) pass medial to the superior costotransverse ligaments (6); ventral rami (8) run in front of these ligaments.

1  Costotransverse ligament
2  Dorsal ramus of spinal nerve
3  Lamina
4  Lateral costotransverse ligament
5  Spinous process
6  Superior costotransverse ligament
7  Transverse process
8  Ventral ramus of spinal nerve

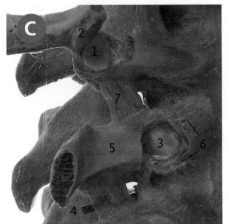

## C Costovertebral joints *disarticulated, from the right*

In the upper part of the figure, the upper rib has been severed through its neck (5) and the part with the tubercle attached has been turned upwards after cutting through the capsule of the costotransverse joint, to show the articular facet of the tubercle (2) and the transverse process (1). The head of the lower rib has been removed after transecting the radiate ligament (6) and underlying capsule of the joint of the head of the rib (3).

1  Articular facet of transverse process
2  Articular facet of tubercle of rib
3  Cavity of joint of head of rib
4  Marker between anterior and posterior parts of superior costotransverse ligament

5  Neck of rib
6  Radiate ligament
7  Superior costotransverse ligament

*Varicella-zoster virus infection – chest wall, see page 220.*

# Cast of the aorta and associated vessels
## A *from the right* B *from the left*

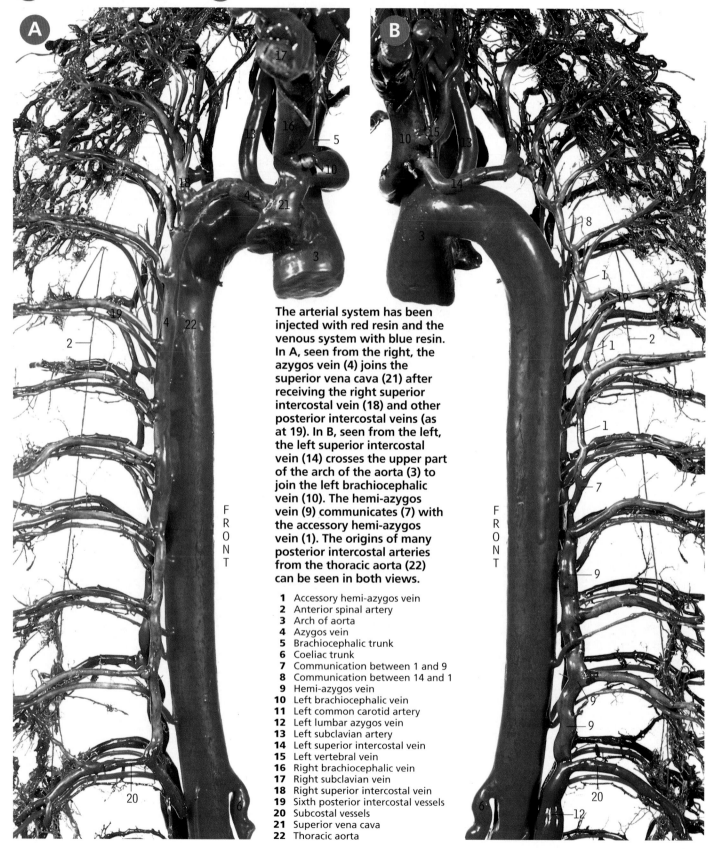

The arterial system has been injected with red resin and the venous system with blue resin. In A, seen from the right, the azygos vein (4) joins the superior vena cava (21) after receiving the right superior intercostal vein (18) and other posterior intercostal veins (as at 19). In B, seen from the left, the left superior intercostal vein (14) crosses the upper part of the arch of the aorta (3) to join the left brachiocephalic vein (10). The hemi-azygos vein (9) communicates (7) with the accessory hemi-azygos vein (1). The origins of many posterior intercostal arteries from the thoracic aorta (22) can be seen in both views.

1 Accessory hemi-azygos vein
2 Anterior spinal artery
3 Arch of aorta
4 Azygos vein
5 Brachiocephalic trunk
6 Coeliac trunk
7 Communication between 1 and 9
8 Communication between 14 and 1
9 Hemi-azygos vein
10 Left brachiocephalic vein
11 Left common carotid artery
12 Left lumbar azygos vein
13 Left subclavian artery
14 Left superior intercostal vein
15 Left vertebral vein
16 Right brachiocephalic vein
17 Right subclavian vein
18 Right superior intercostal vein
19 Sixth posterior intercostal vessels
20 Subcostal vessels
21 Superior vena cava
22 Thoracic aorta

# Diaphragm *from above*

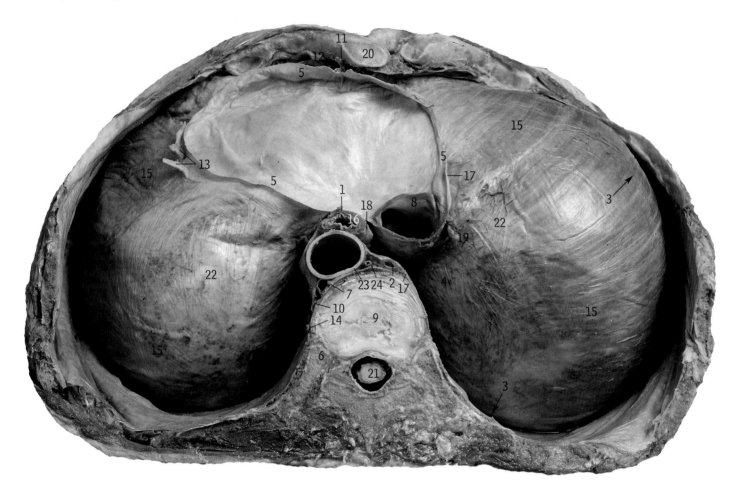

**The thorax has been transected at the level of the disc between the ninth and tenth thoracic vertebrae.**

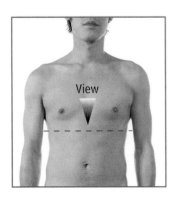

View

1 Anterior vagal trunk
2 Azygos vein
3 Costodiaphragmatic recess
4 Costomediastinal recess
5 Fibrous pericardium (cut edge)
6 Head of left ninth rib
7 Hemi-azygos vein
8 Inferior vena cava
9 Intervertebral disc
10 Left greater splanchnic nerve
11 Left internal thoracic artery
12 Left musculophrenic artery
13 Left phrenic nerve
14 Left sympathetic trunk
15 Muscle of diaphragm
16 Oesophagus
17 Pleura (cut edge)
18 Posterior vagal trunk
19 Right phrenic nerve
20 Seventh left costal cartilage
21 Spinal cord
22 Tendon of diaphragm
23 Thoracic aorta
24 Thoracic duct

According to the standard textbook description, the foramen for the vena cava is at the level of the disc between the eighth and ninth thoracic vertebrae, the oesophageal opening at the level of the tenth thoracic vertebra and the aortic opening opposite the twelfth thoracic vertebra. However, it is common for the oesophageal opening to be nearer the midline, as in this specimen (16), and the vena caval foramen (8) is lower than usual.

The vena caval foramen is in the tendinous part of the diaphragm and the oesophageal opening in the muscular part. The so-called aortic opening is not *in* the diaphragm but behind it (page 261).

The central tendon of the diaphragm has the shape of a trefoil leaf and has no bony attachment.

The right phrenic nerve (19) passes through the vena caval foramen in the tendinous part, but the left phrenic nerve (13) pierces the muscular part in front of the central tendon just lateral to the overlying pericardium.

The phrenic nerves are the *only motor* nerves to the diaphragm, including the crura. The supply from lower thoracic (intercostal and subcostal) nerves is purely sensory. Damage to one phrenic nerve completely paralyses its own half of the diaphragm.

*Gastro-oesophageal reflux, see page 219.*

# Oesophageal radiographs *during a barium swallow*

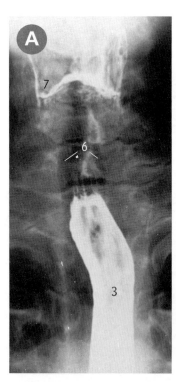

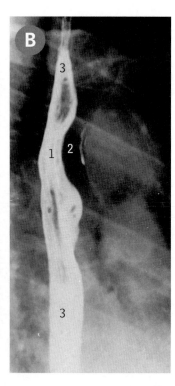

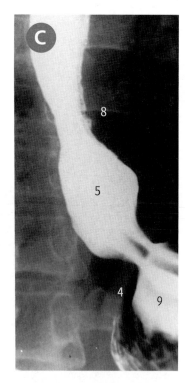

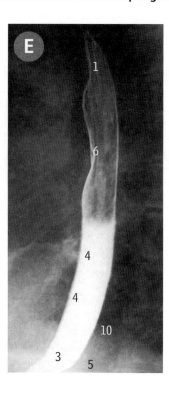

**A** lower pharynx and upper oesophagus

**B** middle part

**C** lower end

1 Aortic impression in oesophagus
2 Arch of aorta with plaque of calcification
3 Barium in oesophagus
4 Diaphragm
5 Lower thoracic oesophagus
6 Margins of trachea (translucent with contained air)
7 Piriform recess in laryngopharynx
8 Position of left atrium
9 Stomach

In A, viewed from the front, some of the barium paste adheres to the pharyngeal wall, outlining the piriform recesses (7), but most of it has passed into the oesophagus (3). In B, viewed obliquely from the left, the oesophagus is indented by the arch of the aorta (2) which shows some calcification in its wall – a useful aid to its identification. In C, there is some dilatation at the lower end of the thoracic oesophagus (5) and it is constricted where it passes through the diaphragm (4) to join the stomach (9). The left atrium of the heart (8) lies in front of the lower thoracic oesophagus (page 214, A8), but only when enlarged does the atrium cause an indentation in the oesophagus.

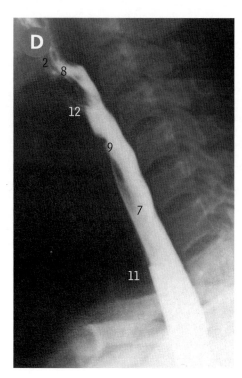

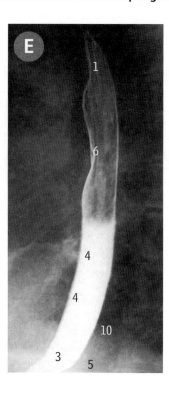

**D** cervical part

**E** thoracic part

1 Aortic arch impression
2 Base of tongue
3 Gastro-oesophageal junction
4 Left atrium position
5 Left hemidiaphragm
6 Left principal bronchus impression
7 Oesophagus
8 Oropharynx
9 Postcricoid venous plexus impression
10 Right hemidiaphragm
11 Trachea
12 Vallecula

# Thorax

**Clinical thumbnails, see DVD Thorax for details and further clinical images**

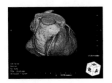

Angina
pectoris

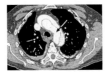

Aortic dissection

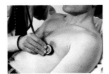

Auscultation of
heart sounds

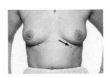

Breast
examination

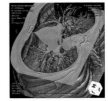

Bronchoscopy

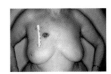

Carcinoma
of the breast

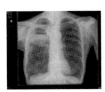

Carcinoma
of the lung

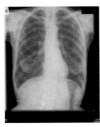

Carcinoma of
the oesophagus

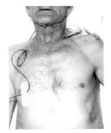

Cardiac
pacemaker

Cardiac
tamponade

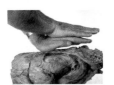

Cardio-
pulmonary
resuscitation
(CPR)

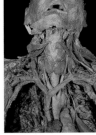

Catheterisa-
tion of the
subclavian vein

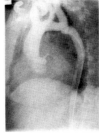

Coarctation
of the aorta

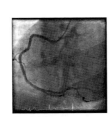

Coronary
angiography

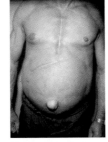

Coronary
artery bypass
grafting (CABG)

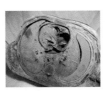

Empyema

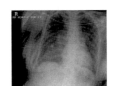

Flail chest

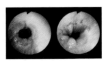

Gastro-
oesophageal
reflux

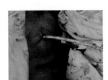

Intercostal
drainage

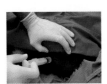

Intercostal
nerve block

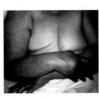

Left
ventricular
enlargement

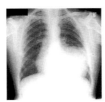

Mastectomy

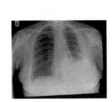

Mesothelioma

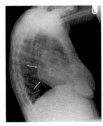

Mitral
valve disease

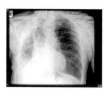

Myocardial
infarction

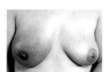

Orange
peel texture
of the skin and
retraction of the
nipple

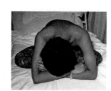

Pancoast
tumour

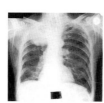

Pericardial
effusion

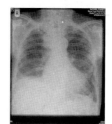

Phrenic
nerve palsy

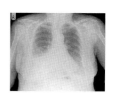

Pleural
effusion

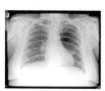

Pneumothorax

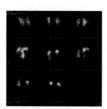

Pulmonary
embolism

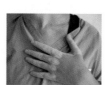

Thoracic
aortic aneurysm

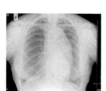

Thoracic
outlet syndromes

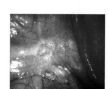

Thymus

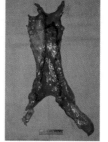

Transthoracic
sympathectomy

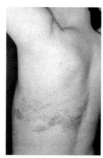

Tuberculosis

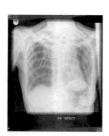

Varicella-
zoster virus
infection –
chest wall

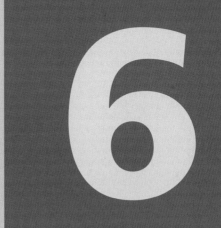
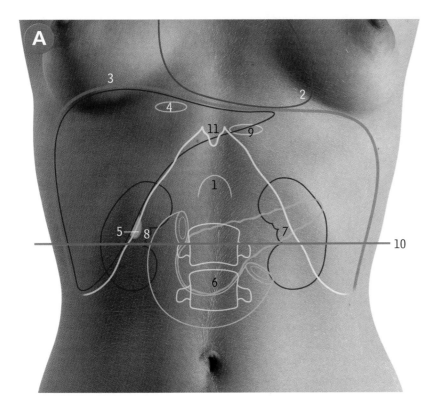

## A Anterior abdominal wall

### surface markings, above the umbilicus

The solid white line indicates the costal margin. The blue line indicates the transpyloric plane. The C-shaped duodenum is outlined in pink, the kidneys and liver in brown and the pancreas in pale green.

1 Aortic opening in diaphragm
2 Apex of heart in fifth intercostal space
3 Dome of diaphragm and upper margin of liver
4 Foramen for inferior vena cava in diaphragm
5 Fundus of gall bladder, and junction of ninth costal cartilage and lateral border of rectus sheath
6 Head of pancreas and level of second lumbar vertebra
7 Hilum of left kidney
8 Hilum of right kidney
9 Oesophageal opening in diaphragm
10 Transpyloric plane
11 Xiphoid process

> The transpyloric plane (10) lies midway between the jugular notch of the sternum and the upper border of the pubic symphysis, or approximately a hand's breadth below the xiphisternal joint (11), and level with the lower part of the body of the first lumbar vertebra.

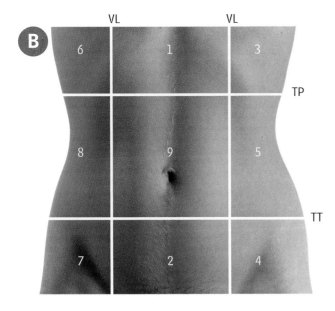

## B Regions of the abdomen

The abdomen may be divided into regions by two vertical and two horizontal lines. The vertical lines (VL) pass through the midinguinal points: the upper horizontal line corresponds to the transpyloric plane (TP, A10), the lower line is drawn between the tubercles of the iliac crests (transtubercular (or supracristal) plane, TT).

1 Epigastric region
2 Hypogastrium or suprapubic
3 Left hypochondrium
4 Left iliac region or iliac fossa
5 Left lumbar region
6 Right hypochondrium
7 Right iliac region or iliac fossa
8 Right lumbar region
9 Umbilical region

# A Anterior abdominal wall

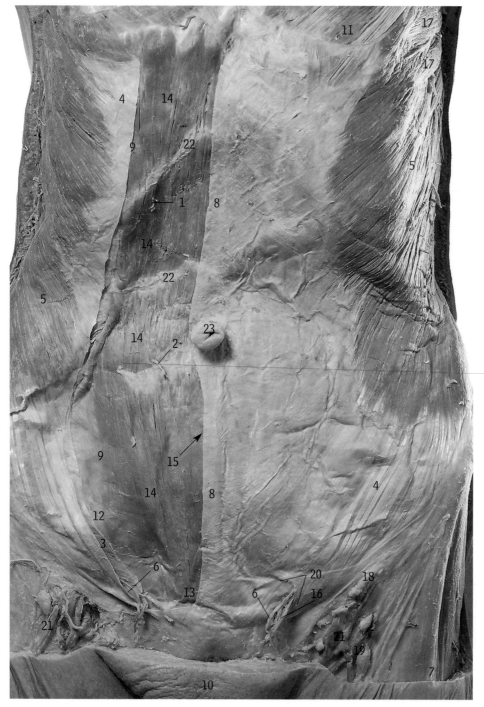

1 Anterior cutaneous nerve (eighth intercostal)
2 Anterior cutaneous nerve (tenth intercostal)
3 Anterior layer internal oblique aponeurosis
4 External oblique aponeurosis
5 External oblique muscle
6 Ilioinguinal nerve
7 Iliotibial tract
8 Linea alba
9 Linea semilunaris
10 Mons pubis
11 Pectoralis major muscle
12 Posterior layer internal oblique aponeurosis
13 Pyramidalis muscle
14 Rectus abdominis
15 Rectus sheath, anterior
16 Round ligament of uterus
17 Serratus anterior muscle
18 Superficial inguinal lymph node (horizontal group)
19 Superficial inguinal lymph node (vertical group)
20 Superficial inguinal ring
21 Superficial inguinal veins
22 Tendinous intersection of rectus abdominis
23 Umbilicus

The rectus sheath (A15) is formed by the internal oblique aponeurosis (A3), which splits at the lateral border of the rectus muscle (A9) into two layers. The posterior (A12) passes behind the muscle to blend with the aponeurosis of transversus abdominis (B19) to form the posterior wall of the sheath (B13), and the anterior layer (A3) passes in front of the muscle to blend with the external oblique aponeurosis (A4) as the anterior wall (A15).

The anterior and posterior walls of the sheath unite at the medial border of the rectus muscle to form the midline linea alba (A8, B11).

*Haematoma of the rectus sheath, Spigelian hernia, see pages 282, 283.*

## B Rectus sheath

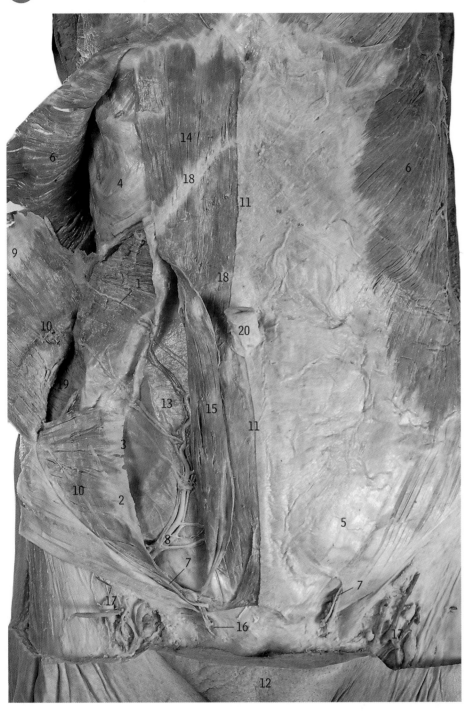

1 Anterior cutaneous nerve (tenth intercostal)
2 Anterior layer of internal oblique aponeurosis
3 Anterior wall of rectus sheath
4 Eighth rib
5 External oblique aponeurosis
6 External oblique muscle
7 Ilioinguinal nerve
8 Inferior epigastric vessels
9 Internal oblique aponeurosis
10 Internal oblique muscle
11 Linea alba
12 Mons pubis
13 Posterior wall of rectus sheath
14 Rectus abdominis
15 Rectus abdominis, reflected
16 Round ligament of uterus
17 Superficial inguinal lymph nodes
18 Tendinous intersection
19 Transversus abdominis
20 Umbilicus

There is no posterior rectus sheath in the lower third of rectus abdominis, below the arcuate line (page 227, A1).

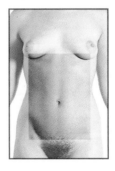

# Groin in the male

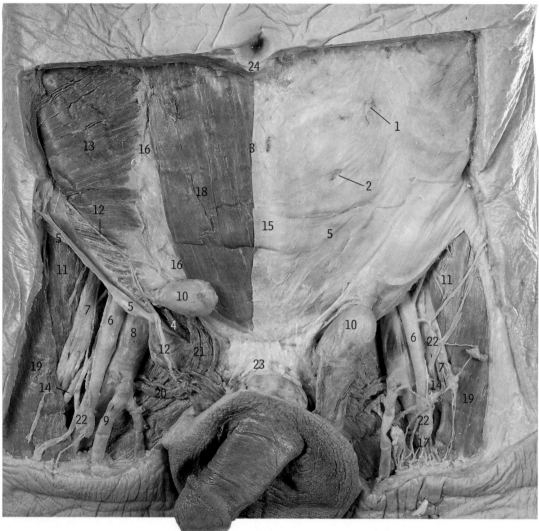

1 Anterior cutaneous nerve (eleventh intercostal)
2 Anterior cutaneous nerve (twelfth intercostal)
3 Anterior rectus sheath (cut edge)
4 Ductus deferens (vas)
5 External oblique aponeurosis
6 Femoral artery
7 Femoral nerve
8 Femoral vein
9 Great saphenous vein
10 Hernial sac (indirect)
11 Iliacus muscle
12 Ilioinguinal nerve
13 Internal oblique muscle
14 Lateral circumflex femoral artery
15 Linea alba
16 Linea semilunaris
17 Lymphatic vessels
18 Rectus abdominis muscle
19 Sartorius muscle
20 Scrotal venous connections
21 Spermatic cord
22 Superficial inguinal lymph node
23 Suspensory ligament of penis
24 Umbilicus

The hernial sacs (10), shown here, are not present in normal subjects.

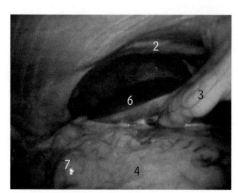

**Laparoscopic view of upper abdominal cavity**

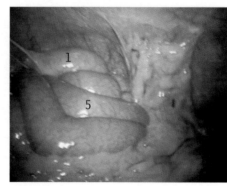

**Laparoscopic view of lower abdominal cavity**

1 Caecum
2 Diaphragm
3 Falciform ligament
4 Greater omentum
5 Ileum
6 Right lobe, liver
7 Transverse colon

*Inguinal hernia repair, varicella zoster virus, see pages 282, 284.*

# Adult anterior abdominal wall in the male *surface markings, right iliac fossa*

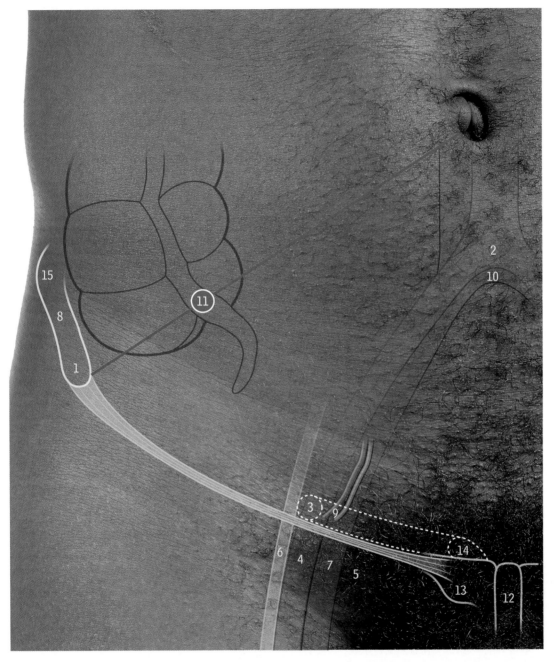

1 Anterior superior iliac spine
2 Bifurcation of aorta (fourth lumbar vertebra)
3 Deep inguinal ring
4 Femoral artery
5 Femoral canal
6 Femoral nerve
7 Femoral vein
8 Iliac crest
9 Inferior epigastric vessels
10 Lower end of inferior vena cava (fifth lumbar vertebra)
11 McBurney's point
12 Pubic symphysis
13 Pubic tubercle
14 Superficial inguinal ring
15 Tubercle of iliac crest

The femoral artery (4, whose pulsation should normally be palpable) enters the thigh midway between the pubic symphysis (12) and the anterior superior iliac spine (1). This is often referred to as the midinguinal point.

The caecum with the appendix opening into it from the left and the ascending colon continuing upwards from it are indicated by the brown line. The inguinal ligament, between the anterior superior iliac spine (1) and the pubic tubercle (13), is indicated by the light blue line. The femoral artery (4) has the femoral vein (7) on its medial side and the femoral nerve (6) on its lateral side. The femoral canal (5) is on the medial side of the vein. The deep inguinal ring (3) and inferior epigastric vessels (9) are above the femoral artery, while the superficial inguinal ring (14) is above and lateral to the pubic tubercle (13). McBurney's point (11) is a site on the surface of the anterior abdominal wall indicating the usual location of the base of the appendix internally. It lies one-third of the way along a line from the right anterior superior iliac spine to the umbilicus (red line).

*Femoral hernia, McBurney's point, see pages 282, 283.*

## **A** Adult anterior abdominal wall *umbilical folds, from behind*

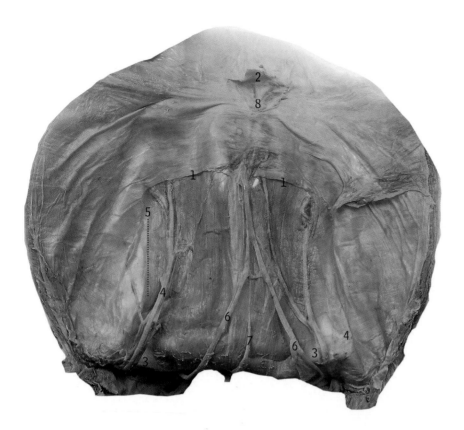

This view of the peritoneal surface of the central region of the anterior abdominal wall shows the peritoneal folds raised by underlying structures. There is one fold above the umbilicus – the falciform ligament – and there are five below it: the median umbilical fold (7) in the midline, and a pair of medial and lateral umbilical folds on each side (6 and 4).

1 Arcuate line
2 Falciform ligament
3 Inguinal triangle (Hesselbach)
4 Lateral umbilical fold which contains the inferior epigastric vessels
5 Linea semilunaris
6 Medial umbilical fold
7 Median umbilical fold
8 Umbilicus

The inguinal triangle of Hesselbach is a naturally weak region between rectus abdominis and the inferior epigastric vessels. Direct inguinal hernias appear through this region.

## **B** Fetal anterior abdominal wall *from behind*

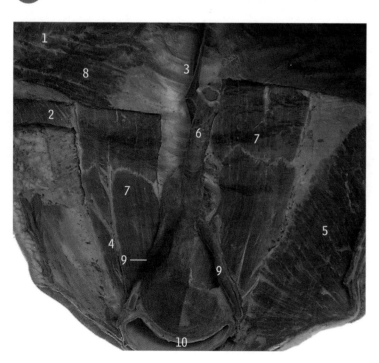

In this at term fetus, the peritoneum and extraperitoneal tissues have been removed from the anterior abdominal wall to show the umbilical arteries (9) and left umbilical vein (6) converging at the back of the (unlabelled) umbilicus.

1 Diaphragm
2 External oblique
3 Falciform ligament
4 Inferior epigastric vessels
5 Internal oblique
6 Left umbilical vein
7 Rectus abdominis
8 Transversus abdominis
9 Umbilical artery
10 Urinary bladder

*Caput medusae, umbilical hernia, see pages 281, 284.*

# **A** Right deep inguinal ring in adult male *laparoscopic view*

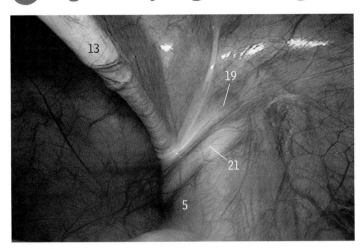

# **B** Anterior abdominal wall *abdominal view*

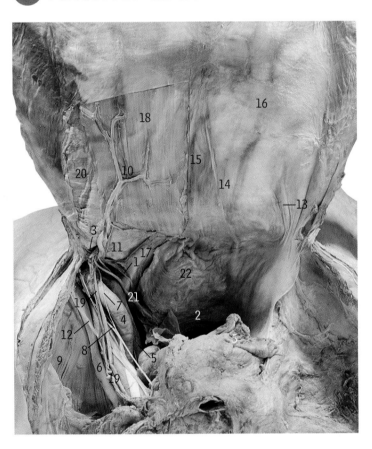

Abdominal viscera have been removed and the anterior abdominal wall detached laterally and reflected anteriorly and inferiorly to reveal the internal surface of the abdominal wall. The parietal peritoneum has been removed from the left side to show deeper structures in the pelvic and abdominal walls.

1   Accessory obturator artery
2   Bladder
3   Deep inguinal ring
4   External iliac artery
5   External iliac vein
6   Femoral nerve
7   Genitofemoral nerve, femoral branch
8   Genitofemoral nerve, genital branch
9   Iliacus
10  Inferior epigastric vessels
11  Inguinal triangle (Hesselbach)
12  Lateral cutaneous nerve of the thigh
13  Lateral umbilical fold (inferior epigastric vessels)
14  Medial umbilical fold (umbilical artery)
15  Median umbilical fold (urachus)
16  Parietal peritoneum
17  Pelvic brim
18  Posterior rectus sheath
19  Testicular vessels
20  Transversus abdominis
21  Vas/ductus deferens
22  Visceral peritoneum

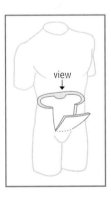

*Inguinal hernia, indirect inguinal hernia, see page 282.*

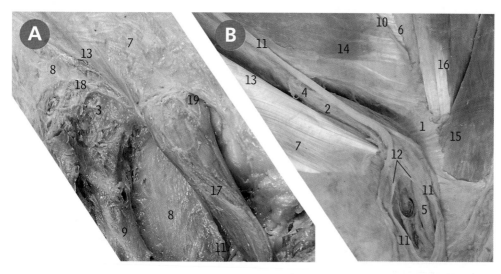

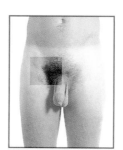

## Right inguinal region *in the male*

**A** superficial dissection

**B** with the external oblique aponeurosis and spermatic cord incised

In A, the spermatic cord (17) is seen emerging from the superficial inguinal ring (19) and covered by the external spermatic fascia. In B, with the external oblique aponeurosis reflected and the anterior wall of the rectus sheath removed, the cord is emerging from the deep inguinal ring (4) with the cremasteric fascia (2) now the most superficial covering. All three coverings of the cord have been incised (12) to show the ductus/vas deferens (5).

1 Conjoint tendon
2 Cremasteric fascia and cremaster muscle over spermatic cord
3 Cribriform fascia
4 Deep inguinal ring
5 Ductus/vas deferens
6 Edge of rectus sheath
7 External oblique aponeurosis
8 Fascia lata
9 Great saphenous vein
10 Iliohypogastric nerve
11 Ilio-inguinal nerve
12 Incised margin of coverings of cord
13 Inguinal ligament
14 Internal oblique
15 Pyramidalis
16 Rectus abdominis
17 Spermatic cord
18 Upper margin of saphenous opening
19 Upper margin of superficial inguinal ring

## Right inguinal region *in the female*

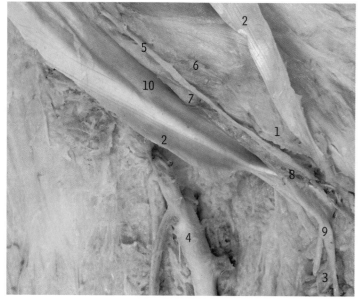

The external oblique aponeurosis (2) has been incised and reflected to show the position of the deep inguinal ring (7) which marks the lateral end of the inguinal canal. The round ligament of the uterus (9) emerges from the superficial inguinal ring (8), which marks the medial end of the canal, and becomes lost in the fat of the labium majus (3). The ilio-inguinal nerve (5) also passes through the canal and out of the superficial ring.

1 Conjoint tendon
2 External oblique aponeurosis
3 Fat of labium majus
4 Great saphenous vein
5 Ilio-inguinal nerve
6 Internal oblique
7 Position of deep inguinal ring
8 Position of superficial inguinal ring
9 Round ligament of uterus
10 Upper surface of inguinal ligament

In the female, the inguinal canal contains the round ligament of the uterus and the ilio-inguinal nerve.

The processus vaginalis is normally obliterated, but if it remains patent within the female inguinal canal, it is sometimes known as the canal of Nuck.

# Abdominal peritoneal folds, after removal of intra-abdominal organs, to show relations of ligaments and mesenteries

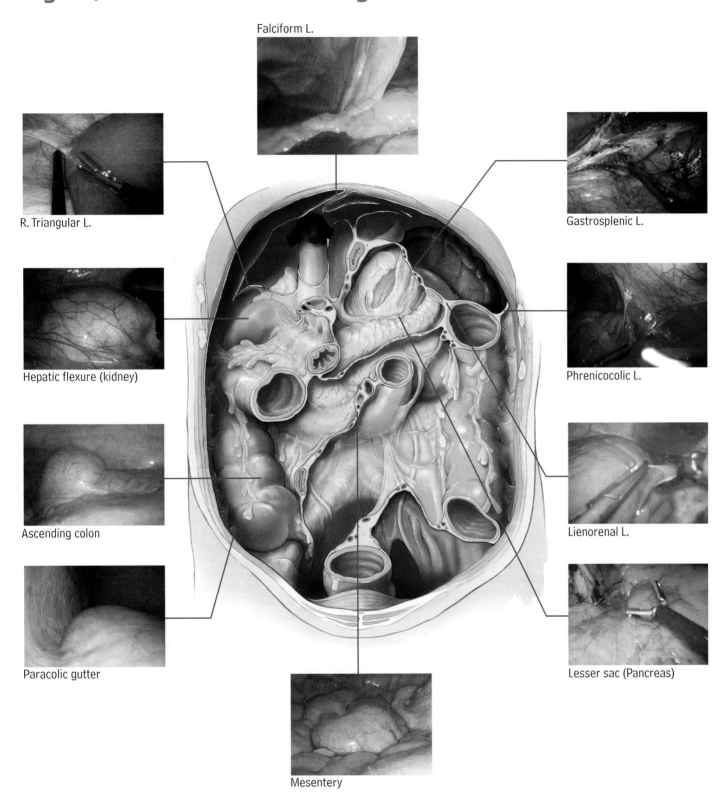

Falciform L.

R. Triangular L.

Hepatic flexure (kidney)

Ascending colon

Paracolic gutter

Gastrosplenic L.

Phrenicocolic L.

Lienorenal L.

Lesser sac (Pancreas)

Mesentery

*Drainage of peritoneal abscesses, see page 282.*

# Upper abdominal viscera *from the front*

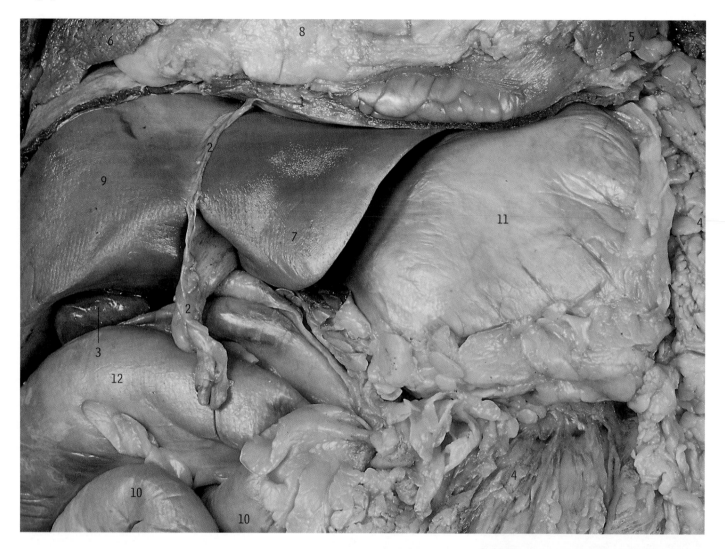

The thoracic and abdominal walls and the anterior part of the diaphragm have been removed to show the undisturbed viscera. The liver (9 and 7) and stomach (11) are immediately below the diaphragm (1). The greater omentum (4) hangs down from the greater curvature (lower margin) of the stomach (11), overlying much of the small and large intestine but leaving some of the transverse colon (12) and small intestine (10) uncovered. The fundus (tip) of the gall bladder (3) is seen between the right lobe of the liver (9) and transverse colon (12).

| | | | |
|---|---|---|---|
| **1** | Diaphragm | **7** | Left lobe of liver |
| **2** | Falciform ligament | **8** | Pericardial fat |
| **3** | Gall bladder | **9** | Right lobe of liver |
| **4** | Greater omentum | **10** | Small intestine |
| **5** | Inferior lobe of left lung | **11** | Stomach |
| **6** | Inferior lobe of right lung | **12** | Transverse colon |

For an explanation of peritoneal structures, see the diagrams on pages 224, 236.

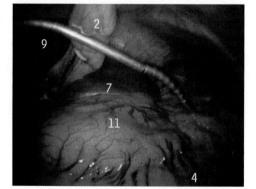

**Laparoscopic view of upper abdominal viscera**

*Liver biopsy, see page 282.*

# Upper abdominal viscera *from the front*

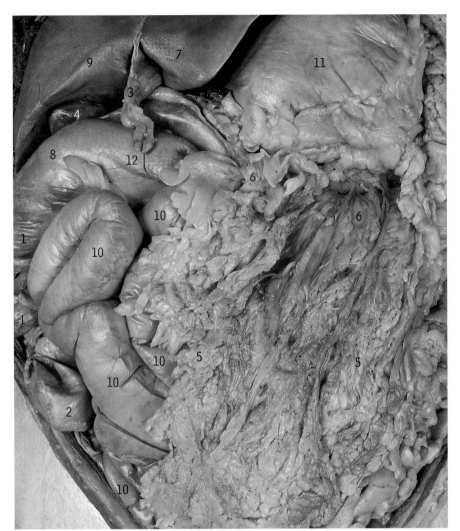

In this view of the undisturbed abdomen, the upper part of the greater omentum (as at 6) overlies much of the transverse colon and mesocolon (with the right part of the transverse colon seen at 12). The lower part of the omentum (5) covers coils of small intestine, some of which (10) are visible beyond the right margin of the omentum. The caecum (2) is at the proximal end of the ascending colon (1) which continues upwards into the right colic flexure (hepatic flexure, 8) and then becomes the transverse colon (12).

1 Ascending colon
2 Caecum
3 Falciform ligament
4 Fundus of gall bladder
5 Greater omentum overlying coils of small intestine
6 Greater omentum overlying transverse colon and mesocolon
7 Left lobe of liver
8 Right colic flexure
9 Right lobe of liver
10 Small intestine
11 Stomach
12 Transverse colon

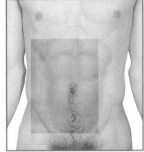

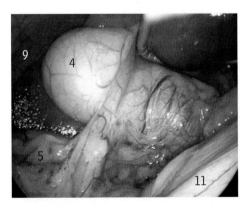

**Laparoscopic view of gall bladder**

*Cholecystectomy, laparoscopy, see pages 281, 282.*

# Upper abdominal viscera *from the front*

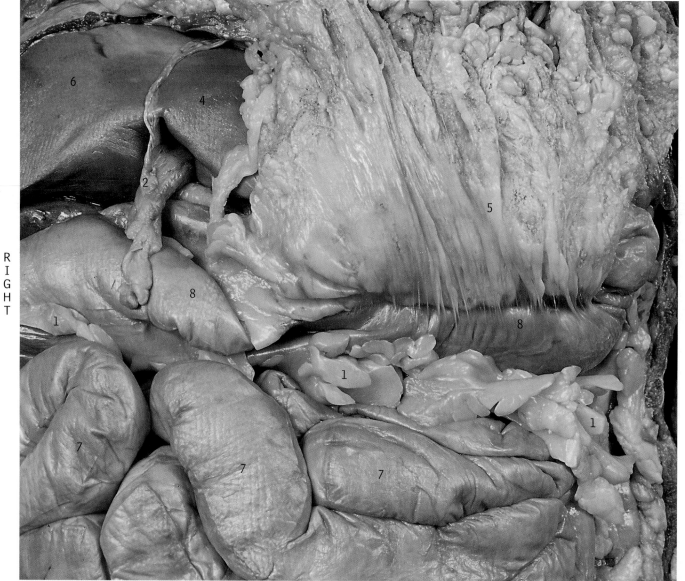

In this view of the same specimen as on page 230, the greater omentum (5) has been lifted upwards to show its adherence to the transverse colon (8) (see page 236, C).

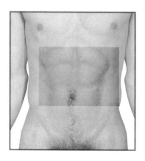

| | |
|---|---|
| **1** | Appendices epiploicae |
| **2** | Falciform ligament |
| **3** | Gall bladder (fundus) |
| **4** | Left lobe of liver |
| **5** | Posterior surface of greater omentum |
| **6** | Right lobe of liver |
| **7** | Small intestine |
| **8** | Transverse colon |

The appendices epiploicae (1) are fat-filled appendages of peritoneum on the various parts of the colon (ascending, transverse, descending and sigmoid). They are not present on the small intestine or the rectum, and may be rudimentary on the caecum and appendix. In abdominal operations, they are one feature that helps to distinguish colon from other parts of the intestine.

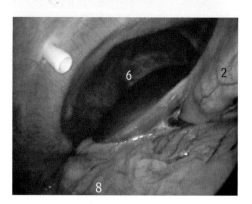

**Laparoscopic view of abdominal viscera**

# Lesser omentum and epiploic foramen

## A *from the front* B *from the front and the right*

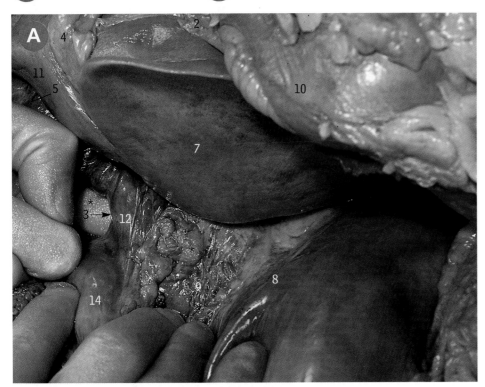

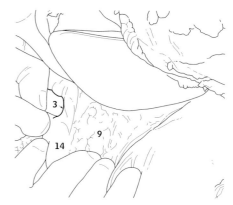

1   Descending (second) part of duodenum
2   Diaphragm
3   Epiploic foramen*
4   Falciform ligament
5   Gall bladder
6   Inferior vena cava
7   Left lobe of liver
8   Lesser curvature of stomach
9   Lesser omentum
10  Pericardium
11  Quadrate lobe of liver
12  Right free margin of lesser omentum
13  Right lobe of liver
14  Superior (first) part of duodenum
15  Upper pole of right kidney

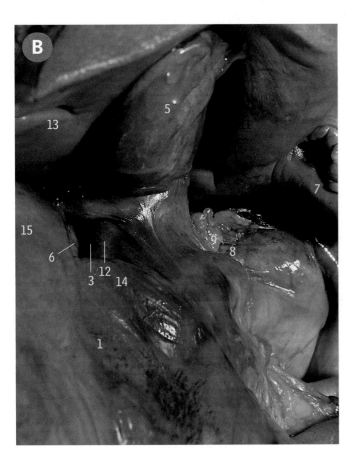

In A, a finger* has been placed in the epiploic foramen (3) behind the right free margin of the lesser omentum (12), and the tip can be seen in the lesser sac, through the transparent lesser omentum (9) which stretches between the liver (7) and the lesser curvature of the stomach (8). In the more lateral view in B, looking into the foramen from the right, the foramen (3) is identified between the right free margin of the lesser omentum (12) in front and the inferior vena cava (6) behind, above the first part of the duodenum (14).

> The epiploic foramen (of Winslow, A3 and B3) is the communication between the general peritoneal cavity (sometimes called the greater sac) and the lesser sac (omental bursa), a space lined by peritoneum behind the stomach (A8 and B8) and lesser omentum (A9 and A12) and in front of parts of the pancreas and left kidney.

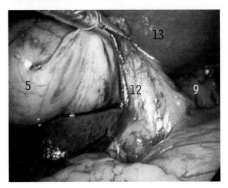

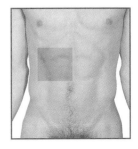

Laparoscopic view of lesser omentum (free margin)

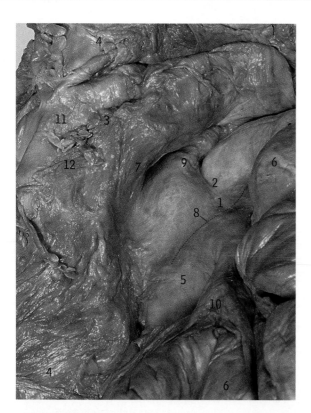

## A Upper abdominal viscera *from the front*

In this view the stomach (3 and 7), transverse colon (11) and greater omentum (4) have been lifted up to show the region of the duodenojejunal flexure (2). The left end of the horizontal (third) part of the duodenum (5) turns upwards as the ascending (fourth) part (1), which is continuous with the jejunum at the duodenojejunal flexure (2) below the lower border of the pancreas (9).

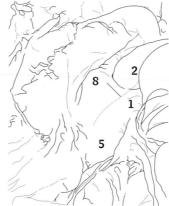

1 Ascending (fourth) part of duodenum
2 Duodenojejunal flexure
3 Greater curvature of stomach
4 Greater omentum (posterior surface)
5 Horizontal (third) part of duodenum
6 Jejunum
7 Lesser curvature of stomach
8 Line of attachment of root of mesentery
9 Lower border of pancreas
10 Mesentery
11 Transverse colon (posterior surface)
12 Transverse mesocolon (posterior surface)

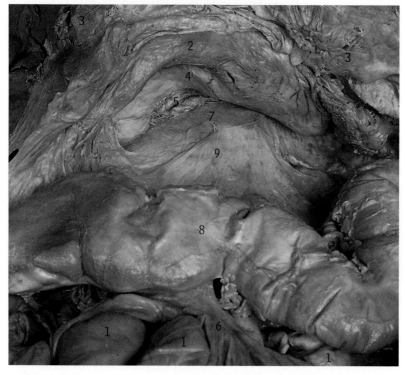

## B Lesser sac and transverse mesocolon *from the front*

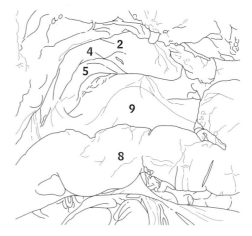

The greater omentum (3) hanging down from the greater curvature of the stomach (2) has been separated from the underlying transverse colon (8) and mesocolon (9) and lifted upwards, and an opening made into the lesser sac (as in D on page 236). This view therefore shows the posterior surface of the greater omentum (3), stomach and lesser omentum (5), and the anterior surface of the transverse mesocolon (9).

1 Coils of jejunum and ileum
2 Greater curvature of stomach
3 Greater omentum (posterior surface)
4 Lesser curvature of stomach
5 Lesser omentum (posterior surface)
6 Mesentery
7 Peritoneum of lesser sac overlying pancreas
8 Transverse colon
9 Transverse mesocolon overlying horizontal (third) part of duodenum

*Ascites, see page 281.*

# Mesentery and descending colon *from the front*

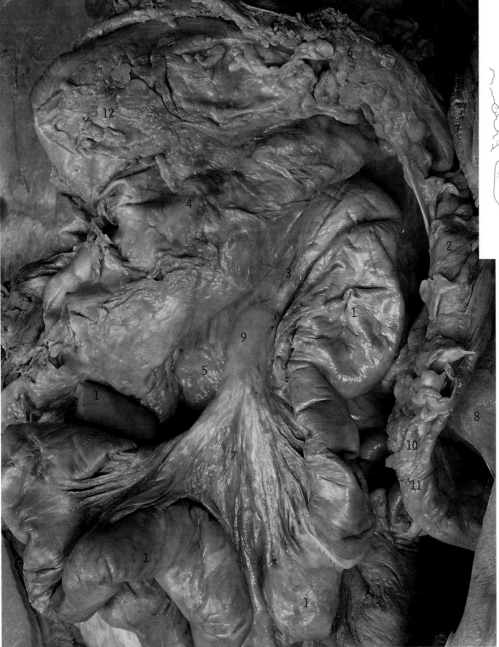

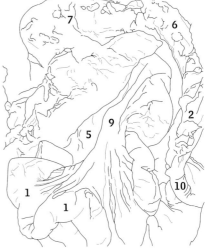

1  Coils of jejunum and ileum
2  Descending colon
3  Duodenojejunal flexure
4  Greater curvature of stomach
5  Horizontal (third) part of
   duodenum
6  Left colic (splenic) flexure
7  Mesentery
8  Peritoneum overlying
   external iliac vessels
9  Root of mesentery
10  Sigmoid colon
11  Sigmoid mesocolon
12  Transverse colon

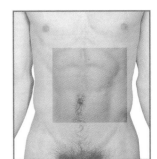

The stomach (4) and transverse colon (12) have been displaced upwards to show the left end of the root of the mesentery (9) at the duodenojejunal flexure (3). The descending colon (2), which is retroperitoneal, becomes the sigmoid colon (10) when it ceases to be retroperitoneal and acquires a mesentery (11).

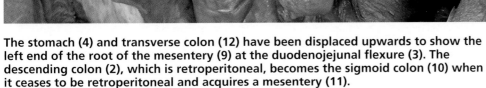

*Volvulus, see page 284.*

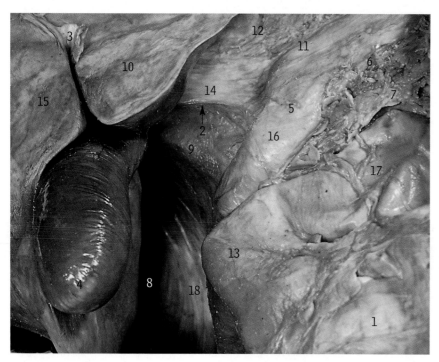

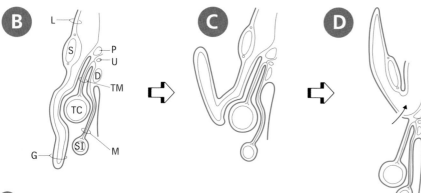

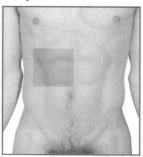

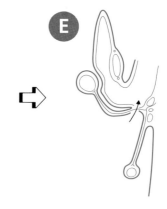

| | | |
|---|---|---|
| **1** Ascending colon | **7** Greater omentum | **13** Right colic (hepatic) flexure |
| **2** Epiploic foramen | **8** Hepatorenal (Morison's) pouch | **14** Right free margin of lesser omentum |
| **3** Falciform ligament | **9** Inferior vena cava | **15** Right lobe of liver |
| **4** Gall bladder | **10** Left lobe of liver | **16** Superior (first) part of duodenum |
| **5** Gastroduodenal junction | **11** Lesser curvature of stomach | **17** Transverse colon |
| **6** Greater curvature of stomach | **12** Lesser omentum overlying pancreas | **18** Upper pole of right kidney |

## Diagrams of peritoneum *(see page 229)*

**B**

**C**

**D**

**E**

**B** normal position

**C** with the lower part of the greater omentum lifted up

**D** with the greater omentum lifted up and separated from the transverse mesocolon and colon, with an opening into the lesser sac

**E** with the greater omentum and transverse mesocolon and colon lifted up, with an opening into the lesser sac through the mesocolon

These drawings of a sagittal section through the middle of the abdomen, viewed from the left, illustrate theoretically how the peritoneum forms the lesser omentum (L, passing down to the stomach, S), greater omentum (G), transverse mesocolon (TM) passing to the transverse colon (TC), and the mesentery (M) of the small intestine (SI). The layer in blue represents the peritoneum of the lesser sac. The superior mesenteric artery passes between the head and uncinate process of the pancreas (P and U), and continues across the duodenum (D) into the mesentery (M) to the small intestine (SI), giving off the middle colic artery which runs in the transverse mesocolon (TM) to the transverse colon (TC). The greater omentum (G) is formed by four layers fused together and also fused with the front of the transverse mesocolon (TM, two layers) and transverse colon. On dissection, no separation between any layers is possible except between the greater omentum and the transverse mesocolon. The six layers between the stomach and transverse colon are sometimes collectively known as the gastrocolic omentum. B corresponds to the dissections on pages 230 and 231, C to page 232, D to page 234B, and E to page 239. The small arrows in D and E indicate the layers cut to make artificial openings into the lesser sac.

# Coeliac trunk

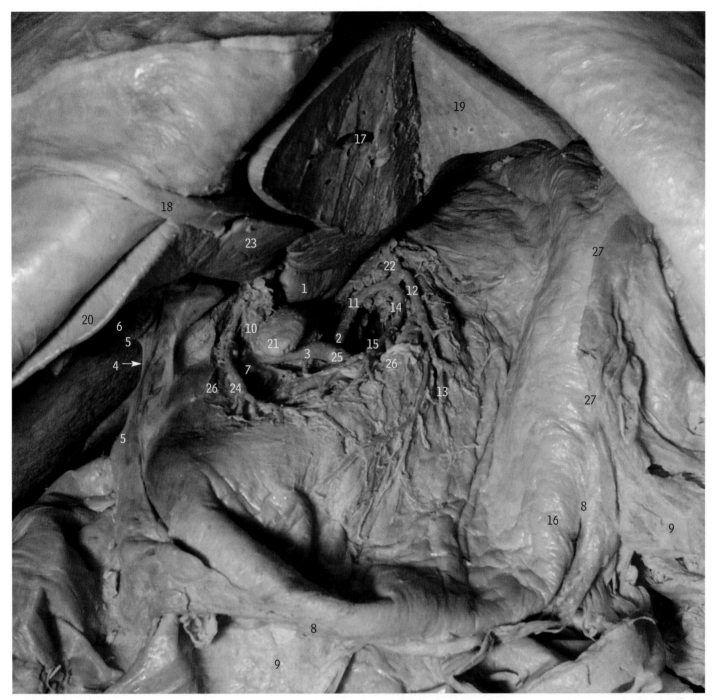

| | |
|---|---|
| **1** Caudate lobe of liver | **15** Left gastric, posterior branch to lesser curvature of stomach |
| **2** Coeliac trunk | **16** Left gastroepiploic vessels |
| **3** Common hepatic artery | **17** Left portal vein |
| **4** Epiploic foramen – arrow | **18** Ligamentum teres within falciform ligament |
| **5** Free edge, lesser omentum | **19** Liver, left lobe |
| **6** Gall bladder | **20** Liver, right lobe |
| **7** Gastroduodenal artery | **21** Lymph node, enlarged coeliac node |
| **8** Greater curvature of stomach | **22** Oesophageal branch of left gastric artery |
| **9** Greater omentum | **23** Quadrate lobe of liver |
| **10** Hepatic artery, proper | **24** Right gastric artery, antral branch |
| **11** Left gastric artery | **25** Splenic artery |
| **12** Left gastric, anterior branch | **26** Stomach, lesser curvature |
| **13** Left gastric, anterior branch to body of stomach | **27** Visceral peritoneum, cut edge |
| **14** Left gastric, posterior branch | |

*Carcinoma of the stomach, see page 281.*

# Superior mesenteric vessels, origins

**A** *duodenum and pancreas in situ*

**B** *duodenum reflected to reveal posterior relations of vessels*

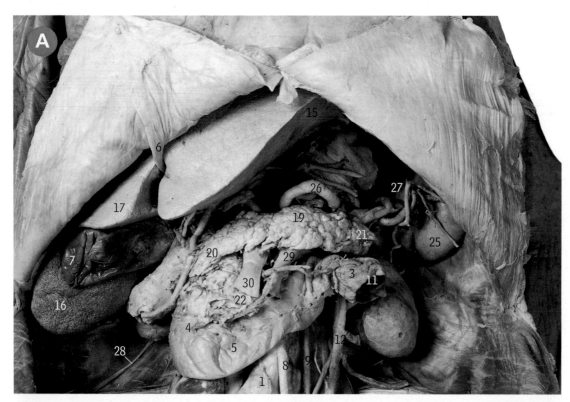

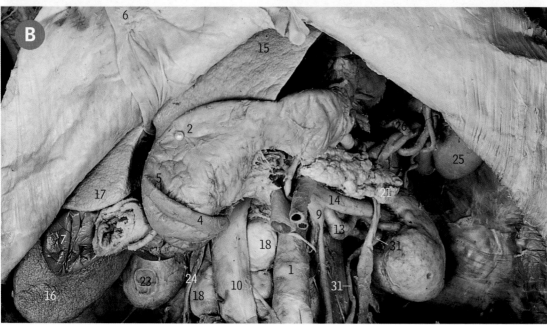

1 Aorta
2 Duodenum reflected and pinned
3 Duodenum, ascending (fourth) part
4 Duodenum, descending (second) part
5 Duodenum, horizontal (third) part
6 Falciform ligament
7 Gall bladder, fundus
8 Inferior mesenteric artery
9 Inferior mesenteric vein
10 Inferior vena cava
11 Jejunum, origin
12 Left gonadal vein
13 Left renal artery
14 Left renal vein
15 Liver, left lobe
16 Liver, Riedel's lobe
17 Liver, right lobe
18 Lymph nodes, moderately enlarged pre and para-aortic
19 Pancreas, body
20 Pancreas, head
21 Pancreas, tail
22 Pancreas, uncinate process
23 Renal cyst, benign
24 Right gonadal vein
25 Spleen
26 Splenic artery
27 Splenic vein
28 Subcostal nerve
29 Superior mesenteric artery
30 Superior mesenteric vein
31 Ureter

*Inferior vena cava (IVC) obstruction, pancreatic pathology, see pages 282, 283.*

# Superior mesenteric vessels

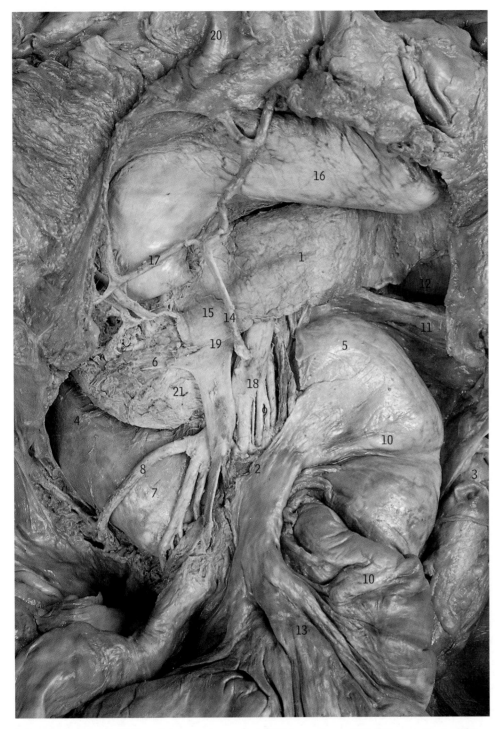

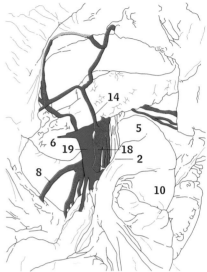

1 Body of pancreas
2 Cut edge of peritoneum at root of mesentery
3 Descending colon
4 Descending (second) part of duodenum
5 Duodenojejunal flexure
6 Head of pancreas
7 Horizontal (third) part of duodenum
8 Ileocolic artery
9 Jejunal and ileal arteries
10 Jejunum
11 Left colic vessels (inferior mesenteric)
12 Left kidney
13 Mesentery
14 Middle colic artery
15 Neck of pancreas
16 Posterior surface of body of stomach
17 Right branch of middle colic artery
18 Superior mesenteric artery
19 Superior mesenteric vein
20 Transverse colon
21 Uncinate process of pancreas

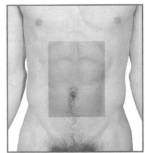

Here the stomach (16) and transverse colon (20) have been lifted upwards, so lifting the middle colic artery (14) upwards also. The root of the mesentery (2) begins at the duodenojejunal flexure (5) and passes obliquely downwards to the right over the horizontal (third) part of the duodenum (7), where the superior mesenteric vessels and their branches (19, 18 and 9) become enclosed between the two layers of the peritoneum that form the mesentery (see B on page 236).

*Meckel's diverticulum, see page 283.*

# Inferior mesenteric vessels *from the front*

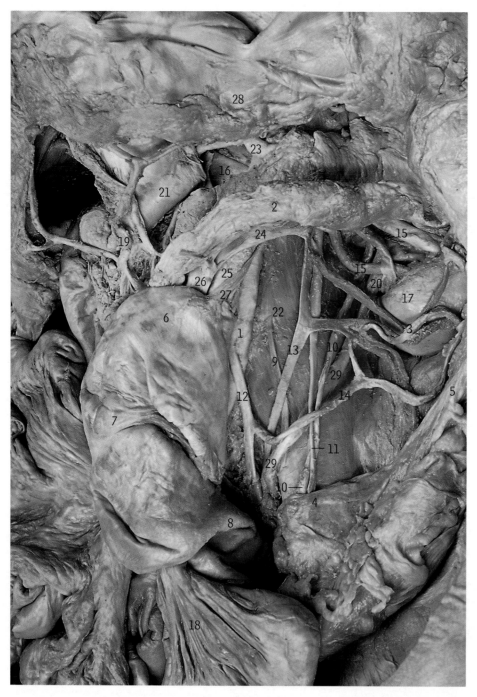

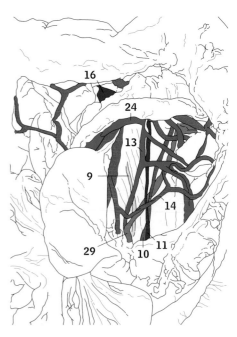

1 Abdominal aorta
2 Body of pancreas
3 Branches of left colic vessels
4 Cut edge of peritoneum
5 Descending colon
6 Duodenojejunal flexure
7 Duodenum: ascending (fourth)
8 Duodenum: horizontal (third)
9 Genitofemoral nerve
10 Gonadal artery
11 Gonadal vein
12 Inferior mesenteric artery
13 Inferior mesenteric vein
14 Left colic artery
15 Left renal artery
16 Left renal vein
17 Lower pole of left kidney
18 Mesentery
19 Middle colic artery
20 Pelvis of kidney
21 Posterior surface of pyloric part of stomach
22 Psoas major
23 Splenic artery
24 Splenic vein
25 Superior mesenteric artery
26 Superior mesenteric vein
27 Suspensory muscle of duodenum (muscle of Treitz)
28 Transverse colon
29 Ureter

The stomach (21) and transverse colon (28) are lifted upwards. The peritoneum of the posterior abdominal wall has been removed and the left-sided parts of the duodenum (7 and 6) reflected towards the right, to show the origin of the inferior mesenteric artery (12) from the aorta (1). The lower border of the pancreas (2) has been lifted up, revealing the splenic vein (24) with the inferior mesenteric (13) running into it. The ureter (29) has the gonadal vessels (10 and 11) in front of it and the genitofemoral nerve (9) behind it, lying on psoas major (22).

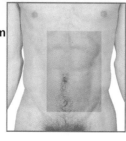

*Bowel ischaemia, see page 281.*

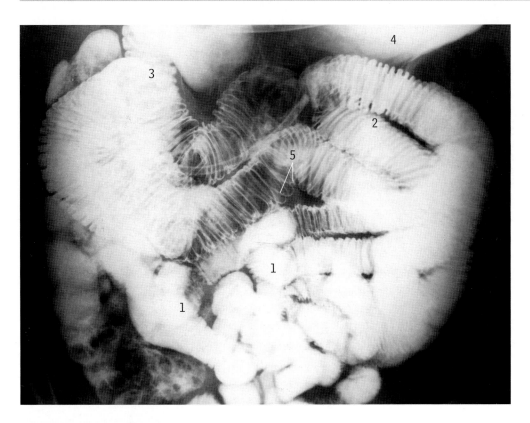

## **A** Small bowel radiograph

### *enema via a tube in the duodenum*

1 Coils of ileum
2 Coils of jejunum
3 Descending (second) part of duodenum
4 Stomach
5 Valvulae conniventes

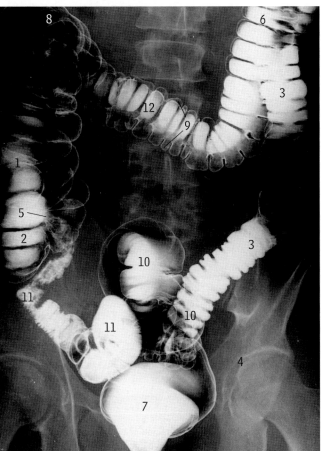

## **B** Large intestine *radiograph*

In this double-contrast barium enema (barium and air), the sacculations (haustrations, 9) of the various parts of the colon allow it to be distinguished from the narrower terminal ileum (11), which has become partly filled by barium flowing into it through the ileocaecal junction (5).

| | |
|---|---|
| 1 Ascending colon | 7 Rectum |
| 2 Caecum | 8 Right colic (hepatic) flexure |
| 3 Descending colon | 9 Sacculations |
| 4 Hip joint | 10 Sigmoid colon |
| 5 Ileocaecal junction | 11 Terminal ileum |
| 6 Left colic (splenic) flexure | 12 Transverse colon |

*Colostomy, see page 281.*

# Stomach *with vessels and vagus nerves, from the front*

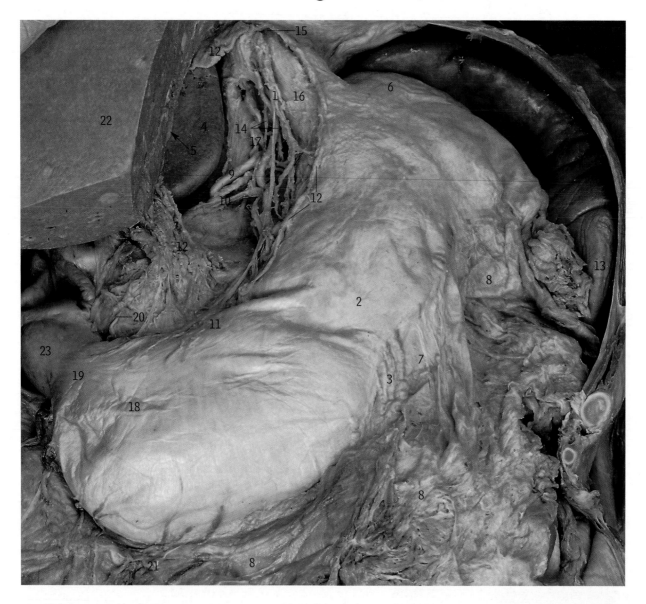

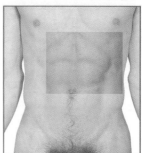

The anterior thoracic and abdominal walls and the left lobe of the liver have been removed, with part of the lesser omentum (12), to show the stomach (6, 2, 18 and 19) in its undisturbed position.

| | | | |
|---|---|---|---|
| **1** | Anterior (left) vagal trunk | **13** | Lower end of spleen |
| **2** | Body of stomach | **14** | Oesophageal branches of left gastric vessels |
| **3** | Branches of left gastro-epiploic vessels | | |
| **4** | Caudate lobe of liver | **15** | Oesophageal opening in diaphragm |
| **5** | Fissure for ligamentum venosum | **16** | Oesophagus |
| **6** | Fundus of stomach | **17** | Posterior (right) vagal trunk |
| **7** | Greater curvature of stomach | **18** | Pyloric antrum |
| **8** | Greater omentum | **19** | Pyloric canal |
| **9** | Left gastric artery | **20** | Right gastric artery |
| **10** | Left gastric vein | **21** | Right gastro-epiploic vessels and branches |
| **11** | Lesser curvature of stomach | **22** | Right lobe of liver |
| **12** | Lesser omentum (cut edge) | **23** | Superior (first) part of duodenum |

*Oesophageal varices, vagotomy, see pages 283, 284.*

# Upper abdomen **A** *stomach – barium meal*

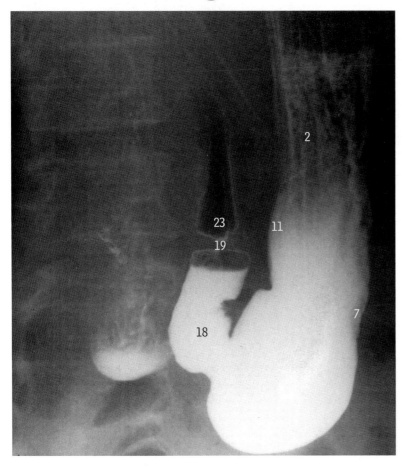

Labels key is shown on opposite page (242).

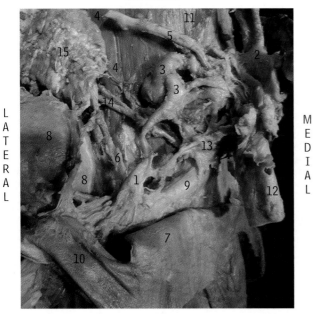

SUPERIOR

LATERAL

MEDIAL

INFERIOR

## **B** *posterior wall – coeliac ganglion and relations*

| | | |
|---|---|---|
| **1** | Aorto-renal ganglion | **8** Kidney, right |
| **2** | Coeliac arterial trunk (reflected anteriorly) | **9** Renal artery, right |
| **3** | Coeliac ganglion | **10** Renal vein (reflected) |
| **4** | Diaphragm | **11** Right crus, diaphragm |
| **5** | Inferior phrenic artery | **12** Superior mesenteric artery |
| **6** | Inferior suprarenal artery | **13** Superior mesenteric ganglion |
| **7** | Inferior vena cava (reflected inferiorly) | **14** Superior suprarenal artery |
| | | **15** Suprarenal gland |

*Coeliac plexus block, hiatus hernia, see pages 281, 282.*

# A Pancreas, duodenum and superior mesenteric vessels. *The stomach with its attached greater omentum has been lifted up.*

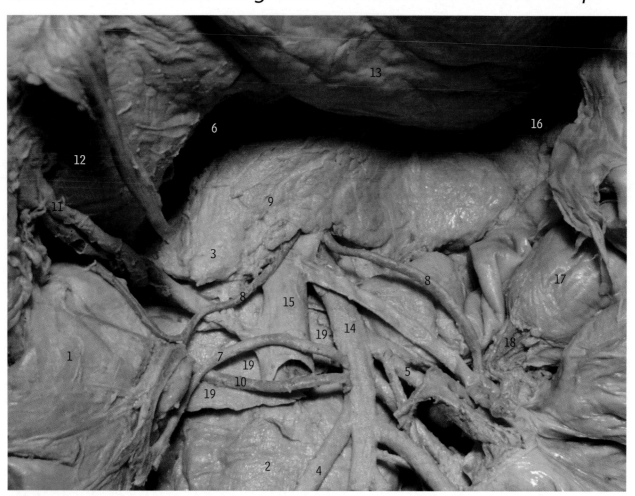

# B Duodenal papilla

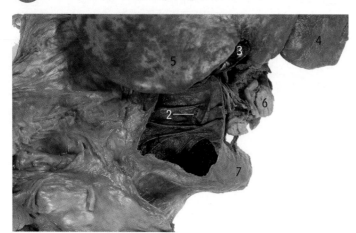

**The anterior wall of the descending (second) part of the duodenum has been removed.**

| | |
|---|---|
| **1** Circular folds of mucous membrane | **4** Liver, left lobe |
| **2** Duodenal papilla | **5** Liver, right lobe |
| **3** Gall bladder | **6** Pancreas |
| | **7** Third part of duodenum |

**The stomach has been retracted superiorly to reveal the 'stomach bed'.**

| | |
|---|---|
| **1** Ascending colon | **11** Right gastroepiploic vessels |
| **2** Duodenum, third part | **12** Stomach, antrum (reflected anteriorly) |
| **3** Head of pancreas | **13** Stomach, body |
| **4** Ileocolic artery | **14** Superior mesenteric artery |
| **5** Jejunal branch of superior mesenteric artery | **15** Superior mesenteric vein |
| **6** Lesser sac | **16** Tail of pancreas |
| **7** Middle colic artery | **17** Transverse colon |
| **8** Middle colic artery, aberrant variation | **18** Transverse colon, artery and vein |
| **9** Neck of pancreas | **19** Uncinate process of pancreas |
| **10** Right colic artery | |

*Pancreatitis, see page 283.*

# Liver *from the front*

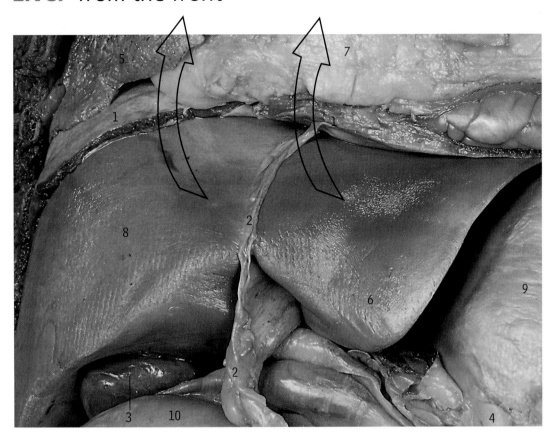

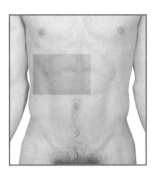

**1** Diaphragm
**2** Falciform ligament
**3** Gall bladder, fundus
**4** Greater omentum
**5** Inferior lobe of right lung
**6** Left lobe of liver
**7** Pericardial fat
**8** Right lobe of liver
**9** Stomach
**10** Transverse colon

For an explanation of peritoneal structures, see the diagrams on pages 224, 236.

The thoracic and abdominal walls and the anterior part of the diaphragm have been removed to show the undisturbed viscera. The liver (6 and 8) and stomach (9) are immediately below the diaphragm (1). The greater omentum (4) hangs down from the greater curvature (lower margin) of the stomach (9), overlying much of the small and large intestine but leaving some of the transverse colon (10) uncovered. The fundus (tip) of the gall bladder (3) is seen between the right lobe of the liver (8) and transverse colon (10). Arrows indicate the direction of liver reflection for the view on following page (page 246).

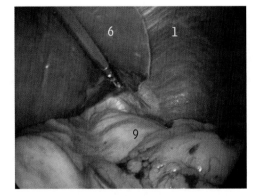

**Laparoscopic view of upper abdominal viscera**

*Liver trauma, see page 282.*

# Liver *from below and behind*

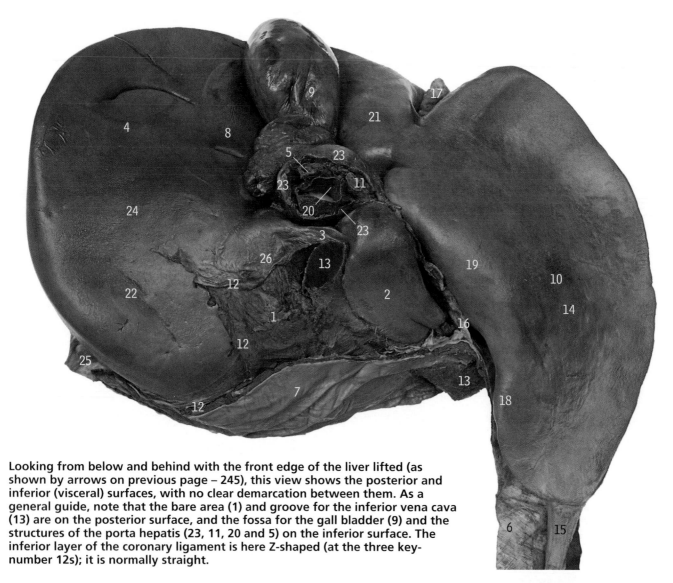

Looking from below and behind with the front edge of the liver lifted (as shown by arrows on previous page – 245), this view shows the posterior and inferior (visceral) surfaces, with no clear demarcation between them. As a general guide, note that the bare area (1) and groove for the inferior vena cava (13) are on the posterior surface, and the fossa for the gall bladder (9) and the structures of the porta hepatis (23, 11, 20 and 5) on the inferior surface. The inferior layer of the coronary ligament is here Z-shaped (at the three key-number 12s); it is normally straight.

| | |
|---|---|
| **1** Bare area | **14** Left lobe |
| **2** Caudate lobe | **15** Left triangular ligament |
| **3** Caudate process | **16** Lesser omentum in fissure for |
| **4** Colic impression | ligamentum venosum |
| **5** Common hepatic duct | **17** Ligamentum teres and |
| **6** Diaphragm | falciform ligament in fissure |
| **7** Diaphragm on part of bare | for ligamentum teres |
| area (obstructing view of | **18** Oesophageal groove |
| superior layer of coronary | **19** Omental tuberosity |
| ligament) | **20** Portal vein |
| **8** Duodenal impression | **21** Quadrate lobe |
| **9** Gall bladder | **22** Renal impression |
| **10** Gastric impression | **23** Right free margin of lesser |
| **11** Hepatic artery | omentum in porta hepatis |
| **12** Inferior layer of coronary | **24** Right lobe |
| ligament | **25** Right triangular ligament |
| **13** Inferior vena cava | **26** Suprarenal impression |

The caudate (2) and quadrate (21) lobes are classified anatomically as part of the right lobe (24), but functionally they belong to the left lobe (14), since they receive blood from the left branches of the hepatic artery and portal vein, and drain bile to the left hepatic duct.

*Liver abscess, Riedel's lobe, see pages 282, 283.*

# Cast of the liver, extrahepatic biliary tract and associated vessels *from below and behind*

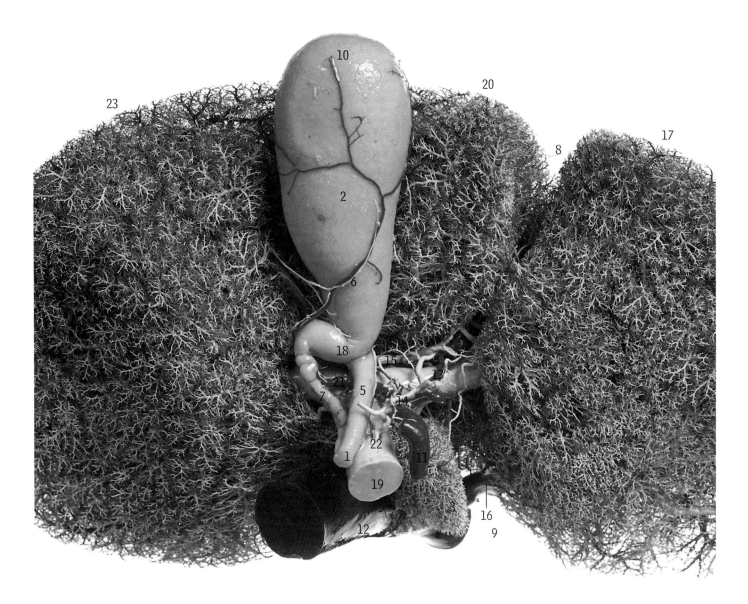

Yellow, gall bladder and biliary tract
Red, hepatic artery and branches
Light blue, portal vein and tributaries
Dark blue, inferior vena cava, hepatic veins and tributaries

This view, like the one opposite, shows the inferior and posterior surfaces, as looking into the abdomen from below with the lower border of the liver pushed up towards the thorax.

**1** Bile duct
**2** Body of gall bladder
**3** Caudate lobe
**4** Caudate process
**5** Common hepatic duct
**6** Cystic artery and veins
**7** Cystic duct
**8** Fissure for ligamentum teres
**9** Fissure for ligamentum venosum
**10** Fundus of gall bladder
**11** Hepatic artery
**12** Inferior vena cava
**13** Left branch of hepatic artery overlying left branch of portal vein

**14** Left gastric vein
**15** Left hepatic duct
**16** Left hepatic vein
**17** Left lobe
**18** Neck of gall bladder
**19** Portal vein
**20** Quadrate lobe
**21** Right branch of hepatic artery overlying right branch of portal vein
**22** Right gastric vein
**23** Right lobe

## Ⓐ Endoscopic retrograde cholangiopancreatogram *ERCP*

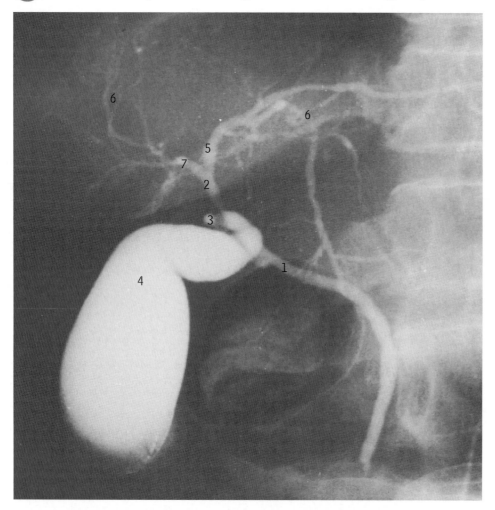

During an ERCP, an endoscope is passed through the mouth, pharynx, oesophagus and stomach into the duodenum, and through it, a cannula is introduced into the major duodenal papilla (page 244B) and bile duct so that contrast medium can be injected up the biliary tract. (The pancreatic duct can also be cannulated in this way – see B).

1 Common bile duct
2 Common hepatic duct
3 Cystic duct
4 Gall bladder
5 Left hepatic duct
6 Liver shadow and tributaries of hepatic ducts
7 Right hepatic duct

## Ⓑ Pancreatic duct *ERCP*

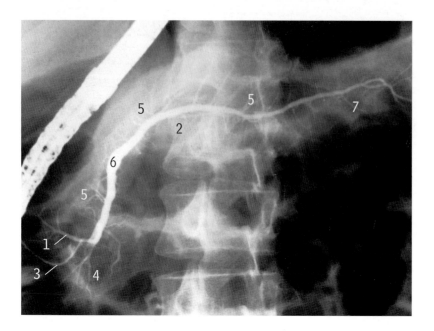

1 Accessory pancreatic duct (Santorini)
2 Body of pancreas
3 Cannula in ampulla (Vater)
4 Head of pancreas
5 Intralobular ducts of the pancreas
6 Pancreatic duct (Wirsung)
7 Tail of pancreas

# Cast of the portal vein and tributaries, and the mesenteric vessels *from behind*

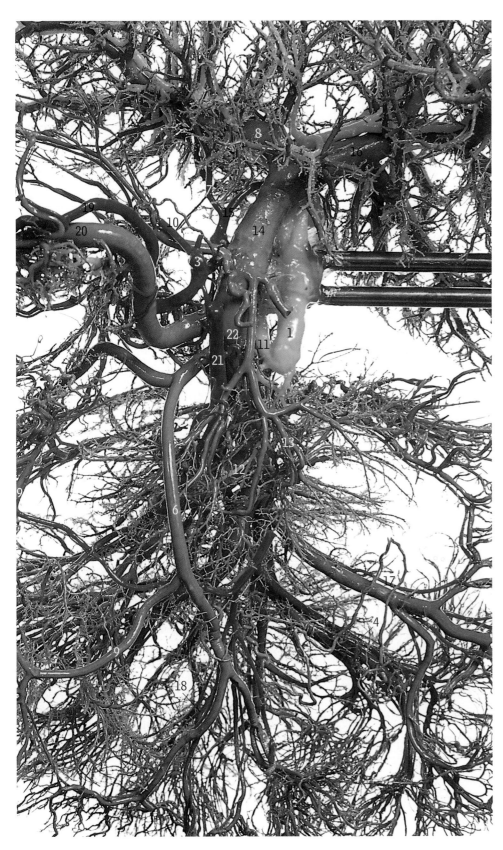

Yellow, biliary tract and pancreatic ducts
Red, arteries
Blue, portal venous system

**In this posterior view (chosen in preference to the anterior view, where the many very small vessels to the intestines would have obscured the larger branches), the superior mesenteric vein (22) is seen continuing upwards to become the portal vein (14) after it has been joined by the splenic vein (20). In the porta hepatis, the portal vein divides into the left and right branches (8 and 16). Owing to removal of the aorta, the upper part of the inferior mesenteric artery (5) has become displaced slightly to the right and appears to have given origin to the ileocolic artery (4), but this is simply an overlap of the vessels; the origin of the ileocolic from the superior mesenteric is not seen in this view.**

**1** Bile duct
**2** Branches of middle colic vessels
**3** Coeliac trunk
**4** Ileocolic vessels
**5** Inferior mesenteric artery
**6** Inferior mesenteric vein
**7** Left branch of hepatic artery
**8** Left branch of portal vein
**9** Left colic vessels
**10** Left gastric artery and vein
**11** Pancreatic duct
**12** Pancreatic ducts in head of pancreas
**13** Pancreaticoduodenal vessels
**14** Portal vein
**15** Right branch of hepatic artery
**16** Right branch of portal vein
**17** Right colic vessels
**18** Sigmoid vessels
**19** Splenic artery
**20** Splenic vein
**21** Superior mesenteric artery
**22** Superior mesenteric vein

## (A) Spleen *from the front*

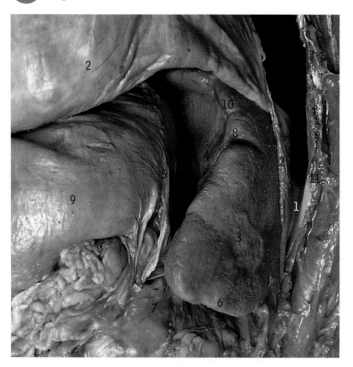

The left upper anterior abdominal and lower anterior thoracic walls have been removed and part of the diaphragm (2) turned upwards to show the spleen in its normal position, lying adjacent to the stomach (9) and colon (7), with the lower part against the kidney (D16 and 9, opposite).

The gastrosplenic ligament contains the short gastric and left gastro-epiploic branches of the splenic vessels.

The lienorenal ligament contains the tail of the pancreas and the splenic vessels.

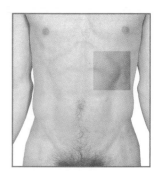

1  Costodiaphragmatic recess
2  Diaphragm
3  Diaphragmatic surface
4  Gastric impression
5  Gastrosplenic ligament
6  Inferior border
7  Left colic flexure
8  Notch
9  Stomach
10 Superior border
11 Thoracic wall

## (B) Spleen *visceral surface*

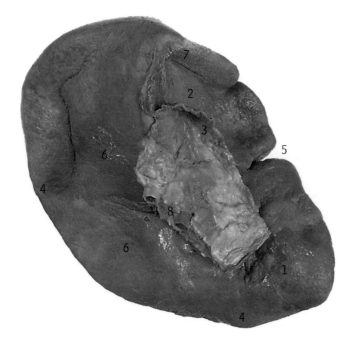

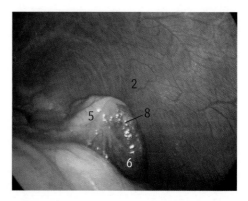

## (C) Laparoscopic view of spleen

**Labels refer to key in A.**

1  Colic impression
2  Gastric impression
3  Gastrosplenic ligament containing short gastric and left gastro-epiploic vessels
4  Inferior border
5  Notch
6  Renal impression
7  Superior border
8  Tail of pancreas and splenic vessels in lienorenal ligament

In B, the spleen has been removed and its visceral or medial surface is shown, with a small part of the gastrosplenic (3) and lienorenal (8) ligaments remaining attached.

*Splenomegaly, splenectomy, see page 283.*

# D Spleen *in a transverse section of the left upper abdomen*

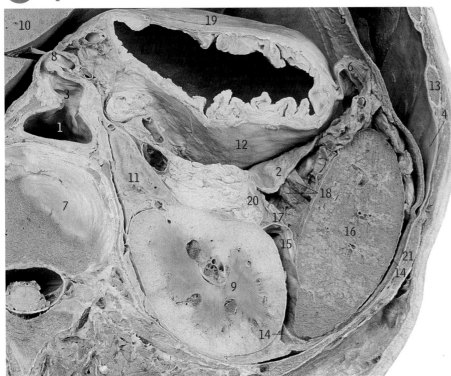

The section is at the level of the disc (7) between the twelfth thoracic and first lumbar vertebrae, and is viewed from below looking towards the thorax.

1 Abdominal aorta
2 Anterior layer of lienorenal ligament
3 Coeliac trunk
4 Costodiaphragmatic recess of pleura
5 Diaphragm
6 Gastrosplenic ligament
7 Intervertebral disc
8 Left gastric artery
9 Left kidney
10 Left lobe of liver
11 Left suprarenal gland
12 Lesser sac
13 Ninth rib
14 Peritoneum of greater sac
15 Posterior layer of lienorenal ligament
16 Spleen
17 Splenic artery
18 Splenic vein
19 Stomach
20 Tail of pancreas
21 Tenth rib

# E Caecum *in sagittal section, interior view*

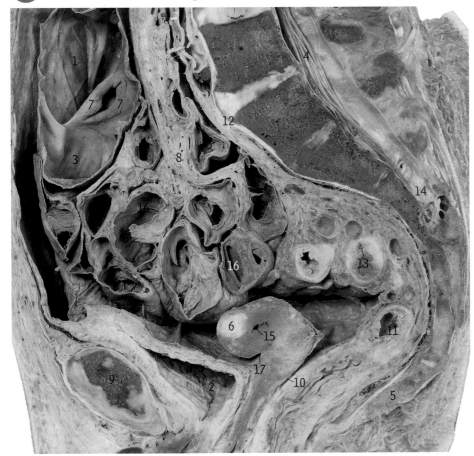

This is a median section of the female pelvis, right side viewed from the left. The caecal anterior wall has been cut open and reflected to show the lips of the

ileocaecal valve (7).
1 Ascending colon
2 Bladder
3 Caecum
4 Cauda equina
5 Coccyx
6 Fibroid in uterine fundus
7 Lips of ileocaecal valve
8 Mesentery of small intestine
9 Pubic symphysis
10 Recto-uterine pouch (of Douglas)
11 Rectum
12 Sacral promontory
13 Sigmoid colon
14 Thecal sac termination
15 Uterine cavity
16 Valvulae conniventes
17 Vesico-uterine pouch

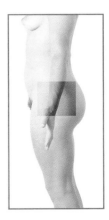

*Carcinoma of the bladder, see page 281.*

## Ⓐ Appendix, ileocolic artery and related structures *from the front*

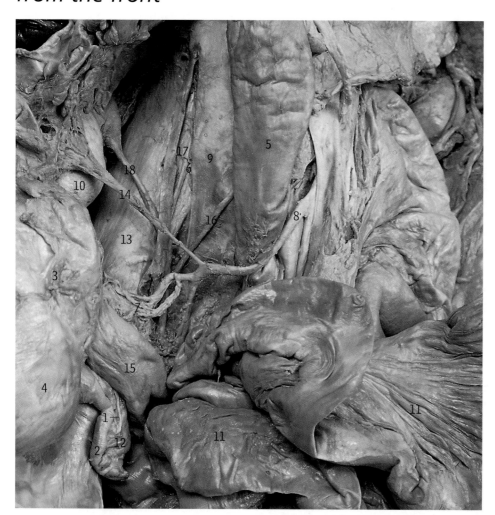

Most of the peritoneum of the mesentery and posterior abdominal wall has been removed, and coils of small intestine (11) have been displaced to the right of the picture, to show the ileocolic artery (8), terminal ileum (15) and appendix (2) with its appendicular artery (1).

1 Appendicular artery in mesoappendix
2 Appendix
3 Ascending colon
4 Caecum
5 Descending (second) part of duodenum
6 Genitofemoral nerve
7 Ileal and caecal vessels
8 Ileocolic artery
9 Inferior vena cava
10 Lower pole of kidney
11 Mesentery and coils of jejunum and ileum
12 Mesoappendix
13 Psoas major
14 Right colic artery
15 Terminal part of ileum
16 Testicular artery
17 Testicular vein
18 Ureter

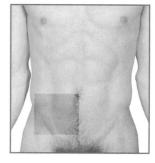

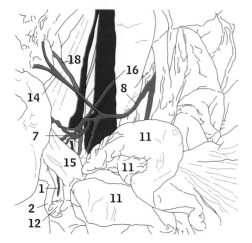

## Ⓑ Caecum and appendix *from the front*

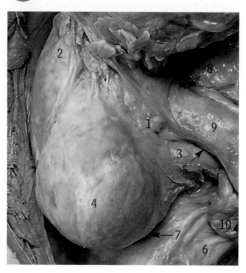

The terminal ileum (9) is seen joining the large intestine at the junction of the caecum (4) and ascending colon (2), and the appendix (3) joins the caecum just below the ileocaecal junction.

1 Anterior taenia coli
2 Ascending colon
3 Base of appendix
4 Caecum
5 Inferior ileocaecal recess
6 Peritoneum overlying external iliac vessels
7 Retrocaecal recess
8 Superior ileocaecal recess
9 Terminal ileum
10 Tip of appendix

*Appendicitis, see page 281.*

# Small intestine

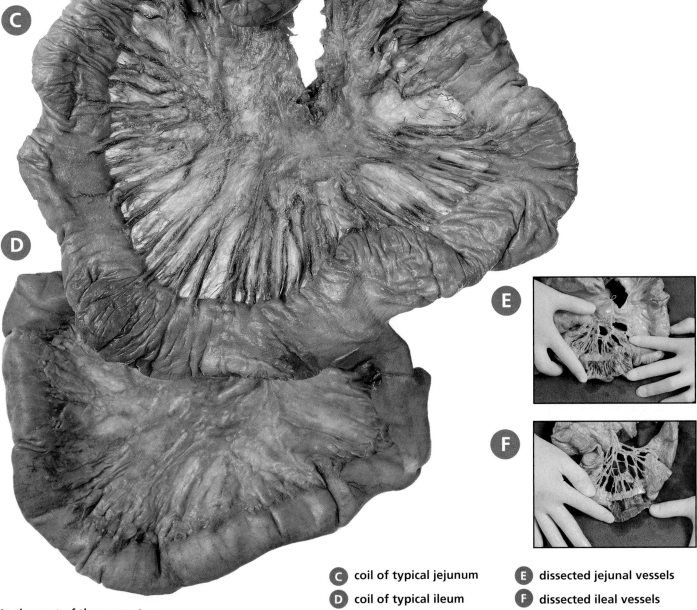

C  coil of typical jejunum
D  coil of typical ileum
E  dissected jejunal vessels
F  dissected ileal vessels

In the part of the mesentery supporting the jejunum in C, the vessels anastomose to form one or perhaps two vascular arcades (E) which give off long straight branches that run to the intestinal wall. The fat in the mesentery tends to be concentrated near the root, leaving areas or 'windows' near the gut wall that are devoid of fat. In the mesentery supporting the ileum in D, the vessels form several arcades with shorter branches (F), and there are no fat-free areas. The jejunal wall (C) is thicker than that of the ileum (D) and has a larger lumen. The jejunum also feels thicker, because the folds of its mucous membrane are more numerous than in the ileum.

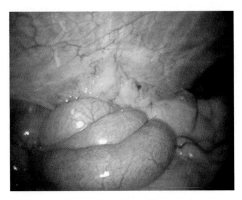

Laparoscopic view of small intestine

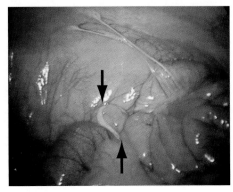

Laparoscopic view of appendix

# Kidneys and suprarenal glands

### A dissection    B right kidney and suprarenal gland, laparoscopic view

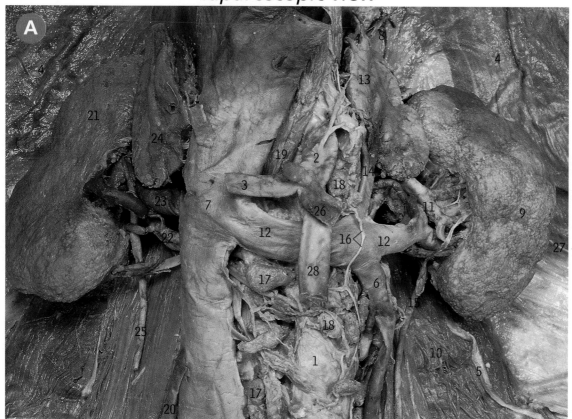

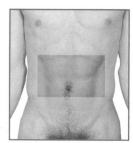

The kidneys (9 and 21) and suprarenal glands (13 and 24) are displayed on the posterior abdominal wall after the removal of all other viscera. The left renal vein (12) receives the left suprarenal (14) and gonadal (6) veins and then passes over the aorta (1) and deep to the superior mesenteric artery (28) to reach the inferior vena cava (7). In the hilum of the right kidney (21) a large branch of the renal artery (22) passes in front of the renal vein (23). The origins of the renal arteries from the aorta are not seen because they underlie the left renal vein (12) and inferior vena cava (7).

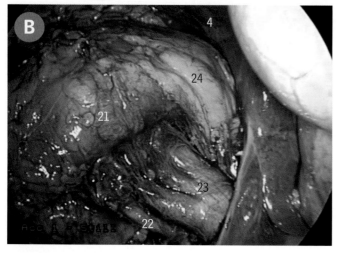

| | | | |
|---|---|---|---|
| **1** | Abdominal aorta and aortic plexus | **15** | Left ureter |
| **2** | Coeliac trunk | **16** | Lymphatic vessels |
| **3** | Common hepatic artery | **17** | Para-aortic lymph nodes |
| **4** | Diaphragm | **18** | Pre-aortic lymph nodes |
| **5** | First lumbar spinal nerve | **19** | Right crus of diaphragm |
| **6** | Gonadal vein, left | **20** | Right gonadal vein |
| **7** | Inferior vena cava | **21** | Right kidney |
| **8** | Left inferior phrenic vessels | **22** | Right renal artery |
| **9** | Left kidney | **23** | Right renal vein |
| **10** | Left psoas major | **24** | Right suprarenal gland |
| **11** | Left renal artery | **25** | Right ureter |
| **12** | Left renal vein | **26** | Splenic artery |
| **13** | Left suprarenal gland | **27** | Subcostal nerve, left |
| **14** | Left suprarenal vein | **28** | Superior mesenteric artery |

*Aortic bruits, see page 281.*

## C Left kidney, suprarenal gland and related vessels *from the front*

## D Right kidney, suprarenal gland and related vessels *from behind*

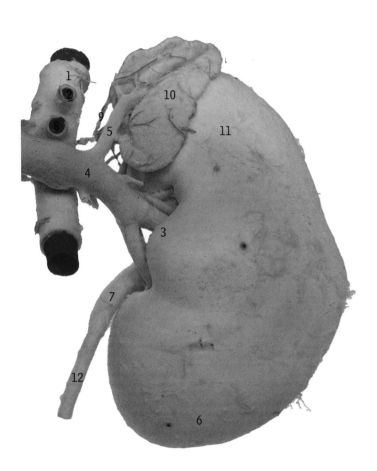

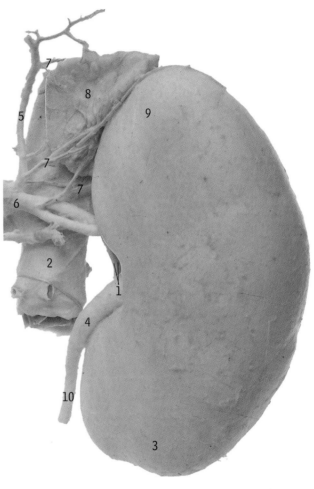

The vessels have been distended by injection of resin, and all fascia has been removed, but the suprarenal gland (10) has been retained in its normal position, lying against the medial side of the upper pole of the kidney (11).

| | |
|---|---|
| **1** Abdominal aorta | **7** Pelvis of kidney |
| **2** Coeliac trunk | **8** Superior mesenteric artery |
| **3** Hilum of kidney | **9** Suprarenal arteries |
| **4** Left renal vein overlying renal artery | **10** Suprarenal gland |
| | **11** Upper pole of kidney |
| **5** Left suprarenal vein | **12** Ureter |
| **6** Lower pole of kidney | |

Similar to B, but note that this is the right kidney from behind, not the left; the hilum of each kidney faces medially.

| | |
|---|---|
| **1** Hilum of kidney | **6** Right renal artery |
| **2** Inferior vena cava | **7** Suprarenal arteries |
| **3** Lower pole of kidney | **8** Suprarenal gland |
| **4** Pelvis of kidney | **9** Upper pole of kidney |
| **5** Right inferior phrenic artery | **10** Ureter |

 *Adrenal gland pathology, see page 281.*

## A Kidney *internal structure in longitudinal section*

The section is through the centre of the kidney and has included the renal pelvis (9) and beginning of the ureter (10). The major vessels in the hilum (2) have been removed.

| | | | |
|---|---|---|---|
| 1 | Cortex | 6 | Minor calix |
| 2 | Hilum | 7 | Renal column |
| 3 | Major calix | 8 | Renal papilla |
| 4 | Medulla | 9 | Renal pelvis |
| 5 | Medullary pyramid | 10 | Ureter |

The two or three major calices (3) unite to form the renal pelvis (9) which passes out through the hilum (2) to become the ureter (10), often with a slight narrowing at the junction. This is known as the pelvi-ureteric junction (PUJ) and is a site of renal stone obstruction.

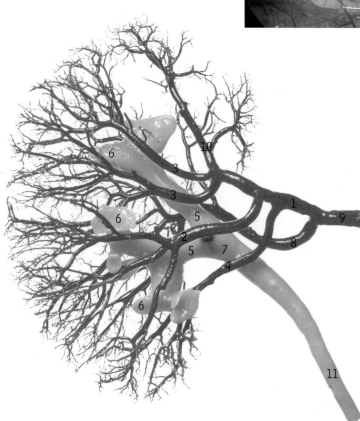

**Laparoscopic view of right kidney NB peritoneal covering**

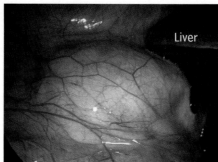

Liver

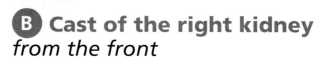

## B Cast of the right kidney *from the front*

Red, renal artery
Yellow, urinary tract

The posterior division (8) of the renal artery (9) here passes behind the pelvis (7) and upper calix (upper 5), but all other vessels are in front of the urinary tract; hence this is a right kidney seen from the front (vein, artery, ureter from front to back, and the hilum on the medial side – see page 255), not a left kidney from behind.

1 Anterior division of the renal artery
2 Anterior inferior segment artery
3 Anterior superior segment artery (double)
4 Inferior segment artery
5 Major calix
6 Minor calix
7 Pelvis of kidney
8 Posterior division (forming posterior segment artery)
9 Renal artery
10 Superior segment artery
11 Ureter

## C Cast of the aorta and kidneys *from the front*

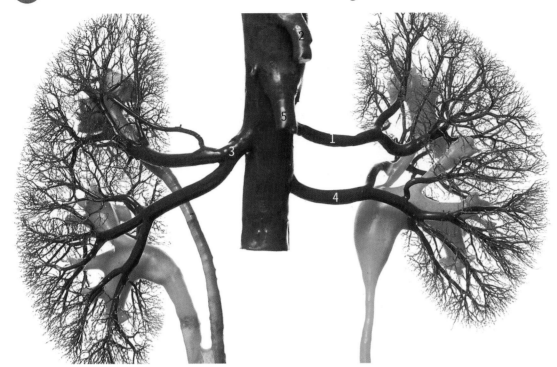

Red, arteries
Yellow, urinary tracts

1 Accessory left renal artery
2 Coeliac trunk
3 Early branching of right
  renal artery
4 Left renal artery
5 Superior mesenteric
  artery

Accessory renal arteries
represent segmental
vessels that arise
directly from the aorta.
In this specimen, the
left accessory vessel (C1)
supplies the superior
and anterior superior
segments, leaving
the 'normal' vessel to
supply the posterior,
anterior inferior and
inferior segments.

On the right side, the ureters (unlabelled) are double, each arising from a separate set of calices. On the left, the arteries are double (1 and 4).

## D Cast of the kidneys and great vessels *from the front*

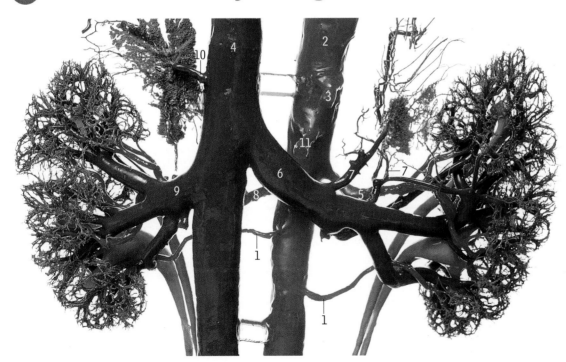

Red, arteries
Blue, veins
Yellow, urinary tracts

1 Accessory renal
  arteries
2 Aorta
3 Coeliac trunk
4 Inferior vena cava
5 Left renal artery
6 Left renal vein
7 Left suprarenal veins
8 Right renal artery
9 Right renal vein
10 Right suprarenal
  vein
11 Superior mesenteric
  artery

Here both kidneys show double ureters (unlabelled), and there are accessory renal arteries (1) to the lower poles of both kidneys. The suprarenal glands (also unlabelled) are outlined by their venous patterns, and the short right suprarenal vein (10) is shown draining directly to the inferior vena cava (4). On the left, there are two suprarenal veins (7), both draining to the left renal vein (6). See also page 258, A14, A9, A12.

# A Left kidney and suprarenal gland *from the front*

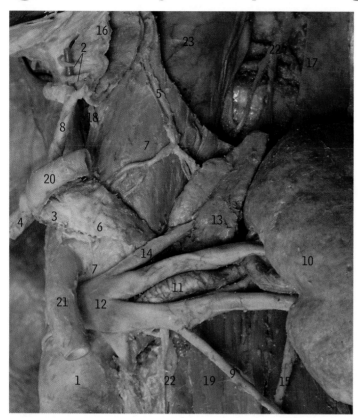

The left kidney (10) and suprarenal gland (13) are seen on the posterior abdominal wall. Much of the diaphragm has been removed but the oesophageal opening remains, with the end of the oesophagus (16) opening out into the cardiac part of the stomach and a (double) anterior vagal trunk (2) overlying the red marker. The posterior vagal trunk (18) is behind and to the right of the oesophagus. Part of the pleura has been cut away (17) to show the sympathetic trunk (22) on the side of the lower thoracic vertebrae. The left coeliac ganglion and the coeliac plexus (6) are at the root of the coeliac trunk (3).

1 Abdominal aorta
2 Anterior vagal trunk (double, over marker)
3 Coeliac trunk
4 Common hepatic artery
5 Inferior phrenic vessels
6 Left coeliac ganglion and coeliac plexus
7 Left crus of diaphragm
8 Left gastric artery
9 Left gonadal vein
10 Left kidney
11 Left renal artery
12 Left renal vein
13 Left suprarenal gland
14 Left suprarenal vein
15 Left ureter
16 Lower end of oesophagus
17 Pleura (cut edge)
18 Posterior vagal trunk
19 Psoas major
20 Splenic artery
21 Superior mesenteric artery
22 Sympathetic trunk
23 Thoracic aorta

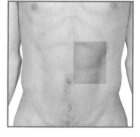

# B Right kidney and renal fascia *in transverse section from below*

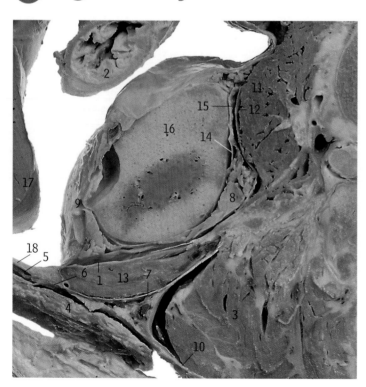

In the transverse section of the lower part of the right kidney (16), seen from below looking towards the thorax, the renal fascia (15) has been dissected out from the perirenal fat (8) and the kidney's own capsule (14). (There was a small cyst on the surface of this kidney.) The section also displays the three layers (10, 7 and 1) of the lumbar fascia (6).

1 Anterior layer of lumbar fascia
2 Coil of small intestine
3 Erector spinae
4 External oblique
5 Internal oblique
6 Lumbar fascia
7 Middle layer of lumbar fascia
8 Perirenal fat
9 Peritoneum
10 Posterior layer of lumbar fascia
11 Psoas major
12 Psoas sheath
13 Quadratus lumborum
14 Renal capsule
15 Renal fascia
16 Right kidney
17 Right lobe of liver
18 Transversus abdominis

Outside the kidney's own capsule (renal capsule, 14), there is a variable amount of fat (perirenal fat, 8) and outside this is a condensation of connective tissue forming the renal fascia (15).

*Nephrectomy, superior mesenteric artery syndrome, see pages 283, 284.*

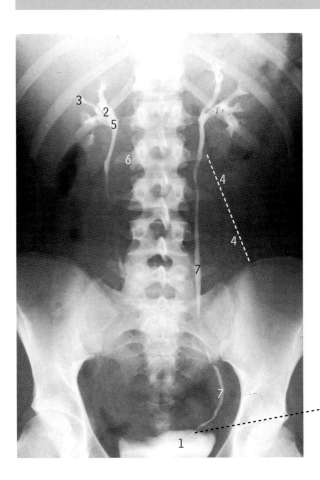

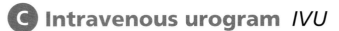

## C Intravenous urogram *IVU*

Contrast medium injected intravenously is excreted by the kidneys to outline the calices (3 and 2), renal pelvis (5) and the ureters (7) which enter the bladder (1) in the pelvis.

**1** Bladder
**2** Major calix
**3** Minor calix
**4** Psoas shadow
**5** Renal pelvis
**6** Transverse processes of lumbar vertebrae
**7** Ureter

The ureters normally lie near the tips of the transverse processes of the lumbar vertebrae and may kink over the psoas when the muscle is hypertrophied, e.g. in rowers.

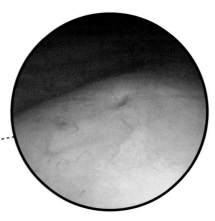

## Cytoscopic view of the ureteric orifice

## D Abdomen *coronal MR image*

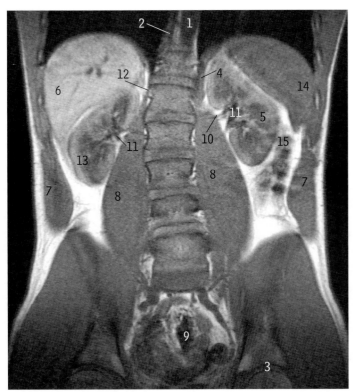

**1** Aorta
**2** Azygos vein
**3** Hip joint
**4** Left crus of diaphragm
**5** Left kidney
**6** Liver
**7** Oblique muscles of abdomen
**8** Psoas major muscle
**9** Rectum
**10** Renal artery
**11** Renal pelvis
**12** Right crus of diaphragm
**13** Right kidney
**14** Spleen
**15** Splenic flexure of colon

*Abdominal aortic aneurysm, urinary tract calculi, see pages 281, 284.*

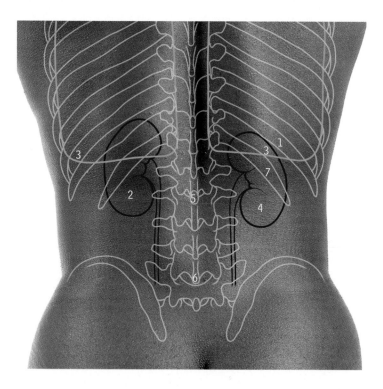

## A Kidneys and ureters

### surface markings, from behind

The upper pole of the left kidney rises to the level of the eleventh rib, but the right kidney is slightly lower (due to the bulk of the liver on the right). The hilum of each kidney is 5 cm (2 in) from the midline. The lower edge of the costodiaphragmatic recess of the pleura crosses the twelfth rib; compare with the dissection below (B6).

1 Eleventh rib
2 Left kidney
3 Lower edge of pleura
4 Right kidney
5 Spinous process of first lumbar vertebra
6 Spinous process of fourth lumbar vertebra
7 Twelfth rib

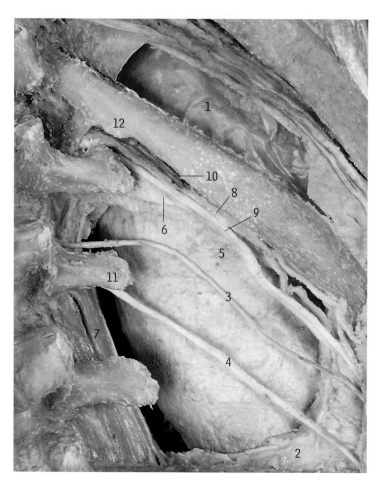

## B Right kidney *from behind*

Most thoracic and abdominal muscles have been removed to show the three nerves (9, 3 and 4) that lie behind the kidney (5). Much more important is the relationship of the upper part of the kidney to the pleura. A window has been cut in the parietal pleura above the twelfth rib (12) to open into the costodiaphragmatic recess (1), whose lower limit (6) runs transversely behind the kidney and in front of the obliquely placed twelfth rib.

1 Costodiaphragmatic recess of pleura
2 Extraperitoneal tissue
3 Iliohypogastric nerve
4 Ilio-inguinal nerve
5 Kidney
6 Lower edge of pleura
7 Psoas major
8 Subcostal artery
9 Subcostal nerve
10 Subcostal vein
11 Transverse process of second lumbar vertebra
12 Twelfth rib

*Lumbar hernia, renal biopsy, see page 283.*

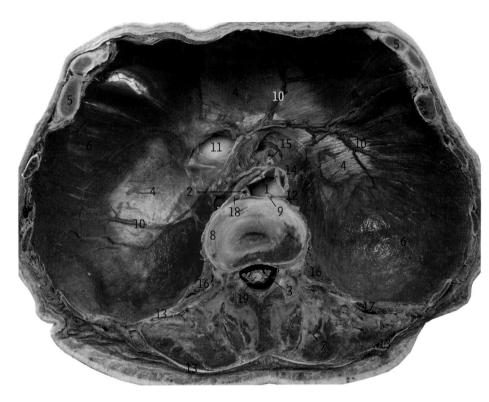

## A Diaphragm *from below*

1 Aorta
2 Azygos vein
3 Cauda equina
4 Central tendon of diaphragm
5 Costal margin
6 Diaphragm
7 Erector spinae muscles
8 First lumbar intervertebral disc
9 Hemi-azygos vein
10 Inferior phrenic vessels
11 Inferior vena caval opening
12 Left crus
13 Lumbar fascia
14 Median arcuate ligament
15 Oesophageal opening (hiatus)
16 Psoas major
17 Quadratus lumborum
18 Right crus
19 Spinal cord

Fibres of the right crus (A18) form the right and left boundaries of the oesophageal opening or hiatus (A15).

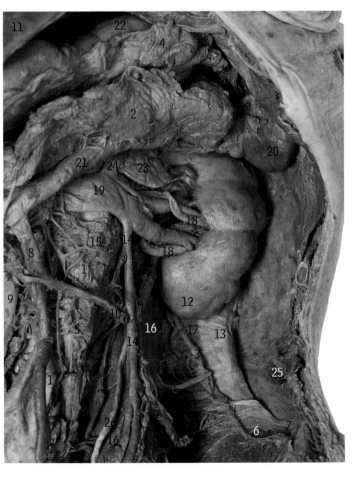

## B Posterior abdominal wall *left side*

The structures on the posterior abdominal wall are here viewed from the front. The body of the pancreas (2) has been turned upwards to expose the splenic vein (21). The suprarenal gland (23) appears detached from the superior pole of the kidney (compared with A13 and 10, page 258).

1 Aorta and aortic plexus
2 Body of pancreas
3 First lumbar spinal nerve
4 Greater omentum
5 Hypogastric plexus
6 Ilio-inguinal nerve
7 Iliohypogastric nerve
8 Inferior mesenteric vein
9 Inferior vena cava
10 Left colic vein
11 Liver
12 Lower pole of kidney
13 Lumbar part of thoracolumbar fascia
14 Ovarian vein
15 Para-aortic lymph node
16 Psoas major
17 Quadratus lumborum
18 Renal artery
19 Renal vein
20 Spleen

21 Splenic vein
22 Stomach
23 Suprarenal gland
24 Suprarenal vein
25 Transversus abdominis
26 Ureter

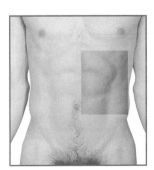

# Posterior abdominal and pelvic walls

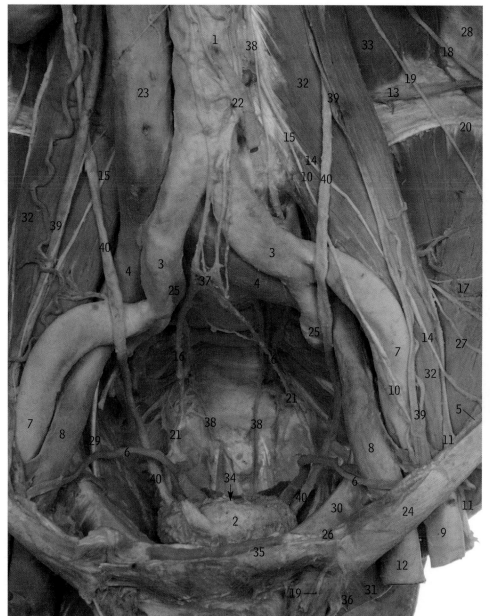

All peritoneum and viscera (except for the bladder, 2, ureter, 40, and ductus deferens or vas deferens, 6) have been removed, to display vessels and nerves.

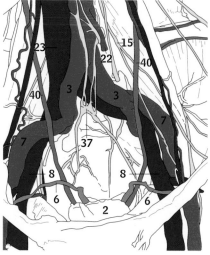

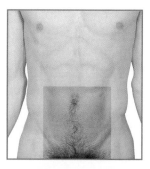

| | | |
|---|---|---|
| **1** Aorta and aortic plexus | **16** Hypogastric nerve | **28** Lumbar part of thoracolumbar fascia |
| **2** Bladder | **17** Iliacus and branches from femoral nerve and iliolumbar artery | **29** Obturator nerve and vessels |
| **3** Common iliac artery | **18** Iliohypogastric nerve | **30** Pectineal ligament |
| **4** Common iliac vein | **19** Ilio-inguinal nerve | **31** Position of femoral canal |
| **5** Deep circumflex iliac artery | **20** Iliolumbar ligament | **32** Psoas major |
| **6** Ductus deferens | **21** Inferior hypogastric (pelvic) plexus and pelvic splanchnic nerves | **33** Quadratus lumborum |
| **7** External iliac artery | **22** Inferior mesenteric artery and plexus | **34** Rectum (cut edge) |
| **8** External iliac vein | **23** Inferior vena cava | **35** Rectus abdominis |
| **9** Femoral artery | **24** Inguinal ligament | **36** Spermatic cord |
| **10** Femoral branch of genitofemoral nerve | **25** Internal iliac artery | **37** Superior hypogastric plexus |
| **11** Femoral nerve | **26** Lacunar ligament | **38** Sympathetic trunk and ganglia |
| **12** Femoral vein | **27** Lateral femoral cutaneous nerve arising from femoral nerve | **39** Testicular vessels |
| **13** Fourth lumbar artery | | **40** Ureter |
| **14** Genital branch of genitofemoral nerve | | |
| **15** Genitofemoral nerve | | |

*Psoas abscess, see page 283.*

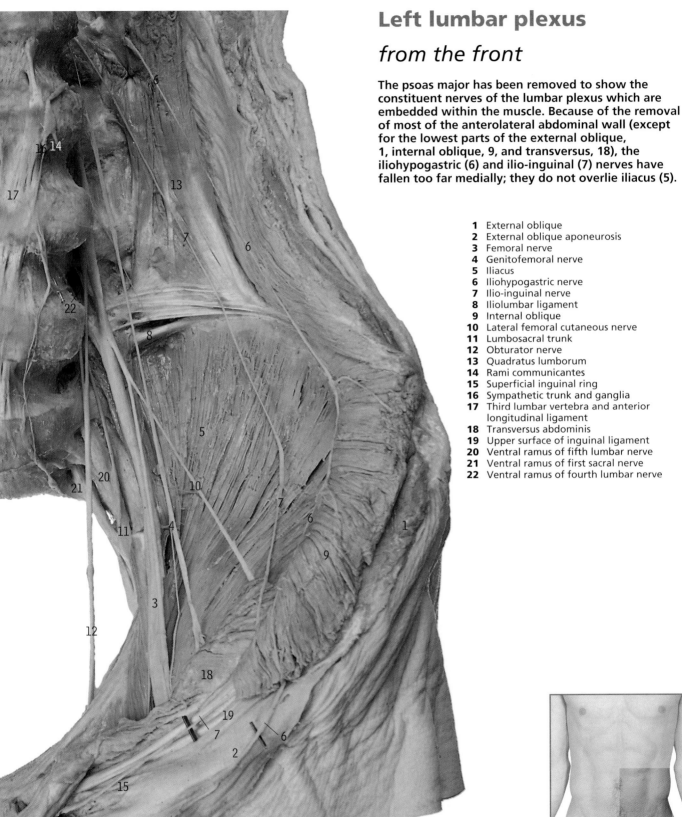

# Left lumbar plexus

## *from the front*

The psoas major has been removed to show the constituent nerves of the lumbar plexus which are embedded within the muscle. Because of the removal of most of the anterolateral abdominal wall (except for the lowest parts of the external oblique, 1, internal oblique, 9, and transversus, 18), the iliohypogastric (6) and ilio-inguinal (7) nerves have fallen too far medially; they do not overlie iliacus (5).

1 External oblique
2 External oblique aponeurosis
3 Femoral nerve
4 Genitofemoral nerve
5 Iliacus
6 Iliohypogastric nerve
7 Ilio-inguinal nerve
8 Iliolumbar ligament
9 Internal oblique
10 Lateral femoral cutaneous nerve
11 Lumbosacral trunk
12 Obturator nerve
13 Quadratus lumborum
14 Rami communicantes
15 Superficial inguinal ring
16 Sympathetic trunk and ganglia
17 Third lumbar vertebra and anterior longitudinal ligament
18 Transversus abdominis
19 Upper surface of inguinal ligament
20 Ventral ramus of fifth lumbar nerve
21 Ventral ramus of first sacral nerve
22 Ventral ramus of fourth lumbar nerve

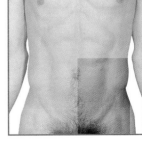

*Lumbar sympathectomy, see page 283.*

# Ⓐ Muscles of the left pelvis and proximal thigh
*slightly oblique anterior view*

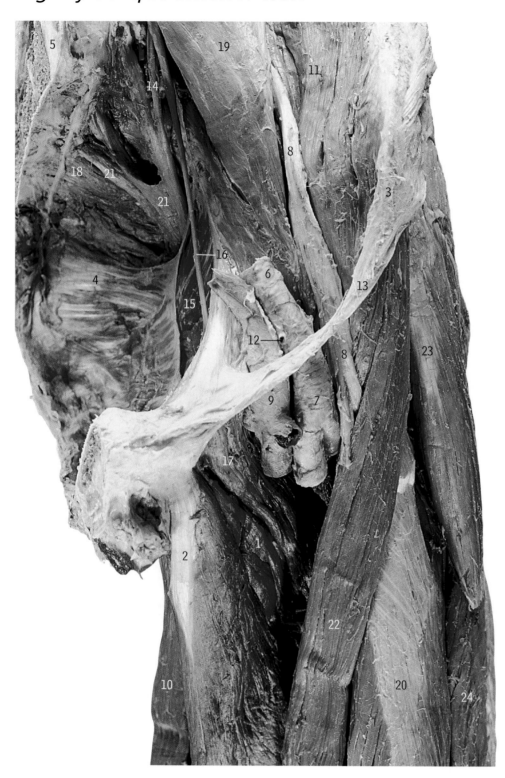

1 Adductor brevis
2 Adductor longus
3 Anterior superior iliac spine
4 Coccygeus
5 Disc, fifth lumbar
6 External iliac artery
7 Femoral artery
8 Femoral nerve
9 Femoral vein
10 Gracilis
11 Iliacus
12 Inferior epigastric artery, origin
13 Inguinal ligament
14 Lumbosacral trunk
15 Obturator internus
16 Obturator nerve
17 Pectineus
18 Piriformis
19 Psoas major
20 Rectus femoris
21 Sacral plexus
22 Sartorius
23 Tensor fasciae latae
24 Vastus lateralis

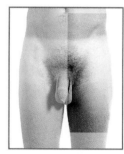

The anterior superior iliac spine
(3) and the pubic tubercle, which
give attachment to the ends of
the inguinal ligament (13), are
important palpable landmarks in
the inguinal region (see page
229).

The part of obturator internus
(15) *above* the attachment of
levator ani is part of the lateral
wall of the pelvic cavity, while the
part *below* the attachment is in
the perineum and forms part of
the lateral wall of the ischio-anal
(ischiorectal) fossa (pages 279
and 280).

Piriformis (18) passes out of the
pelvis into the gluteal region
through the *greater* sciatic
foramen *above* the ischial spine,
while obturator internus (15)
passes out through the *lesser*
sciatic foramen *below* the ischial
spine.

**The anterior abdominal wall, most viscera and fasciae have been removed. Segments
of the external iliac/femoral vessels and the inferior margin of the external oblique
aponeurosis (inguinal ligament) have been retained to assist orientation.**

# Muscles of the left half of the pelvis

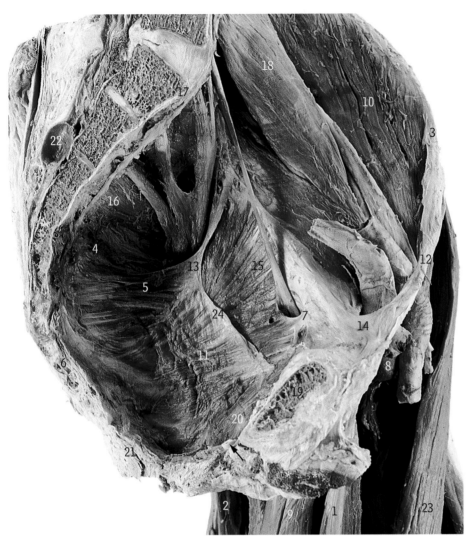

## B Male pelvis

The fascia overlying the obturator internus (15) has been removed down to the tendinous origin of the levator ani (11 and 20), a urethral catheter (arrow) indicates the position of the sphincter urethrae, and the plane of section passes through the bulbocavernosus (asterisks).

1 Adductor longus
2 Adductor magnus
3 Anterior superior iliac spine
4 Branch of fourth sacral nerve
5 Coccygeus
6 Coccyx
7 Fascia over obturator internus
8 Femoral vein
9 Gracilis
10 Iliacus
11 Iliococcygeus part of levator ani
12 Inguinal ligament
13 Ischial spine
14 Lacunar ligament
15 Obturator internus, pierced by obturator nerve
16 Piriformis
17 Promontory of sacrum
18 Psoas major
19 Pubic symphysis
20 Pubococcygeus part of levator ani
21 Rectum
22 Sacral canal with cyst
23 Sartorius
24 Arcus tendinous (white line)

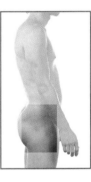

## Ⓐ Right spermatic cord and testis

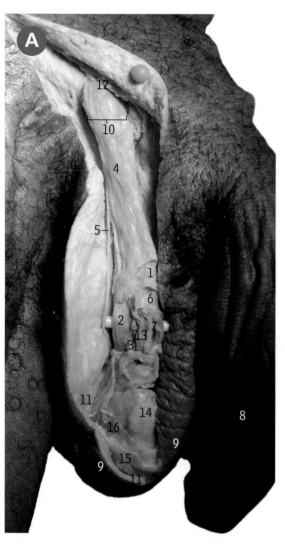

## Ⓑ Right testis, epididymis and penis *from the right*

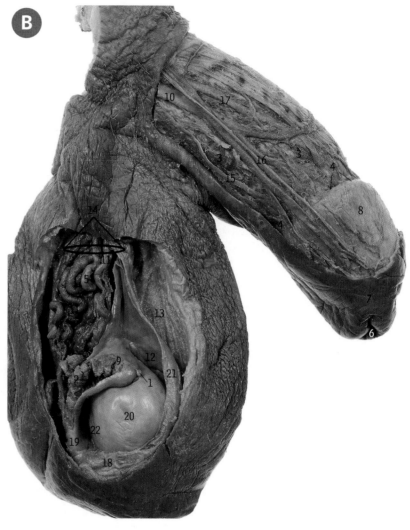

| | |
|---|---|
| **1** Cremasteric fascia | |
| **2** Ductus deferens | |
| **3** Ductus deferens, artery | |
| **4** External spermatic fascia | |
| **5** Ilio-inguinal nerve | |
| **6** Internal spermatic fascia | |
| **7** Pampiniform venous plexus | |
| **8** Penis | |
| **9** Scrotal sac | |
| **10** Spermatic cord | |
| **11** Superficial fascia with dartos muscle fibres | |
| **12** Superficial inguinal ring | |
| **13** Testicular artery | |
| **14** Tunica albuginea | |
| **15** Tunica vaginalis, parietal layer | |
| **16** Tunica vaginalis, visceral layer | |

| | |
|---|---|
| **1** Appendix epididymis | **13** Scrotal sac |
| **2** Body of epididymis | **14** Spermatic cord |
| **3** Body of penis | **15** Superficial dorsal artery |
| **4** Corona of glans | **16** Superficial dorsal nerve |
| **5** Ductus deferens | **17** Superficial dorsal vein |
| **6** External urethral orifice | **18** Superficial scrotal (dartos) fascia |
| **7** Foreskin | **19** Tail of epididymis |
| **8** Glans penis | **20** Testis |
| **9** Head of epididymis | **21** Tunica vaginalis, parietal |
| **10** Lateral superficial vein | **22** Tunica vaginalis, visceral, overlying tunica albuginea |
| **11** Pampiniform venous plexus | |
| **12** Sac of tunica vaginalis | |

*Circumcision, hydrocoele, phimosis and paraphimosis, scrotal swellings, varicocoeles, vasectomy, see pages 281–284.*

# Male pelvis *left half of a midline sagittal section*

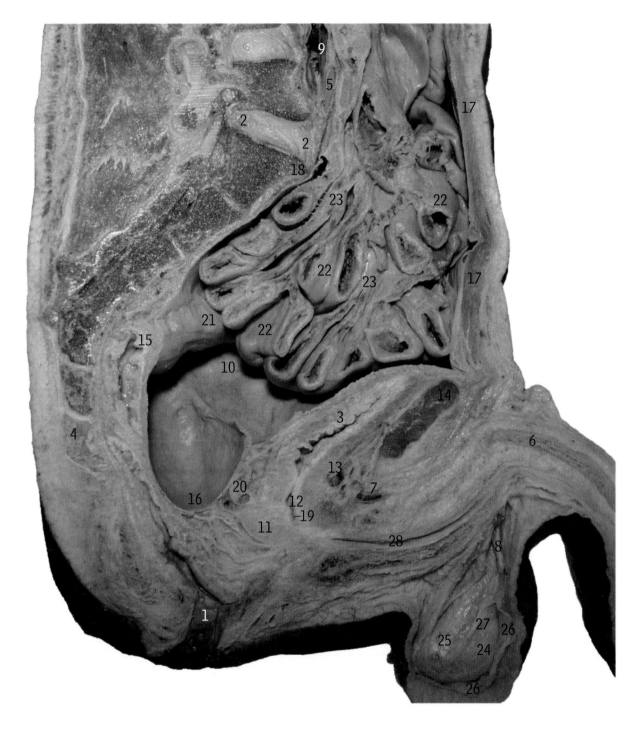

| | | |
|---|---|---|
| **1** Anal canal | **11** Prostate | **21** Sigmoid colon |
| **2** Annulus fibrosus | **12** Prostatic urethra | **22** Small intestine, multiple coils |
| **3** Bladder | **13** Prostatic venous plexus | **23** Superior mesenteric vessels, jejunal and |
| **4** Coccyx | **14** Pubic symphysis | ileal branches |
| **5** Common iliac artery | **15** Rectosigmoid junction | **24** Testis |
| **6** Corpus cavernosum | **16** Rectovesical pouch of pelvic peritoneum | **25** Tunica albuginea |
| **7** Deep dorsal vein of penis | **17** Rectus abdominis | **26** Tunica vaginalis, parietal layer |
| **8** Ductus deferens | **18** Sacral promontory | **27** Tunica vaginalis, visceral layer |
| **9** Inferior vena cava | **19** Seminal colliculus | **28** Urethra, bulbous |
| **10** Parietal peritoneum | **20** Seminal vesicle | |

*Extravasation of urine, proctoscopy and sigmoidoscopy, testicular torsion, see pages 282, 283, 284.*

## A Right deep inguinal ring and inguinal triangle *internal view*

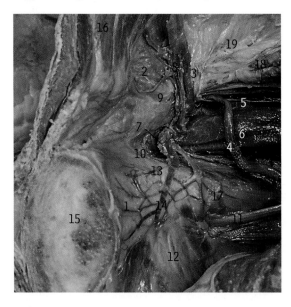

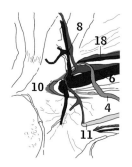

This is the view looking into the right half of the pelvis from the left, showing the posterior surface of the lower part of the anterior abdominal wall, above the pubic symphysis. The femoral ring (7), the entrance to the femoral canal, is below the medial end of the inguinal ligament (9). The inferior epigastric vessels (8) lie medial to the deep inguinal ring (3).

The inguinal triangle (Hesselbach's triangle) is the area bounded laterally by the inferior epigastric vessels (A8), medially by the lateral border of rectus abdominis (A16) and below by the inguinal ligament (A9). A direct inguinal hernia passes forwards through this triangle, medial to the inferior epigastric vessels.

An indirect inguinal hernia passes through the deep inguinal ring (A3) lateral to the inferior epigastric vessels (A8).

## B Right deep inguinal ring in male *internal peritoneal view*

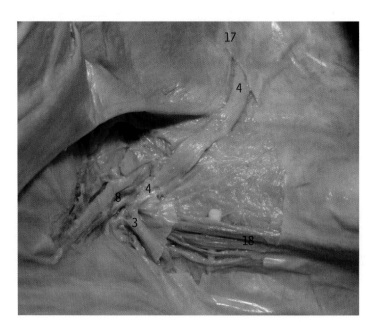

1 Body of pubis
2 Conjoint tendon
3 Deep inguinal ring
4 Ductus deferens
5 External iliac artery
6 External iliac vein
7 Femoral ring
8 Inferior epigastric vessels
9 Inguinal ligament
10 Lacunar ligament
11 Obturator nerve
12 Origin of levator ani from fascia overlying obturator internus
13 Pectineal ligament
14 Pubic branches of inferior epigastric vessels
15 Pubic symphysis
16 Rectus abdominis
17 Superior ramus of pubis
18 Testicular vessels
19 Transversalis fascia overlying transversus abdominis

# Pelvis, right inguinal region and penis *from above*

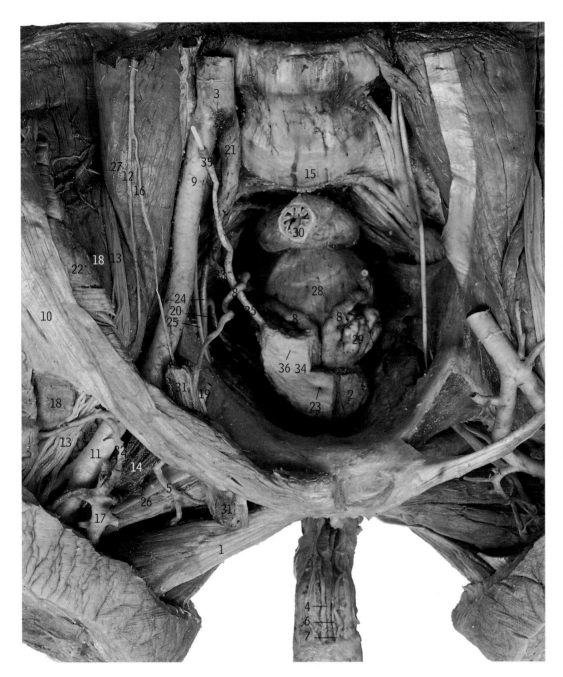

In the pelvis, most of the bladder (34) has been removed to show part of the basal surface of the prostate (2), and the left seminal vesicle (29) lying lateral to the ductus deferens (8). The ductus in the pelvis crosses superficial to the ureter (35). The external iliac artery (9) passes under the inguinal ligament (10) to become the femoral artery (11). On the dorsum of the penis, the fascia has been removed, showing the single midline deep dorsal vein (4) with a dorsal artery (6) and dorsal nerve (7) on each side.

The trigone of the bladder (34), at the lower part of the base or posterior surface, is the relatively fixed area with smooth mucous membrane between the internal urethral orifice (23) and the two ureteral openings (36 on the right side).

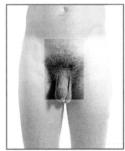

| | | |
|---|---|---|
| **1** Adductor longus | **13** Femoral nerve | **26** Pectineus |
| **2** Base of prostate | **14** Femoral vein | **27** Psoas major |
| **3** Common iliac artery | **15** Fifth lumbar intervertebral disc | **28** Rectum |
| **4** Deep dorsal vein of penis | **16** Genital branch of genitofemoral | **29** Seminal vesicle |
| **5** Deep external pudendal artery | nerve | **30** Sigmoid colon (cut lower end) |
| **6** Dorsal artery of penis | **17** Great saphenous vein | **31** Spermatic cord |
| **7** Dorsal nerve of penis | **18** Iliacus | **32** Superficial circumflex iliac vein |
| **8** Ductus deferens | **19** Inferior epigastric artery | **33** Superior vesical artery |
| **9** External iliac artery | **20** Inferior vesical artery | **34** Trigone of bladder |
| **10** External oblique aponeurosis | **21** Internal iliac artery | **35** Ureter |
| and inguinal ligament | **22** Internal oblique | **36** Ureteral orifice |
| **11** Femoral artery | **23** Internal urethral orifice | |
| **12** Femoral branch of | **24** Obturator artery | |
| genitofemoral nerve | **25** Obturator nerve | |

*Carcinoma of the large bowel, cystoscopy, see pages 281, 282.*

# A Bladder and prostate *from behind*

1 Base of bladder
2 Ductus deferens
3 Left ejaculatory duct
4 Posterior surface of prostate
5 Seminal vesicle
6 Ureter

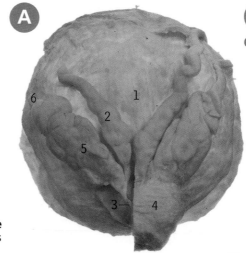

# B Left side of the male pelvis *from the right*

In this midline sagittal section, the prostate (24) is enlarged, lengthening the prostatic urethra (25) and accentuating the trabeculae of the bladder. The mucous membrane of the bladder (whose trigone is labelled at 36) has been removed to show muscular trabeculae in the wall. Variations in the branches of the internal iliac artery (14) are common, and here the obturator artery (22) gives origin to the superior vesical (34) and inferior vesical (13) as well as the middle rectal (20) arteries.

# C Cytoscopy of bladder

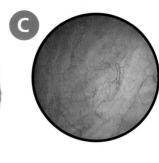

# D Cytoscopy of prostate (TURP)

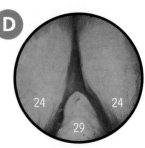

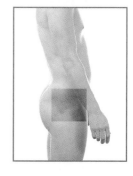

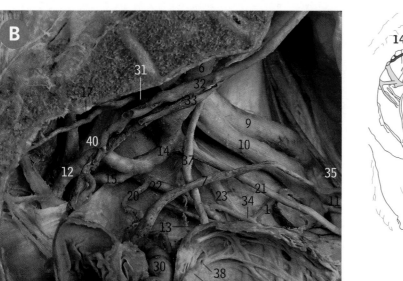

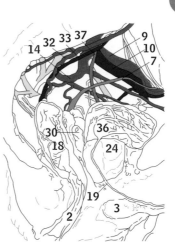

| | | |
|---|---|---|
| 1 | Accessory obturator vein | |
| 2 | Anal canal | |
| 3 | Bulb of penis | |
| 4 | Bulbar part of spongy urethra | |
| 5 | Bulbospongiosus | |
| 6 | Common iliac artery | |
| 7 | Ductus deferens | |
| 8 | External anal sphincter | |
| 9 | External iliac artery | |
| 10 | External iliac vein | |
| 11 | Inferior epigastric vessels | |
| 12 | Inferior gluteal artery | |
| 13 | Inferior vesical artery | |
| 14 | Internal iliac artery | |
| 15 | Internal pudendal artery | |
| 16 | Internal urethral orifice | |
| 17 | Lateral sacral artery | |
| 18 | Lower end of rectum | |
| 19 | Membranous part of urethra | |
| 20 | Middle rectal artery | |
| 21 | Obliterated umbilical artery | |
| 22 | Obturator artery | |
| 23 | Obturator nerve | |
| 24 | Prostate (enlarged) | |
| 25 | Prostatic part of urethra | |
| 26 | Pubic symphysis | |
| 27 | Puborectalis part of levator ani | |
| 28 | Rectovesical fascia | |
| 29 | Seminal colliculus | |
| 30 | Seminal vesicle | |
| 31 | Superior gluteal artery | |
| 32 | Superior rectal artery | |
| 33 | Superior rectal vein | |
| 34 | Superior vesical artery | |
| 35 | Testicular vessels and deep inguinal ring | |
| 36 | Trigone of bladder | |
| 37 | Ureter | |
| 38 | Ureteral orifice | |
| 39 | Urogenital diaphragm | |
| 40 | Ventral ramus of first sacral nerve | |
| 41 | Vesicoprostatic venous plexus | |

*Benign prostatic hyperplasia, carcinoma of the prostate, transurethral resection of prostate (TURP), see pages 281, 284.*

# A Arteries and nerves of the pelvis *from the right*

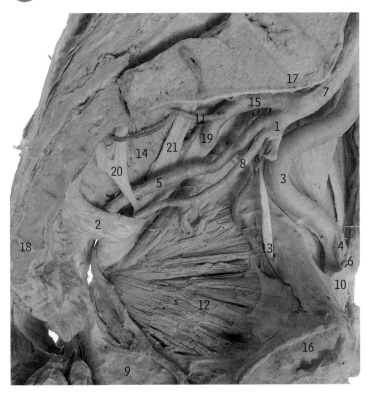

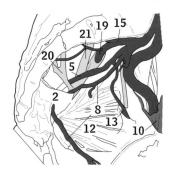

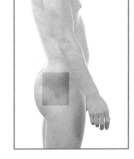

| | |
|---|---|
| **1** Anterior trunk of internal iliac artery | **13** Obturator nerve and artery |
| **2** Coccygeus and sacrospinous ligament | **14** Piriformis |
| **3** External iliac artery | **15** Posterior trunk of internal iliac artery |
| **4** Inferior epigastric artery | **16** Pubic symphysis |
| **5** Inferior gluteal artery | **17** Sacral promontory |
| **6** Inguinal ligament | **18** Sacrococcygeal joint |
| **7** Internal iliac artery | **19** Superior gluteal artery piercing lumbosacral trunk |
| **8** Internal pudendal artery | **20** Union of ventral rami of second and third sacral nerves |
| **9** Ischial tuberosity | |
| **10** Lacunar ligament | **21** Ventral ramus of first sacral nerve |
| **11** Lateral sacral artery | |
| **12** Obturator internus | |

In this left half section of the pelvis, all peritoneum, fascia, veins and visceral arteries have been removed together with the left levator ani, so displaying the whole of the internal surface of obturator internus (12). On the posterior pelvic wall, the vessels in general lie superficial to the nerves.

In this specimen, the external iliac artery (3) is unusually tortuous, and the anterior trunk of the internal iliac artery (1) has divided unusually high up into its terminal branches, the internal pudendal (8) and the inferior gluteal (5). The superior gluteal artery (19) has perforated the lumbosacral trunk.

# B Left inferior hypogastric plexus *from the right*

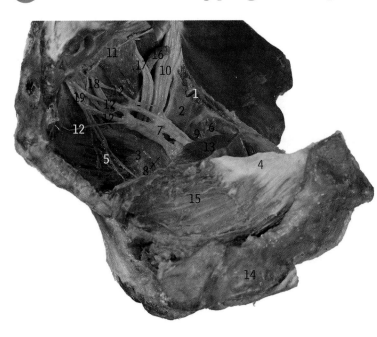

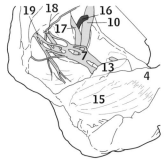

| | |
|---|---|
| **1** Arcuate line of ilium | |
| **2** Fascia overlying obturator internus | |
| **3** Ischial spine | |
| **4** Lateral surface of fascia overlying right obturator internus | |
| **5** Left coccygeus and nerves to levator ani | |
| **6** Left ductus deferens | |
| **7** Left inferior hypogastric plexus | |
| **8** Left levator ani | |
| **9** Left seminal vesicle | |
| **10** Lumbosacral trunk | |
| **11** Part of left sympathetic trunk | |
| **12** Pelvic splanchnic nerves (nervi erigentes) | |
| **13** Rectum | |
| **14** Right ischiopubic ramus | |
| **15** Right levator ani and ischio-anal (ischiorectal) fossa | |
| **16** Superior gluteal artery | |
| **17** Ventral ramus of first sacral nerve | |
| **18** Ventral ramus of second sacral nerve | |
| **19** Ventral ramus of third sacral nerve | |

In this view of the left side of the pelvis from the right, the right pelvic wall has been removed but the right levator ani (15) forming part of the pelvic floor (pelvic diaphragm) has been preserved and is seen from its right (perineal) side. Pelvic splanchnic nerves (12) arise from the ventral rami of the second and third sacral nerves (18 and 19) and contribute to the inferior hypogastric plexus (7).

# Internal Iliac artery *branches and relationships, left side female pelvis*

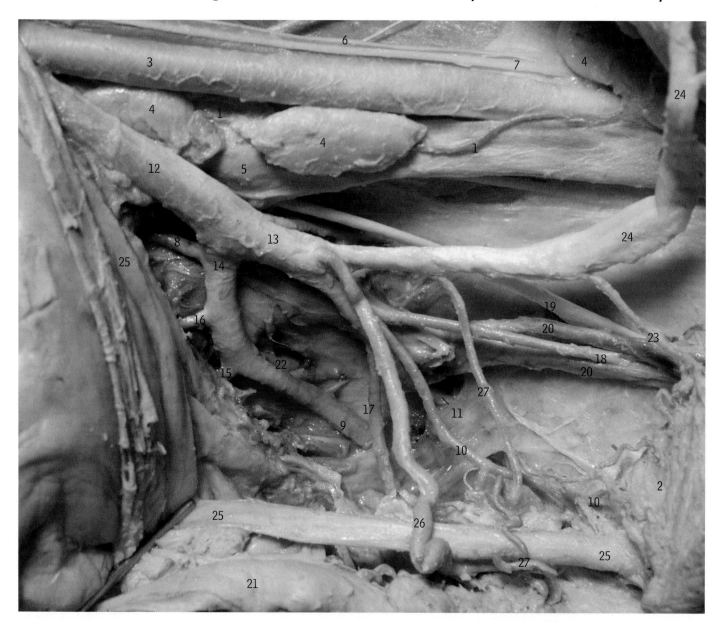

| | | |
|---|---|---|
| **1** Artery to iliac nodes | **10** Inferior vesical artery | **19** Obturator nerve |
| **2** Bladder | **11** Internal pudendal artery | **20** Obturator veins |
| **3** External iliac artery | **12** Internal iliac artery | **21** Round ligament of the uterus (reflected) |
| **4** External iliac lymph nodes (enlarged) | **13** Internal iliac artery, anterior division | **22** Superior gluteal artery |
| **5** External iliac vein | **14** Internal iliac artery, posterior division | **23** Superior vesical artery |
| **6** Genitofemoral nerve, femoral branch | **15** Lateral sacral artery, inferior | **24** Umbilical artery remnant |
| **7** Genitofemoral nerve, genital branch | **16** Lateral sacral artery, superior | **25** Ureter (retracted) |
| **8** Iliolumbar artery | **17** Middle rectal artery | **26** Uterine artery |
| **9** Inferior gluteal artery | **18** Obturator artery | **27** Vaginal artery |

# A Pelvic skeleton and ligaments *left side*

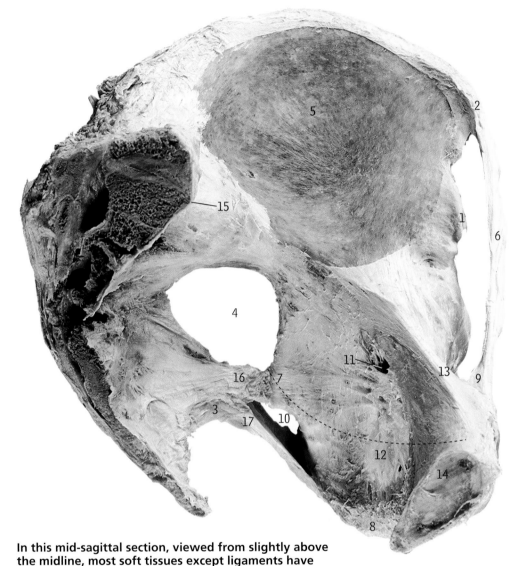
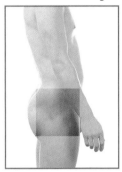

1 Anterior inferior iliac spine and origin of straight head of rectus femoris
2 Anterior superior iliac spine
3 Falciform process of sacrotuberous ligament
4 Greater sciatic foramen
5 Iliac fossa
6 Inguinal ligament
7 Ischial spine
8 Ischial tuberosity
9 Lacunar ligament
10 Lesser sciatic foramen
11 Obturator foramen with obturator nerve and vessels
12 Obturator membrane
13 Pectineal ligament
14 Pubic symphysis
15 Sacral promontory
16 Sacrospinous ligament
17 Sacrotuberous ligament

The ligaments classified as 'the ligaments of the pelvis' (vertebropelvic ligaments) are the sacrotuberous (17), sacrospinous (16) and iliolumbar (seen in the posterior view on page 325, C7).

The lacunar ligament (9) passes backwards from the medial end of the inguinal ligament (6) to the medial end of the pectineal line of the pubis, to which the pectineal ligament (13) is attached.

In this mid-sagittal section, viewed from slightly above the midline, most soft tissues except ligaments have been removed.

# B Greater sciatic foramen, sacral plexus and levator ani *left side*

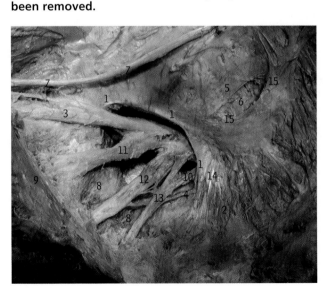

1 Greater sciatic foramen
2 Levator ani
3 Lumbosacral trunk (with S1)
4 Nerve to levator ani
5 Obturator internus fascia
6 Obturator internus muscle
7 Obturator nerve
8 Piriformis muscle fibres (muscle bulk removed)
9 Posterior longitudinal ligament, overlying sacrum
10 Pudendal nerve
11 Sacral nerve, S2
12 Sacral nerve, S3 and S4
13 Sacral nerve, S5
14 Sacrospinous ligament
15 Tendinous arch of levator ani, an origin of levator

*Bone marrow aspiration, see page 281.*

# Female pelvis *left half with arterial injection, viewed from right*

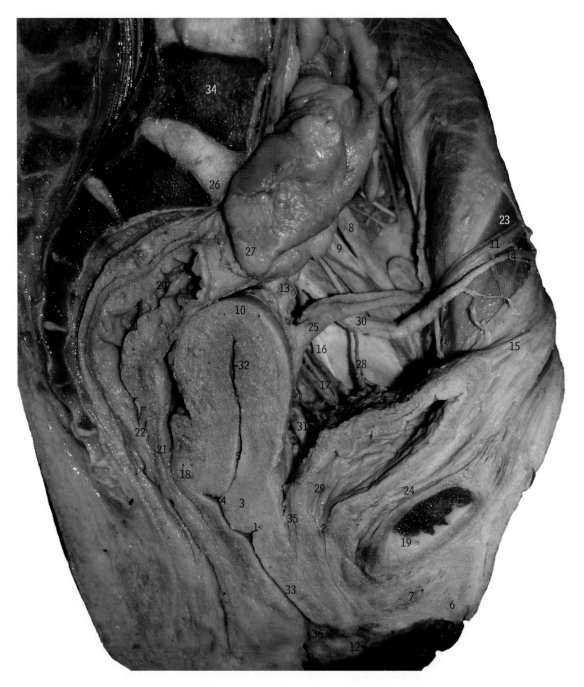

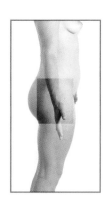

| | | |
|---|---|---|
| **1** Anterior vaginal fornix | **15** Median umbilical ligament (urachus) | **27** Sigmoid colon |
| **2** Bladder neck | **16** Obturator nerve | **28** Superior vesical artery |
| **3** Cervix | **17** Obturator vessels | **29** Trigone of bladder |
| **4** Cervix, external os | **18** Posterior vaginal fornix | **30** Umbilical artery (remnant) |
| **5** Cervix, internal os | **19** Pubic symphysis | **31** Ureter |
| **6** Clitoris | **20** Rectosigmoid junction | **32** Uterine cavity |
| **7** Crus of clitoris | **21** Rectouterine peritoneal space | **33** Vagina |
| **8** External iliac artery | **22** Rectum | **34** Vertebral body, L5 |
| **9** External iliac vein | **23** Rectus abdominis | **35** Vesicouterine peritoneal pouch |
| **10** Fundus uterus | **24** Retropubic space | **36** Vestibule of vagina |
| **11** Inferior epigastric vessels | **25** Round ligament of uterus | |
| **12** Labium minus | **26** Sacral promontory | **NB: retroverted uterus – a common normal variant.** |
| **13** Ligament of ovary | | |
| **14** Medial umbilical ligament | | |

*Faecal continence, haemorrhoids, rectal examination, rectal prolapse, uterine fibroids, see pages 282, 283, 284.*

# Female pelvis

## A sagittal MR image during menstruation    B coronal MR image

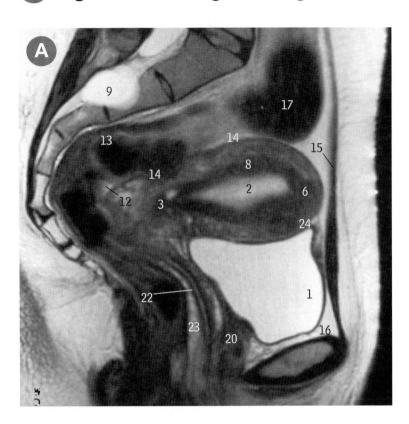

1 Bladder
2 Blood clot in endometrial cavity
3 Cervix of uterus
4 Corpus luteum
5 Endometrial cavity
6 Fundus of uterus
7 Levator ani
8 Myometrium
9 Nerve root cyst (Tarlov)
10 Ovary
11 Perineal muscles
12 Posterior fornix of vagina
13 Rectosigmoid junction
14 Recto-uterine pouch (Douglas)
15 Rectus abdominis muscle
16 Retropubic space (Retzius)
17 Sigmoid colon
18 Small intestine
19 Trigone
20 Urethra
21 Uterine (Fallopian) tube
22 Vaginal cavity
23 Vaginal wall
24 Vesico-uterine pouch

**Looking down into the pelvis from the front, the fundus of the uterus (6) overlies the bladder (1) with the peritoneum of the vesico-uterine pouch (24) intervening. These relationships are seen in this MR image.**

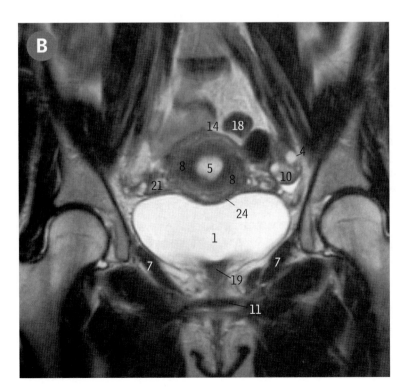

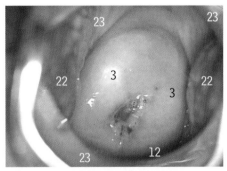

**Speculum examination of cervix**

*Cervical smear, cystitis, ovarian dermoid, vaginal examination (PV), see pages 281–284.*

# Female pelvis

## **A** *uterus and ovaries, from above and in front* **B** *hysterosalpingogram*

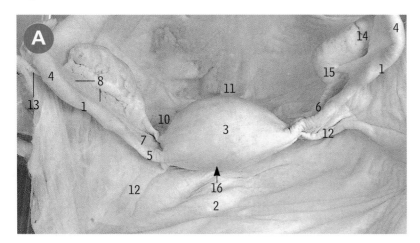

| | |
|---|---|
| **1** Ampulla of uterine tube | **10** Posterior surface of broad |
| **2** Bladder | ligament |
| **3** Fundus of uterus | **11** Recto-uterine space |
| **4** Infundibulum of uterine tube | **12** Round ligament of uterus |
| **5** Isthmus of uterine tube | **13** Suspensory ligament of ovary |
| **6** Ligament of ovary | with ovarian vessels |
| **7** Mesosalpinx | **14** Tubal extremity of ovary |
| **8** Mesovarium | **15** Uterine extremity of ovary |
| **9** Overspill of contrast into the | **16** Vesico-uterine pouch |
| peritoneal cavity | |

**Looking down into the pelvis from the front in A, the fundus of the uterus (3) overlies the bladder (2) with the peritoneum of the vesico-uterine pouch (16) intervening. In B, contrast medium has filled the uterus and tubes (3, 5, 1 and 4) and spilled out into the peritoneal cavity (9).**

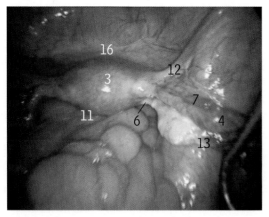

**Laparoscopic view of female pelvis**

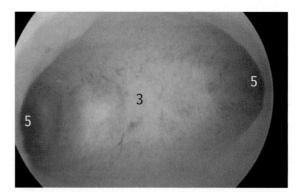

**Hysteroscopic view of uterine cavity and uterine tubes**

*Acute salpingitis, carcinoma of the ovary, ectopic pregnancy rupture, intrauterine contraceptive devices (IUCD), see pages 281, 282.*

# Female pelvis *left half, obliquely from the front*

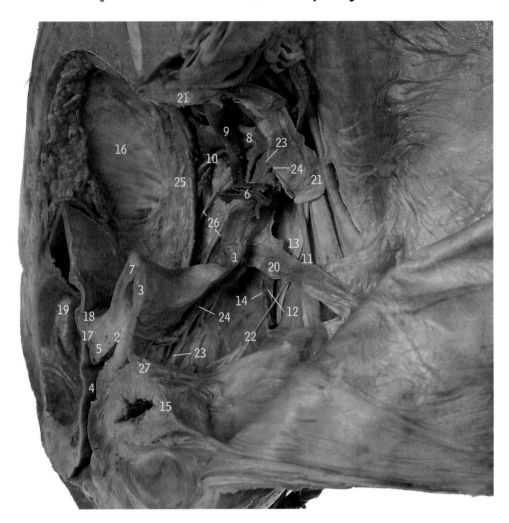

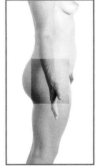

1 Ampulla of uterine tube
2 Anterior fornix of vagina
3 Body of uterus
4 Cavity of vagina
5 Cervix of uterus
6 Fimbriated end of uterine tube
7 Fundus of uterus
8 Internal iliac artery
9 Internal iliac vein
10 Middle rectal artery
11 Obliterated umbilical artery
12 Obturator artery
13 Obturator nerve
14 Obturator vein
15 Peritoneum overlying bladder
16 Peritoneum overlying piriformis
17 Posterior fornix of vagina
18 Recto-vaginal pouch
19 Rectum
20 Round ligament of uterus
21 Sigmoid mesocolon
22 Superior vesical artery
23 Ureter
24 Uterine artery
25 Uterosacral ligament
26 Vaginal artery (double)
27 Vesico-uterine pouch

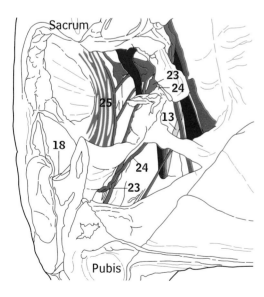

Looking obliquely into the left half of the pelvis from the front, with the anterior abdominal wall turned forwards, the peritoneum of the vesico-uterine pouch (27) has been incised and the uterus (3) displaced backwards. This shows the ureter (23) running towards the bladder and being crossed by the uterine artery (24). The uterosacral ligament (25) passes backwards at the side of the rectum (19) towards the pelvic surface of the sacrum. The root of the sigmoid mesocolon (21) has been left in place to emphasise that the left ureter (23) passes from the abdomen into the pelvis beneath it.

*Anorectal abscesses, carcinoma of the uterus, supports of pelvic viscera, see pages 281, 284.*

# Female perineum   Ⓐ *Surface features*

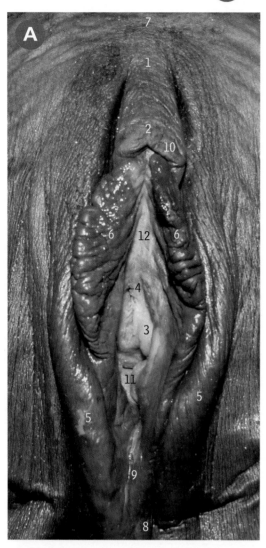

1 Anterior commissure of labia majora
2 Clitoris
3 Cystocoele (prolapse of bladder)
4 External urethral orifice (urinary meatus)
5 Labium majus
6 Labium minus
7 Mons pubis
8 Perineal body
9 Posterior commissure of labia majora
10 Prepuce of clitoris
11 Vaginal orifice (introitus)
12 Vestibule

# Ⓑ *Ischio-anal fossae from behind*

1 Anal margin
2 Anococcygeal body
3 Biceps femoris, long head
4 Coccyx
5 External anal sphincter
6 Gluteal maximus
7 Gluteus medius
8 Gracilis
9 Inferior gemellus
10 Inferior gluteal artery
11 Inferior rectal nerve
12 Ischial tuberosity
13 Ischio-anal fossa, fat removed
14 Levator ani
15 Obturator internus and fascia

16 Obturator internus tendon
17 Piriformis
18 Posterior femoral cutaneous nerve, perineal branch
19 Posterior labial nerve
20 Pudendal artery
21 Pudendal nerve
22 Quadratus femoris
23 Sacrotuberous ligament
24 Sacrum
25 Sciatic nerve
26 Semimembranosus and semitendinosus
27 Superficial transverse perineal muscle
28 Superior gluteal artery

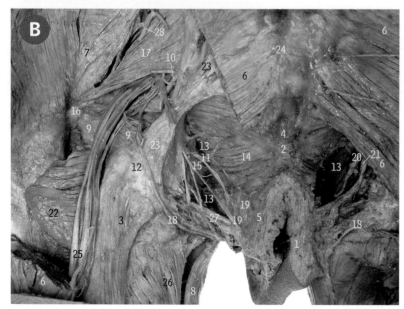

The ischiorectal fossa is now properly and more correctly called the ischio-anal fossa; the anal canal, not the rectum, is its lower medial boundary. The walls and contents are similar in both sexes.

*Episiotomy, female genital cutting, pudendal block, see pages 282, 283.*

# A Male perineum

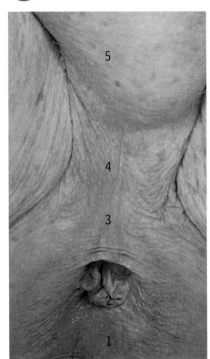

The central area is shown, with the scrotum (5) pulled upwards and forwards.

1 Anococcygeal body
2 Margin of anus, with skin tags
3 Perineal body
4 Raphe overlying bulb of penis
5 Scrotum overlying right testis

> Skin tags are often the remnants of previous haemorrhoids.

## Cytoscopic view of urethra

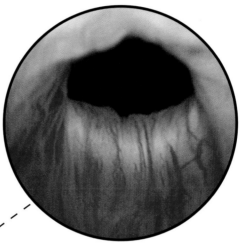

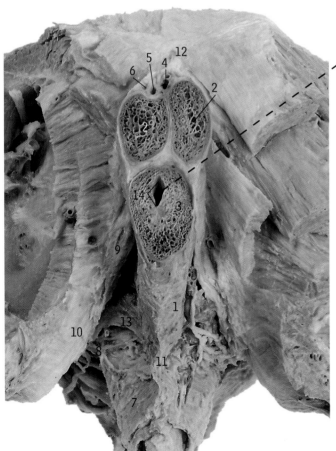

## B Root of the penis
### from below and in front

The front part of the penis has been removed to show the root, formed by the two corpora cavernosa dorsally (2) and the single corpus spongiosum ventrally (3) containing the urethra (14).

1 Bulbospongiosus
2 Corpus cavernosum
3 Corpus spongiosum
4 Deep dorsal vein of penis
5 Dorsal artery of penis
6 Dorsal nerve of penis
7 External anal sphincter
8 Inferior rectal vessels and nerve crossing ischio-anal fossa
9 Ischiocavernosus
10 Ischiopubic ramus
11 Perineal body
12 Pubic symphysis
13 Superficial transverse perineal muscle overlying perineal membrane
14 Urethra

*Carcinoma of the anus, hypospadias, imperforate anus, see pages 281, 282, 283.*

# Male perineum and ischio-anal (ischiorectal) fossae from below

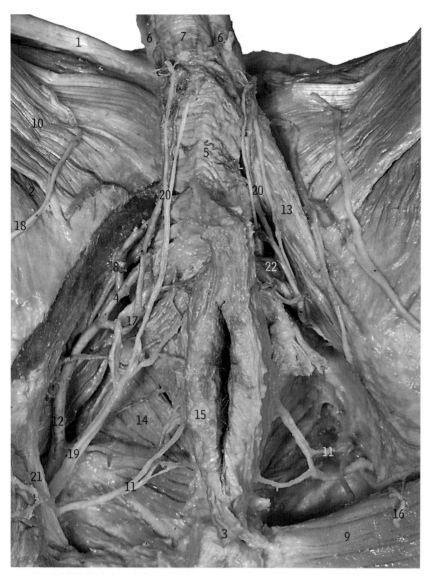

All the fat has been removed from the ischio-anal fossae so that a clear view is obtained of the perineal surface of levator ani (14) and of the vessels and nerves within the fossae. On the left side (right of the picture) the perineal membrane (22) is intact but on the right side it, and the underlying muscle (urogenital diaphragm), have been removed.

1 Adductor longus
2 Adductor magnus
3 Anococcygeal body
4 Artery to bulb
5 Bulbospongiosus overlying bulb of penis
6 Corpus cavernosum of penis
7 Corpus spongiosum of penis
8 Dorsal nerve and artery of penis
9 Gluteus maximus
10 Gracilis
11 Inferior rectal vessels and nerve in ischio-anal fossa
12 Internal pudendal artery
13 Ischiocavernosus overlying crus of penis
14 Levator ani
15 Margin of anus
16 Perforating cutaneous nerve
17 Perineal artery
18 Perineal branch of posterior femoral cutaneous nerve
19 Perineal nerve
20 Posterior scrotal vessels and nerves
21 Sacrotuberous ligament
22 Superficial transverse perineal muscle overlying posterior border of perineal membrane

In both sexes, the ischio-anal (ischiorectal) fossa has the pudendal canal in its lateral wall. The canal has been opened up to display its contents: the internal pudendal artery (12) and the terminal branches of the pudendal nerve – the perineal nerve (19) and the dorsal nerve of the penis (8) or clitoris.

## Lithotomy position

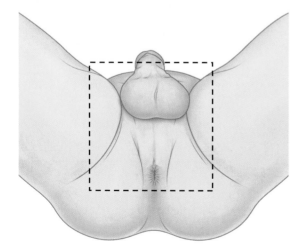

*Priapism, see page 283.*

# Abdomen and pelvis

Clinical thumbnails, see DVD Abdomen and pelvis for details and further clinical images

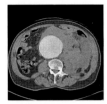
Abdominal aortic aneurysm

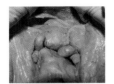
Acute salpingitis

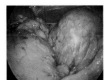
Adrenal gland pathology

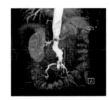
Anorectal abscesses

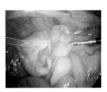
Aortic bruits

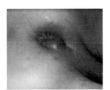
Appendicitis

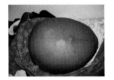
Ascites

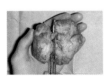
Benign prostatic hyperplasia

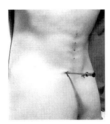
Bone marrow aspiration

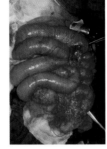
Bowel ischaemia

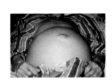
Caput medusae

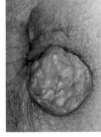
Carcinoma of the anus

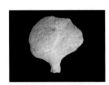
Carcinoma of the bladder

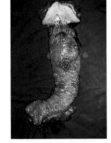
Carcinoma of the large bowel

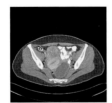
Carcinoma of the ovary

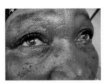
Carcinoma of the pancreas

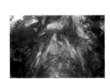
Carcinoma of the prostate

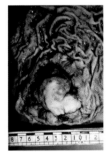
Carcinoma of the stomach

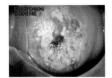
Carcinoma of the uterus

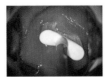
Cervical smear

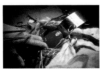
Cholecystectomy

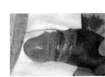
Circumcision

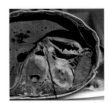
Coeliac plexus block

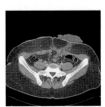
Colostomy

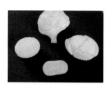

Cystitis

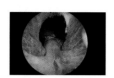

Cystoscopy

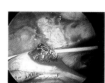

Drainage of peritoneal abscesses

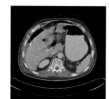

Ectopic pregnancy rupture

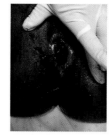

Episiotomy

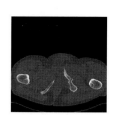

Extravasation of urine

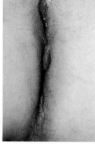

Faecal continence

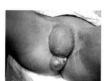

Female genital cutting

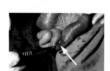

Femoral hernia

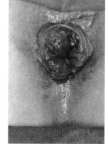

Haematoma of the rectus sheath

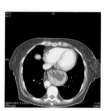

Haemorrhoids

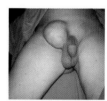

Hiatus hernia

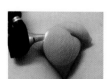

Hydrocoele

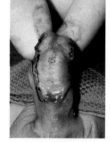

Hypospadias

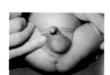

Imperforate anus

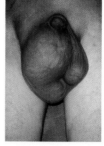

Indirect inguinal hernia

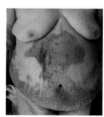

Inferior vena cava (IVC) obstruction

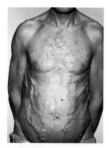

Inguinal hernia

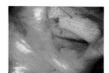

Inguinal hernia repair

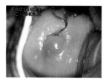

Intrauterine contraceptive devices (IUCDs)

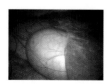

Laparoscopy

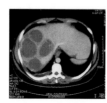

Liver abscess

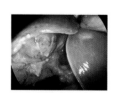

Liver biopsy

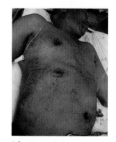

Liver trauma

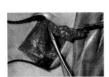

Lumbar hernia

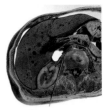

Lumbar sympathectomy

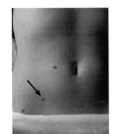

McBurney's point

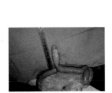

Meckel's diverticulum

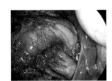

Nephrectomy

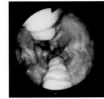

Oesophageal varices

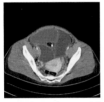

Ovarian dermoid

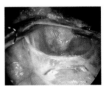

Pancreatic pathology

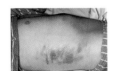

Pancreatitis

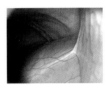

Peritoneal lavage

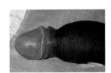

Peritonitis

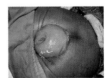

Phimosis and paraphimosis

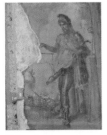

Priapism

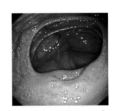

Proctoscopy and sigmoidoscopy

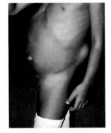

Psoas abscess

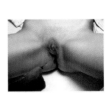

Pudendal block

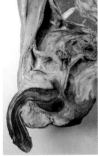

Rectal (PR) examination

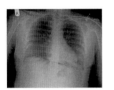

Rectal prolapse

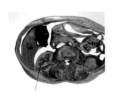

Renal biopsy

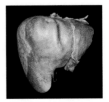

Riedel's lobe

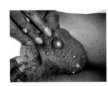

Scrotal swellings

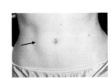

Spigelian hernia

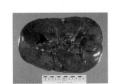

Splenectomy

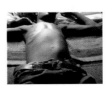

Splenomegaly

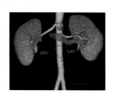
Superior mesenteric artery syndrome

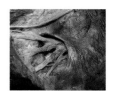
Support of the pelvic viscera

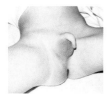
Testicular torsion

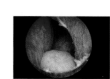
Transurethral resection of the prostate (TURP)

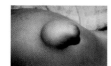
Umbilical and paraumbilical hernia

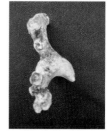
Urinary tract calculi

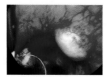
Uterine fibroids

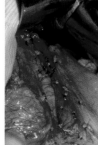
Vaginal examination

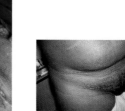
Vagotomy

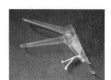
Varicella-zoster virus infection – abdominal wall

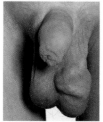
Varicocoeles

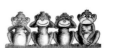
Vasectomy

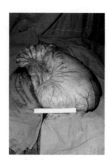
Volvulus

# Lower limb

**Lower limb A** *surface anatomy, from the front*
**B** *dissection, from the front* **C** *dissection, from behind*
**D** *dissection, from the lateral side* **E** *skeleton, from the lateral side*

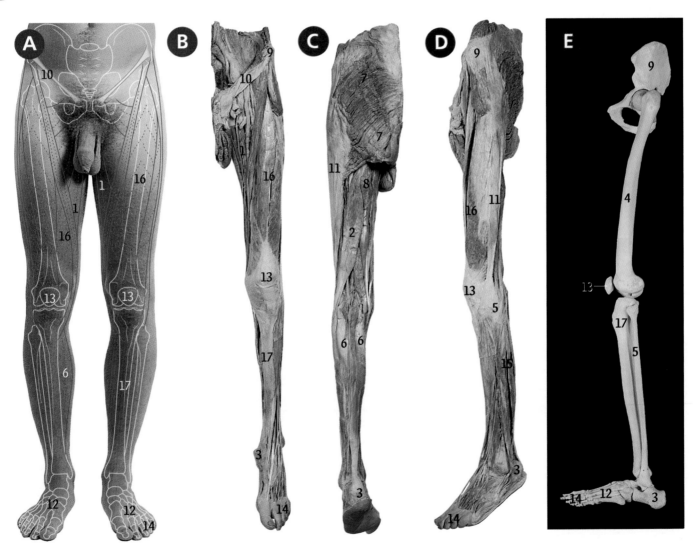

| | | | | |
|---|---|---|---|---|
| **1** Adductors | **5** Fibula | **9** Hip bone | **12** Metatarsal bones | **15** Peroneus (fibularis) |
| **2** Biceps femoris | **6** Gastrocnemius | **10** Inguinal ligament | **13** Patella | **16** Quadriceps |
| **3** Calcaneus | **7** Gluteus maximus | **11** Iliotibial tract | **14** Phalanges of toes | **17** Tibia |
| **4** Femur | **8** Hamstrings | | | |

# Left hip bone *lateral surface*

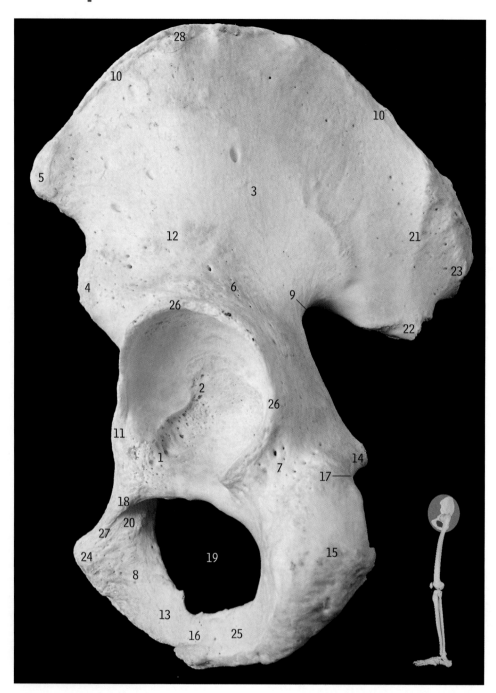

1 Acetabular notch
2 Acetabulum
3 Anterior gluteal line
4 Anterior inferior iliac spine
5 Anterior superior iliac spine
6 Body of ilium
7 Body of ischium
8 Body of pubis
9 Greater sciatic notch
10 Iliac crest
11 Iliopubic eminence
12 Inferior gluteal line
13 Inferior ramus of pubis
14 Ischial spine
15 Ischial tuberosity
16 Junction of 25 and 13
17 Lesser sciatic notch
18 Obturator crest
19 Obturator foramen
20 Obturator groove
21 Posterior gluteal line
22 Posterior inferior iliac spine
23 Posterior superior iliac spine
24 Pubic tubercle
25 Ramus of ischium
26 Rim of acetabulum
27 Superior ramus of pubis
28 Tubercle of iliac crest

The hip (innominate) bone is formed by the union of the ilium (6), ischium (7) and pubis (8).

The two hip bones articulate in the midline anteriorly at the pubic symphysis; posteriorly they are separated by the sacrum, forming the sacro-iliac joints. The two hip bones with the sacrum and coccyx constitute the pelvis (see page 102).

# Left hip bone *attachments, lateral surface*

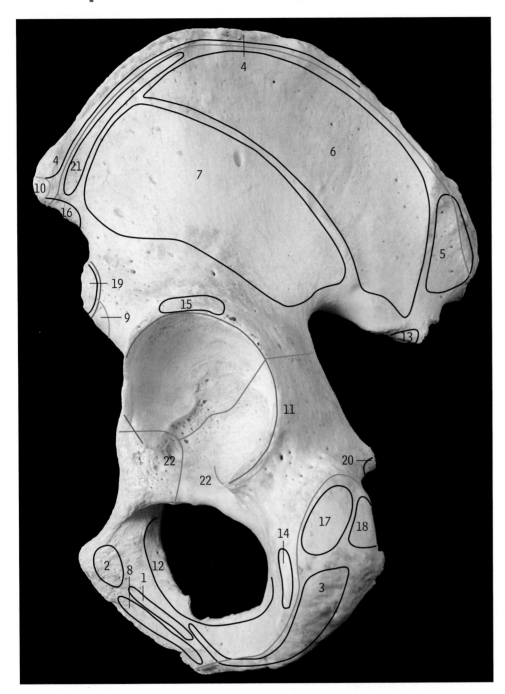

Blue lines, epiphysial lines
Green lines, capsular attachment
of hip joint
Pale green lines, ligament
attachments

**1** Adductor brevis
**2** Adductor longus
**3** Adductor magnus
**4** External oblique
**5** Gluteus maximus
**6** Gluteus medius
**7** Gluteus minimus
**8** Gracilis
**9** Iliofemoral ligament
**10** Inguinal ligament
**11** Ischiofemoral ligament
**12** Obturator externus
**13** Piriformis
**14** Quadratus femoris
**15** Reflected head of rectus femoris
**16** Sartorius
**17** Semimembranosus
**18** Semitendinosus and long head of
biceps
**19** Straight head of rectus femoris
**20** Superior gemellus
**21** Tensor fasciae latae
**22** Transverse ligament

# Left hip bone *medial surface*

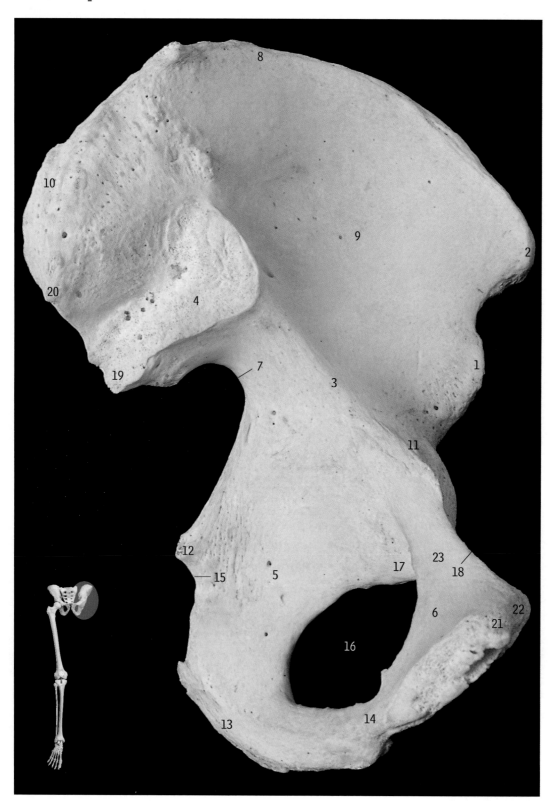

1. Anterior inferior iliac spine
2. Anterior superior iliac spine
3. Arcuate line
4. Auricular surface
5. Body of ischium
6. Body of pubis
7. Greater sciatic notch
8. Iliac crest
9. Iliac fossa
10. Iliac tuberosity
11. Iliopubic eminence
12. Ischial spine
13. Ischial tuberosity
14. Ischiopubic ramus
15. Lesser sciatic notch
16. Obturator foramen
17. Obturator groove
18. Pecten of pubis (pectineal line)
19. Posterior inferior iliac spine
20. Posterior superior iliac spine
21. Pubic crest
22. Pubic tubercle
23. Superior ramus of pubis

The auricular surface of the ilium (4) is the articular surface for the sacro-iliac joint.

The greater sciatic notch (7) is more hooked (J-shaped) in the male, whereas the female notch is more right-angled (L-shaped).

# Left hip bone *attachments, medial surface*

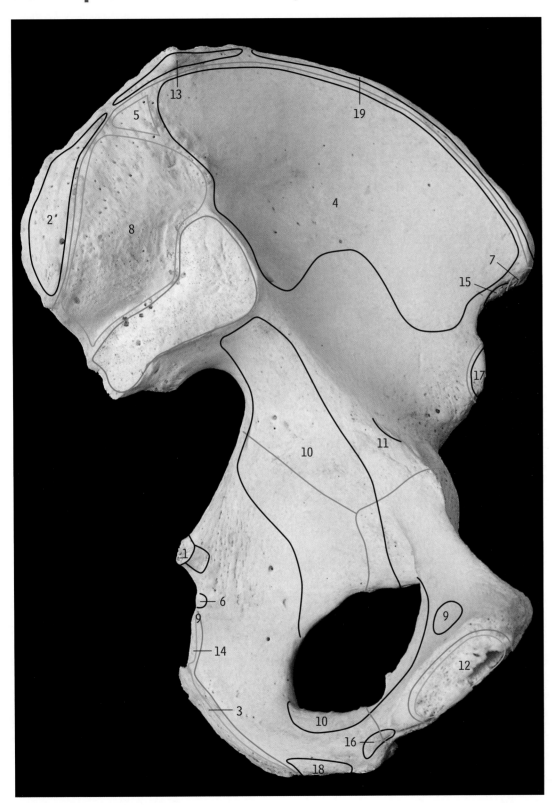

Blue lines, epiphysial lines
Green line, capsular attachment of sacro-iliac joint
Pale green lines, ligament attachments

1  Coccygeus and sacrospinous ligament
2  Erector spinae
3  Falciform process of sacrotuberous ligament
4  Iliacus
5  Iliolumbar ligament
6  Inferior gemellus
7  Inguinal ligament
8  Interosseous sacro-iliac ligament
9  Levator ani
10 Obturator internus
11 Psoas minor
12 Pubic symphysis
13 Quadratus lumborum
14 Sacrotuberous ligament
15 Sartorius
16 Sphincter urethrae
17 Straight head of rectus femoris
18 Superficial transverse perineal and ischiocavernosus
19 Transversus abdominis

# Left hip bone *from above*

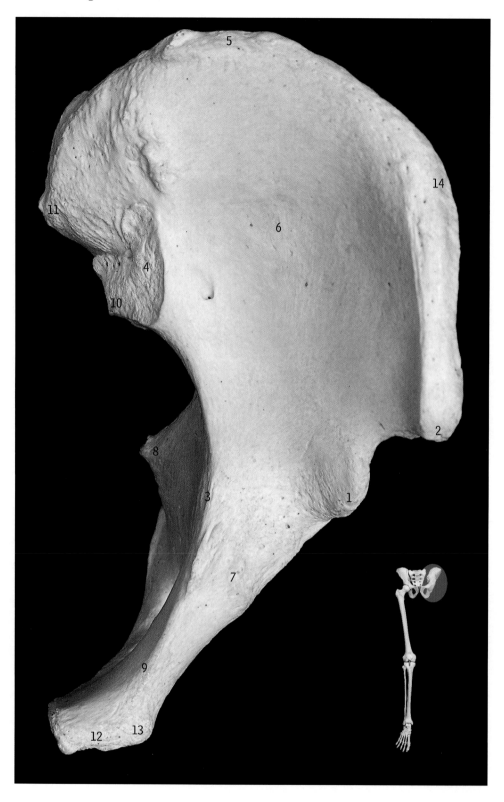

1 Anterior inferior iliac spine
2 Anterior superior iliac spine
3 Arcuate line
4 Auricular surface
5 Iliac crest
6 Iliac fossa
7 Iliopubic eminence
8 Ischial spine
9 Pecten of pubis (pectineal line)
10 Posterior inferior iliac spine
11 Posterior superior iliac spine
12 Pubic crest
13 Pubic tubercle
14 Tubercle of iliac crest

The arcuate line on the ilium (3) and the pecten and crest of the pubis (9 and 12) form part of the brim of the pelvis (the rest of the brim being formed by the promontory and upper surface of the lateral part of the sacrum – see pages 100 and 102).

The pecten of the pubis (9) is more commonly called the pectineal line.

# Left hip bone *attachments, from above*

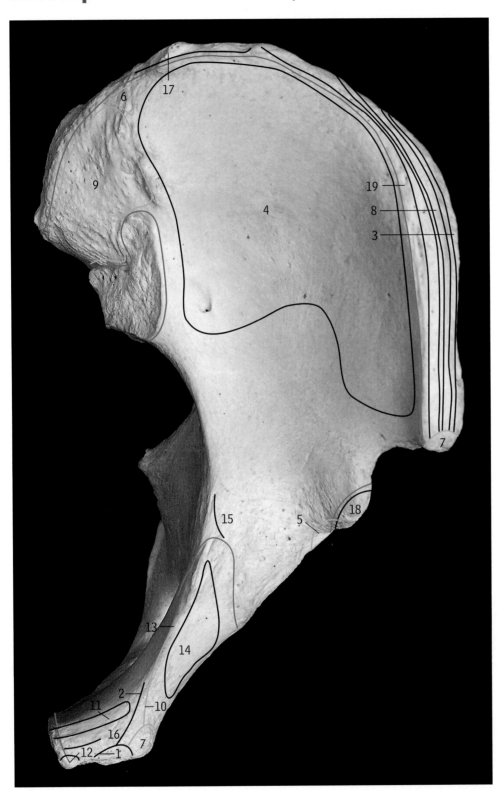

Blue lines, epiphysial lines
Green line, capsular attachment
of sacro-iliac joint
Pale green lines, ligament
attachments

  **1** Anterior wall of rectus sheath
  **2** Conjoint tendon
  **3** External oblique
  **4** Iliacus
  **5** Iliofemoral ligament
  **6** Iliolumbar ligament
  **7** Inguinal ligament
  **8** Internal oblique
  **9** Interosseous sacro-iliac ligament
 **10** Lacunar ligament
 **11** Lateral head of rectus abdominis
 **12** Medial head of rectus abdominis
 **13** Pectineal ligament
 **14** Pectineus
 **15** Psoas minor
 **16** Pyramidalis
 **17** Quadratus lumborum
 **18** Straight head of rectus femoris
 **19** Transversus abdominis

The inguinal ligament (7) is formed
by the lower border of the
aponeurosis of the external oblique
muscle, and extends from the
anterior superior iliac spine to the
pubic tubercle.

The lacunar ligament (10, sometimes
called the pectineal part of the
inguinal ligament) is the part of
the inguinal ligament that extends
backwards from the medial end of
the inguinal ligament to the pecten
of the pubis.

The pectineal ligament (13) is the
lateral extension of the lacunar
ligament along the pecten. It is not
classified as a part of the inguinal
ligament, and must not be confused
with the alternative name for the
lacunar ligament, i.e. with the
pectineal part of the inguinal
ligament.

The conjoint tendon (2) is formed
by the aponeuroses of the internal
oblique and transversus muscles,
and is attached to the pubic crest
and the adjoining part of the
pecten, blending medially with the
anterior wall of the rectus sheath.

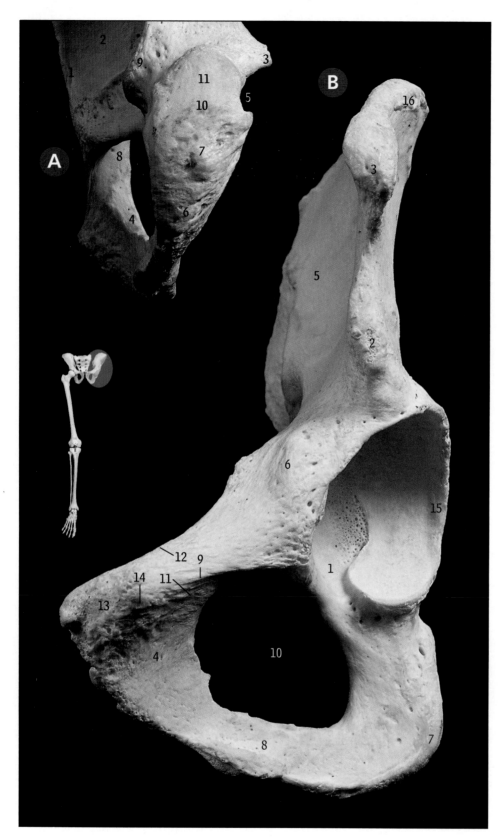

## A Left hip bone

### *ischial tuberosity, from behind and below*

1 Acetabular notch
2 Acetabulum
3 Ischial spine
4 Ischiopubic ramus
5 Lesser sciatic notch
6 Longitudinal ridge
7 Lower part of tuberosity
8 Obturator groove
9 Rim of acetabulum
10 Transverse ridge
11 Upper part of tuberosity

## B Left hip bone

### *from the front*

1 Acetabular notch
2 Anterior inferior iliac spine
3 Anterior superior iliac spine
4 Body of pubis
5 Iliac fossa
6 Iliopubic eminence
7 Ischial tuberosity
8 Ischiopubic ramus
9 Obturator crest
10 Obturator foramen
11 Obturator groove
12 Pecten of pubis (pectineal line)
13 Pubic crest
14 Pubic tubercle
15 Rim of acetabulum
16 Tubercle of iliac crest

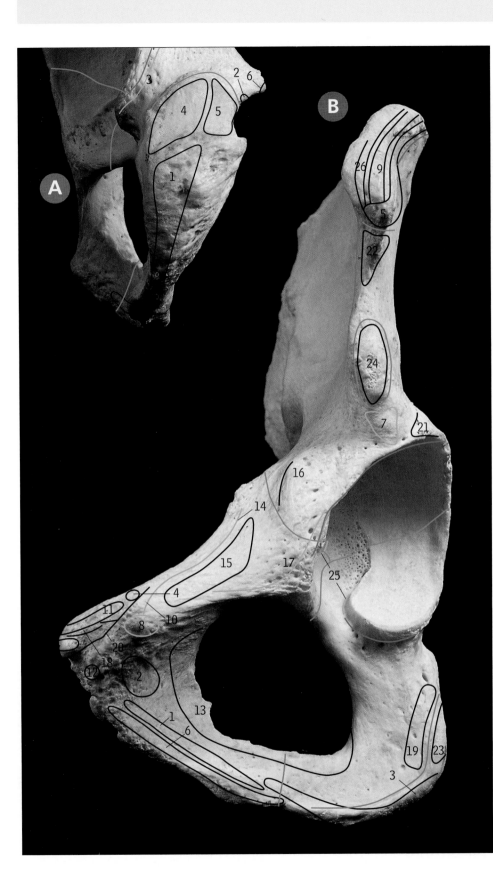

## A Left hip bone attachments, ischial tuberosity, from behind and below

Blue lines, epiphysial lines
Green line, capsular attachment of hip joint
Pale green lines, ligament attachments

1 Adductor magnus
2 Inferior gemellus
3 Ischiofemoral ligament
4 Semimembranosus
5 Semitendinosus and long head of biceps
6 Superior gemellus

> The area on the ischial tuberosity medial to the adductor magnus attachment (1) is covered by fibrofatty tissue and the ischial bursa underlying gluteus maximus.

## B Left hip bone attachments, from the front

Blue lines, epiphysial lines
Green line, capsular attachment of hip joint
Pale green lines, ligament attachments

1 Adductor brevis
2 Adductor longus
3 Adductor magnus
4 Conjoint tendon
5 External oblique and inguinal ligament
6 Gracilis
7 Iliofemoral ligament
8 Inguinal ligament
9 Internal oblique
10 Lacunar ligament
11 Lateral head of rectus abdominis
12 Medial head of rectus abdominis
13 Obturator externus
14 Pectineal ligament
15 Pectineus
16 Psoas minor
17 Pubofemoral ligament
18 Pyramidalis
19 Quadratus femoris
20 Rectus sheath
21 Reflected head of rectus femoris
22 Sartorius
23 Semimembranosus
24 Straight head of rectus femoris
25 Transverse ligament
26 Transversus abdominis

# Left femur *upper end*

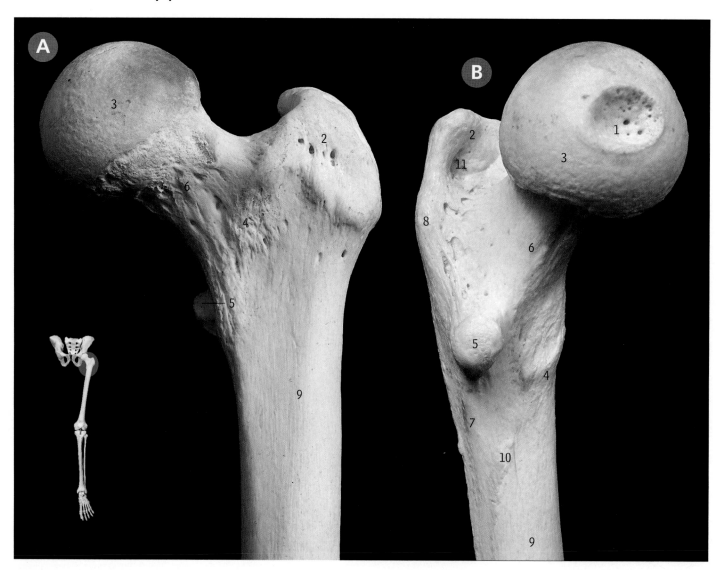

**1**  Fovea of head
**2**  Greater trochanter
**3**  Head
**4**  Intertrochanteric line
**5**  Lesser trochanter
**6**  Neck
**7**  Pectineal line
**8**  Quadrate tubercle on intertrochanteric crest
**9**  Shaft
**10**  Spiral line
**11**  Trochanteric fossa

The intertrochanteric *line* (4) is at the junction of the neck (6) and shaft (9) on the anterior surface; the intertrochanteric *crest* is in a similar position on the posterior surface (8, and page 296, A5).

The neck makes an angle with the shaft of about 125° in an adult.

The pectineal line of the femur (7) must not be confused with the pectineal line (pecten) of the pubis (9, page 290), nor with the spiral line of the femur (10) which is usually more prominent than the pectineal line.

# Left femur *attachments, upper end*

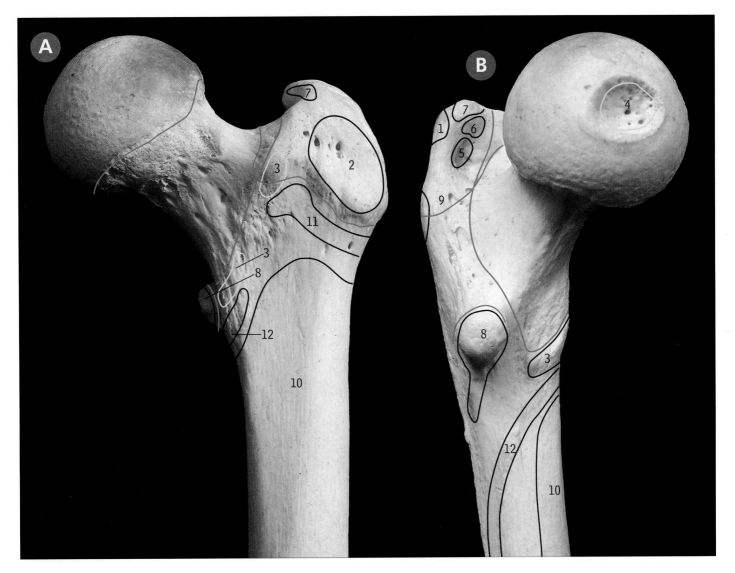

**A** from the front

**B** from the medial side

Blue lines, epiphysial lines
Green line, capsular
attachment of hip joint
Pale green lines, ligament
attachments

| | |
|---|---|
| **1** | Gluteus medius |
| **2** | Gluteus minimus |
| **3** | Iliofemoral ligament |
| **4** | Ligament of head of femur |
| **5** | Obturator externus |
| **6** | Obturator internus and gemelli |
| **7** | Piriformis |
| **8** | Psoas major and iliacus |
| **9** | Quadratus femoris |
| **10** | Vastus intermedius |
| **11** | Vastus lateralis |
| **12** | Vastus medialis |

The iliofemoral ligament has the shape of an inverted V, with the stem attached to the anterior inferior iliac spine of the hip bone (page 293, B7), and the lateral and medial bands attached to the upper (lateral) and lower (medial) ends of the intertrochanteric line (page 296, 6), blending with the capsule of the hip joint.

The tendon of psoas major is attached to the lesser trochanter (page 296, 8); many of the muscle fibres of iliacus are inserted into the psoas tendon but some reach the femur below the trochanter.

*Intertrochanteric fracture of the femur, see page 355.*

# Left femur *upper end*

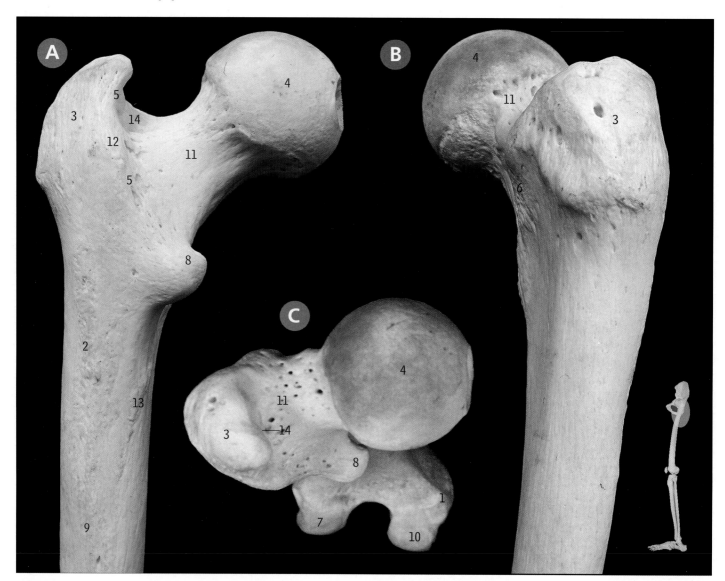

**A** from behind

**B** from the lateral side

**C** from above

1  Adductor tubercle at lower end
2  Gluteal tuberosity
3  Greater trochanter
4  Head
5  Intertrochanteric crest
6  Intertrochanteric line
7  Lateral condyle at lower end
8  Lesser trochanter
9  Linea aspera
10  Medial condyle at lower end
11  Neck
12  Quadrate tubercle
13  Spiral line
14  Trochanteric fossa

The neck of the femur passes forwards as well as upwards and medially (C11), making an angle of about 15° with the transverse axis of the lower end (the angle of femoral torsion).

The lesser trochanter (8) projects backwards and medially.

# Left femur *attachments, upper end*

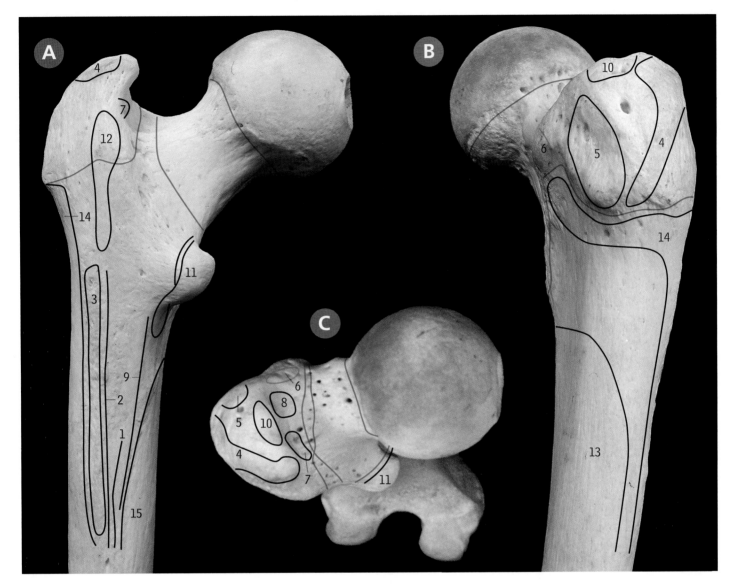

**A** from behind

**B** from the lateral side

**C** from above

Blue lines, epiphysial lines
Green line, capsular
attachment of hip joint
Pale green lines, ligament
attachments

1 Adductor brevis
2 Adductor magnus
3 Gluteus maximus
4 Gluteus medius
5 Gluteus minimus
6 Iliofemoral ligament
  (lateral band)
7 Obturator externus
8 Obturator internus
  and gemelli

9 Pectineus
10 Piriformis
11 Psoas major and iliacus
12 Quadratus femoris
13 Vastus intermedius
14 Vastus lateralis
15 Vastus medialis

On the front of the femur (page
295) the capsule of the hip joint is
attached to the intertrochanteric
line, but at the back the capsule
is attached to the neck of the
femur and does not extend as far
laterally as the intertrochanteric
crest (page 296, A5).

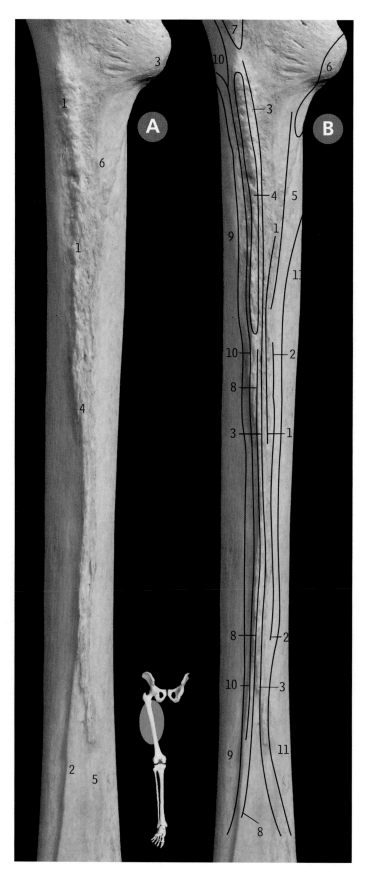

### A Left femur *shaft, from behind*

| | | | |
|---|---|---|---|
| **1** | Gluteal tuberosity | **4** | Linea aspera |
| **2** | Lateral supracondylar line | **5** | Medial supracondylar line |
| **3** | Lesser trochanter | **6** | Pectineal line |

The rough linea aspera (4) often shows distinct medial and lateral lips; the lateral lip continues upwards as the gluteal tuberosity (1).

### B Left femur *attachments, shaft, from behind*

| | | | |
|---|---|---|---|
| **1** | Adductor brevis | **7** | Quadratus femoris |
| **2** | Adductor longus | **8** | Short head of biceps |
| **3** | Adductor magnus | **9** | Vastus intermedius |
| **4** | Gluteus maximus | **10** | Vastus lateralis |
| **5** | Pectineus | **11** | Vastus medialis |
| **6** | Psoas and iliacus | | |

For diagrammatic clarity, the muscle attachments to the linea aspera have been slightly separated.

### C Left femur *upper end, from the front*

**This is the posterior half of a cleared and bisected specimen, to show the major groups of bone trabeculae.**

**1** Calcar femorale
**2** From lateral surface of shaft to greater trochanter
**3** From lateral surface of shaft to head
**4** From medial surface of shaft to greater trochanter
**5** From medial surface of shaft to head
**6** Triangular area of few trabeculae

The calcar femorale (1) is a dense concentration of trabeculae passing from the region of the lesser trochanter to the under-surface of the neck.

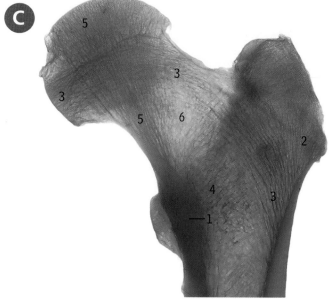

*Fracture of the femoral shaft, see page 355.*

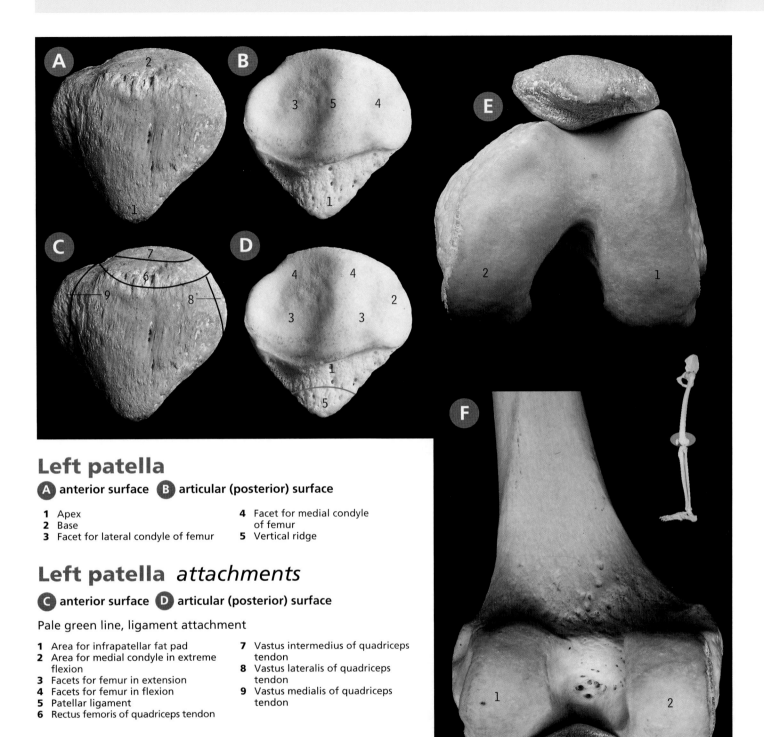

# Left patella

**A** anterior surface    **B** articular (posterior) surface

**1** Apex
**2** Base
**3** Facet for lateral condyle of femur

**4** Facet for medial condyle of femur
**5** Vertical ridge

# Left patella *attachments*

**C** anterior surface    **D** articular (posterior) surface

Pale green line, ligament attachment

**1** Area for infrapatellar fat pad
**2** Area for medial condyle in extreme flexion
**3** Facets for femur in extension
**4** Facets for femur in flexion
**5** Patellar ligament
**6** Rectus femoris of quadriceps tendon

**7** Vastus intermedius of quadriceps tendon
**8** Vastus lateralis of quadriceps tendon
**9** Vastus medialis of quadriceps tendon

# Left femur and patella *articulated*

**E** from below with knee extended

**F** from below and behind with knee flexed

In flexion, note the increased area of contact between the medial condyle of the femur (2) and the patella.

**1** Lateral condyle      **2** Medial condyle

The most medial facet of the patella (D2) only comes into contact with the medial condyle in extreme flexion as in F.

*Bipartite patella, dislocation of the patella, see page 355.*

# Left femur *lower end*

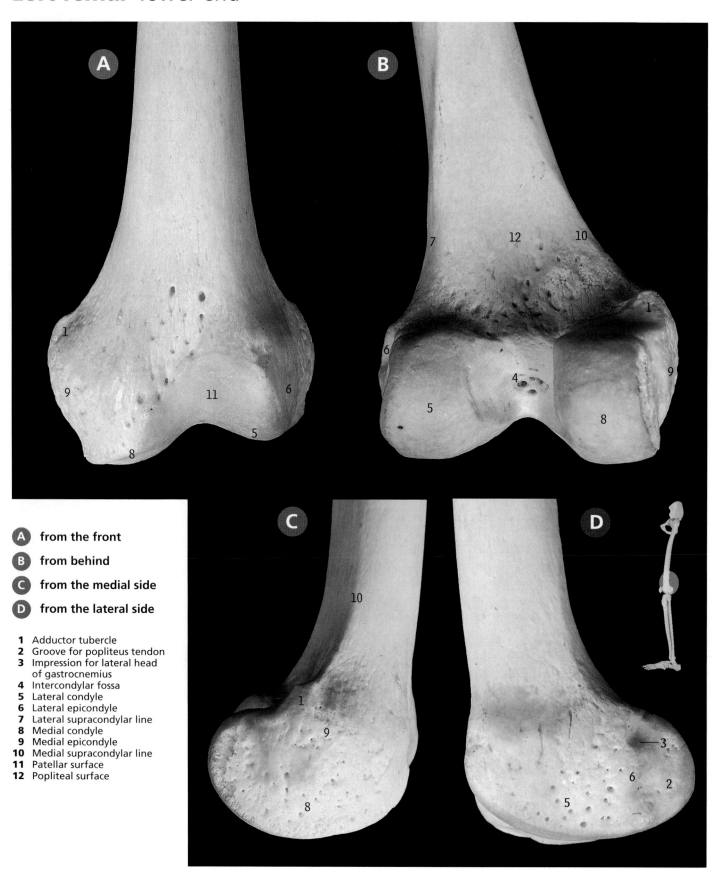

**A** from the front

**B** from behind

**C** from the medial side

**D** from the lateral side

1 Adductor tubercle
2 Groove for popliteus tendon
3 Impression for lateral head
   of gastrocnemius
4 Intercondylar fossa
5 Lateral condyle
6 Lateral epicondyle
7 Lateral supracondylar line
8 Medial condyle
9 Medial epicondyle
10 Medial supracondylar line
11 Patellar surface
12 Popliteal surface

# Left femur *attachments, lower end*

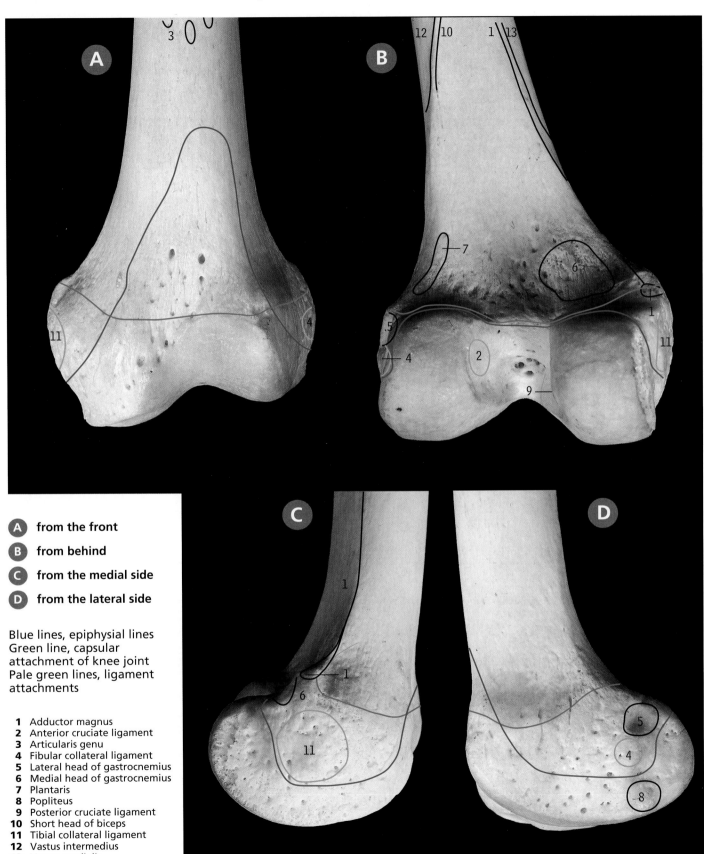

A from the front

B from behind

C from the medial side

D from the lateral side

Blue lines, epiphysial lines
Green line, capsular
attachment of knee joint
Pale green lines, ligament
attachments

 1  Adductor magnus
 2  Anterior cruciate ligament
 3  Articularis genu
 4  Fibular collateral ligament
 5  Lateral head of gastrocnemius
 6  Medial head of gastrocnemius
 7  Plantaris
 8  Popliteus
 9  Posterior cruciate ligament
10  Short head of biceps
11  Tibial collateral ligament
12  Vastus intermedius
13  Vastus medialis

# Left tibia *upper end*

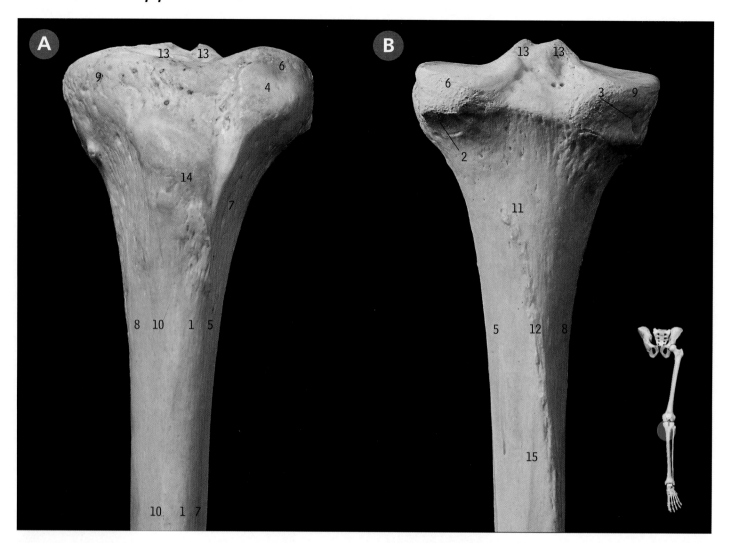

**from the front**

**from behind**

1 Anterior border
2 Articular facet for fibula
3 Groove for semimembranosus
4 Impression for iliotibial tract
5 Interosseous border
6 Lateral condyle
7 Lateral surface
8 Medial border
9 Medial condyle
10 Medial surface
11 Posterior surface
12 Soleal line
13 Tubercles of intercondylar eminence
14 Tuberosity
15 Vertical line

The shaft of the tibia has three borders: anterior (1), medial (8) and interosseous (5) – and three surfaces: medial (10), lateral (7) and posterior (11).

Much of the anterior border (1) forms a slightly curved crest commonly known as the shin. Most of the smooth medial surface (10) is subcutaneous. The posterior surface contains the soleal and vertical lines (12 and 15).

The tuberosity (14) is at the upper end of the anterior border.

# Left tibia *attachments, upper end*

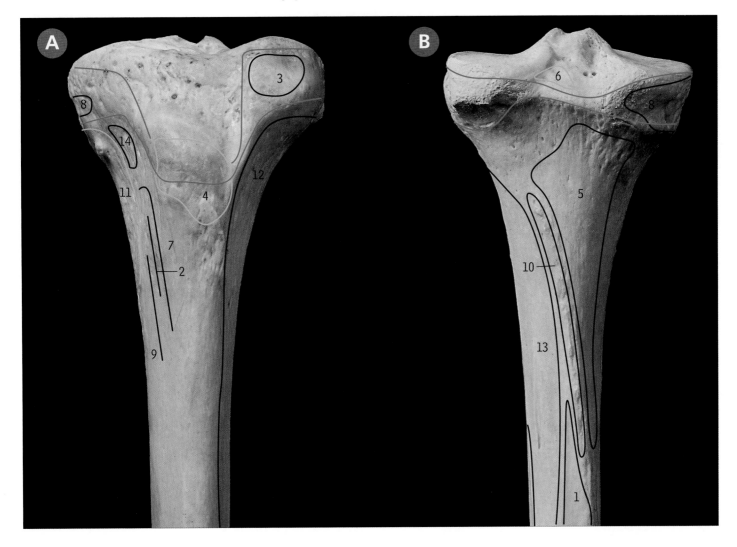

Blue lines, epiphysial lines
Green line, capsular attachment
of knee joint
Pale green lines, ligament
attachments

| | | | |
|---|---|---|---|
| **1** | Flexor digitorum longus | **8** | Semimembranosus |
| **2** | Gracilis | **9** | Semitendinosus |
| **3** | Iliotibial tract | **10** | Soleus |
| **4** | Patellar ligament | **11** | Tibial collateral ligament |
| **5** | Popliteus | **12** | Tibialis anterior |
| **6** | Posterior cruciate ligament | **13** | Tibialis posterior |
| **7** | Sartorius | **14** | Vastus medialis |

# Left tibia *upper end*

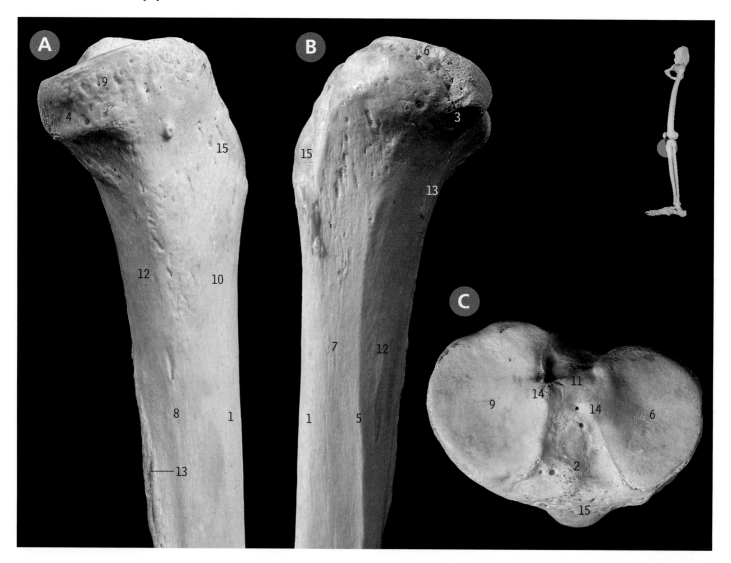

**A** from the medial side

**B** from the lateral side

**C** from above

| | |
|---|---|
| **1** Anterior border | **9** Medial condyle |
| **2** Anterior intercondylar area | **10** Medial surface |
| **3** Articular facet for fibula | **11** Posterior intercondylar |
| **4** Groove for |     area |
|     semimembranosus | **12** Posterior surface |
| **5** Interosseous border | **13** Soleal line |
| **6** Lateral condyle | **14** Tubercles of intercondylar |
| **7** Lateral surface |     eminence |
| **8** Medial border | **15** Tuberosity |

The medial condyle (C9) is larger than the lateral condyle (C6).

The articular facet for the fibula is on the postero-inferior aspect of the lateral condyle (B3).

*Osgood-Schlatter's disease, see page 356.*

# Left tibia *attachments, upper end*

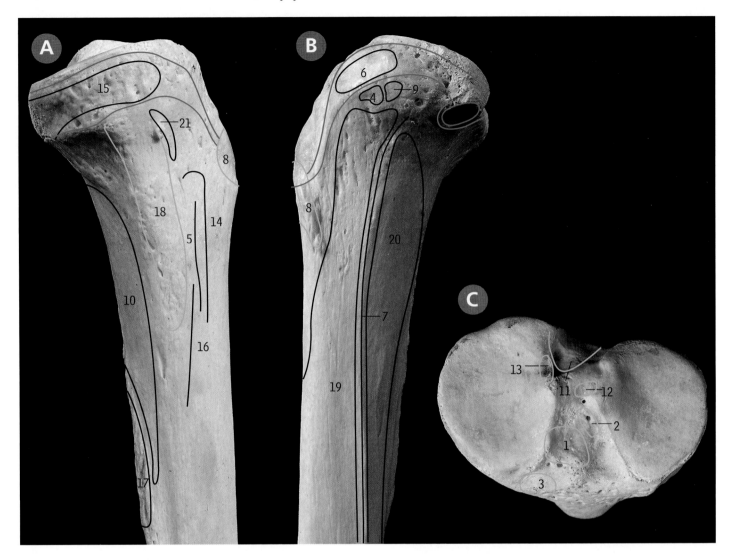

**A** from the medial side

**B** from the lateral side

**C** from above

Blue lines, epiphysial lines
Green lines, capsular
attachments of knee
joint and superior
tibiofibular joint
Pale green lines, ligament
attachments

1 Anterior cruciate ligament
2 Anterior horn of lateral
  meniscus
3 Anterior horn of medial
  meniscus
4 Extensor digitorum longus
5 Gracilis
6 Iliotibial tract
7 Interosseous membrane
8 Patellar ligament
9 Peroneus (fibularis) longus
10 Popliteus
11 Posterior cruciate ligament

12 Posterior horn of lateral
   meniscus
13 Posterior horn of medial
   meniscus
14 Sartorius
15 Semimembranosus
16 Semitendinosus
17 Soleus
18 Tibial collateral ligament
19 Tibialis anterior
20 Tibialis posterior
21 Vastus medialis

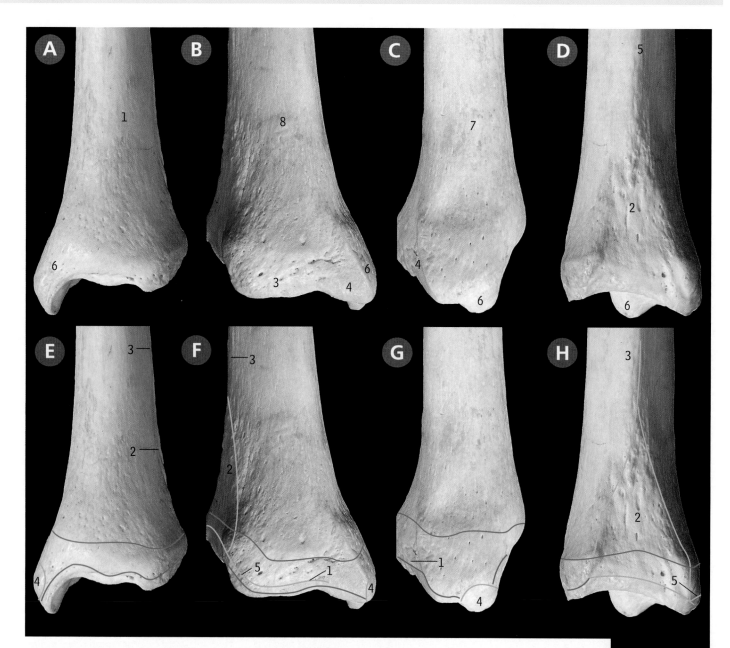

# Left tibia *lower end*

(A) **from the front**

(B) **from behind**

(C) **from the medial side**

(D) **from the lateral side**

1 Anterior surface
2 Fibular notch
3 Groove for flexor hallucis longus
4 Groove for tibialis posterior
5 Interosseous border
6 Medial malleolus
7 Medial surface
8 Posterior surface

# Left tibia *attachments, lower end*

(E) **from the front**

(F) **from behind**

(G) **from the medial side**

(H) **from the lateral side**

Blue line, epiphysial line
Green line, capsular attachment of ankle joint
Pale green lines, ligament attachments

1 Inferior transverse ligament
2 Interosseous ligament
3 Interosseous membrane
4 Medial collateral ligament
5 Posterior tibiofibular ligament

> The medial collateral ligament (G4) is commonly known as the deltoid ligament.

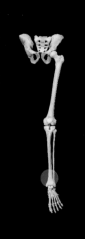

# Left tibia and fibula *articulated*

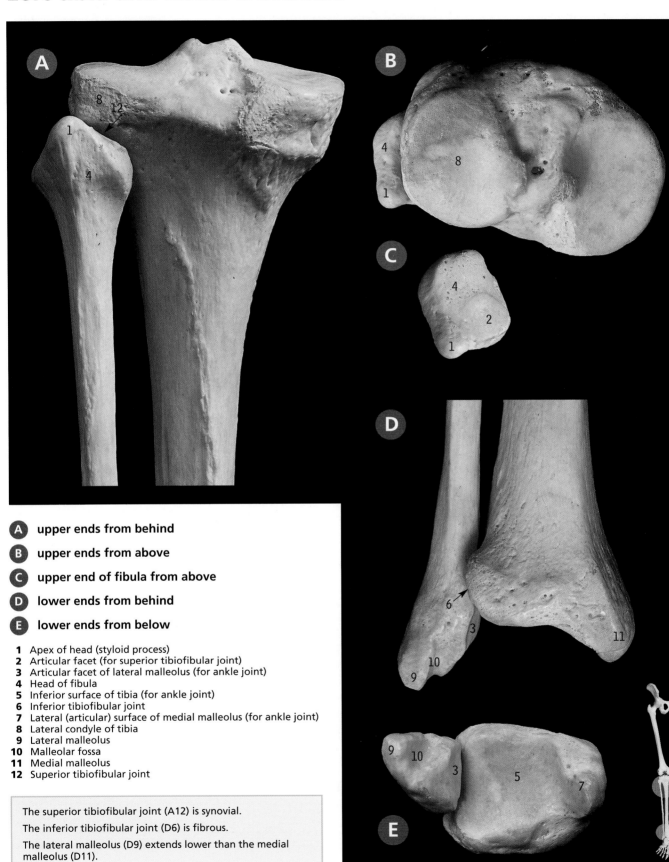

**A** upper ends from behind

**B** upper ends from above

**C** upper end of fibula from above

**D** lower ends from behind

**E** lower ends from below

1 Apex of head (styloid process)
2 Articular facet (for superior tibiofibular joint)
3 Articular facet of lateral malleolus (for ankle joint)
4 Head of fibula
5 Inferior surface of tibia (for ankle joint)
6 Inferior tibiofibular joint
7 Lateral (articular) surface of medial malleolus (for ankle joint)
8 Lateral condyle of tibia
9 Lateral malleolus
10 Malleolar fossa
11 Medial malleolus
12 Superior tibiofibular joint

The superior tibiofibular joint (A12) is synovial.

The inferior tibiofibular joint (D6) is fibrous.

The lateral malleolus (D9) extends lower than the medial malleolus (D11).

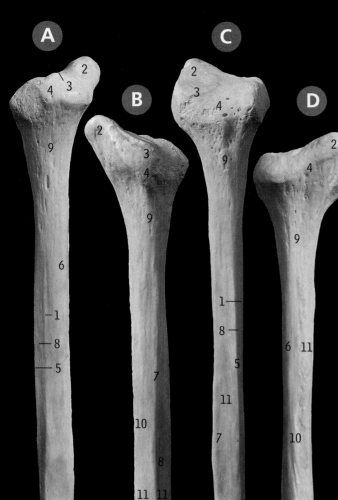

# Left fibula *upper end*

**Ⓐ** from the front     **Ⓒ** from the medial side

**Ⓑ** from behind     **Ⓓ** from the lateral side

1 Anterior border
2 Apex (styloid process)
3 Articular facet on upper surface
4 Head
5 Interosseous border
6 Lateral surface
7 Medial crest
8 Medial surface
9 Neck
10 Posterior border
11 Posterior surface

> The fibula has three borders: anterior (A1), interosseous (A5) and posterior (B10) – and three surfaces: medial (A8), lateral (A6) and posterior (B11).
>
> At first sight, much of the shaft appears to have four borders and four surfaces, but this is because the posterior surface (B11) is divided into two parts (medial and lateral) by the medial crest (B7).

# Left fibula *lower end*

**Ⓔ** from the front

**Ⓕ** from behind

**Ⓖ** from the medial side

**Ⓗ** from the lateral side

1 Anterior border
2 Articular surface of lateral malleolus
3 Groove for peroneus (fibularis) brevis
4 Interosseous border
5 Lateral malleolus
6 Lateral surface
7 Malleolar fossa
8 Medial crest
9 Medial surface
10 Posterior border
11 Posterior surface
12 Surface for interosseous ligament
13 Triangular subcutaneous area

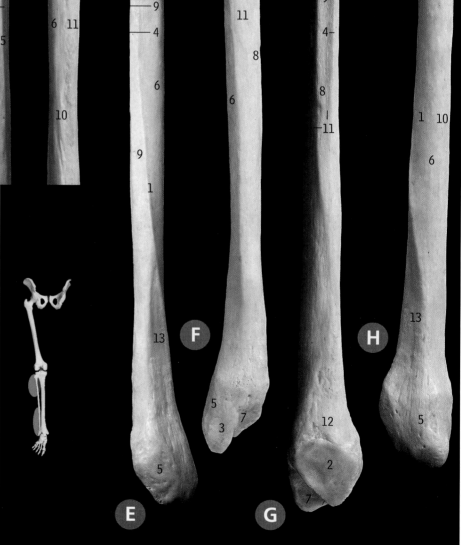

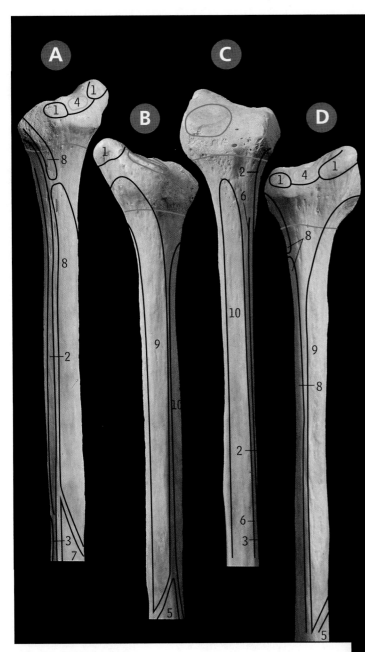

## Left fibula
### attachments, upper end

**A** from the front     **C** from the medial side

**B** from behind     **D** from the lateral side

Blue line, epiphysial line
Green line, capsular attachment of superior tibiofibular joint
Pale green lines, ligament attachments

| | | | |
|---|---|---|---|
| **1** | Biceps | **6** | Interosseous membrane |
| **2** | Extensor digitorum longus | **7** | Peroneus (fibularis) brevis |
| **3** | Extensor hallucis longus | **8** | Peroneus (fibularis) longus |
| **4** | Fibular collateral ligament | **9** | Soleus |
| **5** | Flexor hallucis longus | **10** | Tibialis posterior |

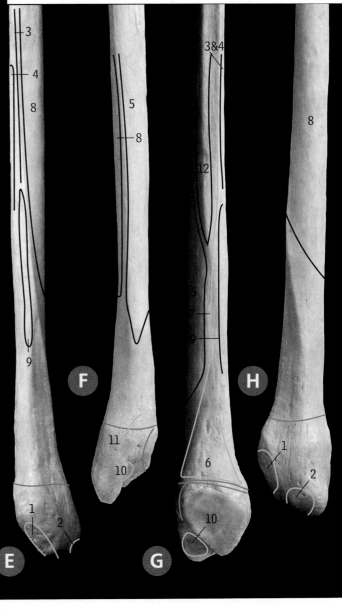

## Left fibula
### attachments, lower end

**E** from the front     **G** from the medial side

**F** from behind     **H** from the lateral side

Blue line, epiphysial line
Green line, capsular attachment of ankle joint
Pale green lines, ligament attachments

| | | | |
|---|---|---|---|
| **1** | Anterior talofibular ligament | **8** | Peroneus (fibularis) brevis |
| **2** | Calcaneofibular ligament | **9** | Peroneus (fibularis) tertius |
| **3** | Extensor digitorum longus | **10** | Posterior talofibular ligament |
| **4** | Extensor hallucis longus | **11** | Posterior tibiofibular ligament |
| **5** | Flexor hallucis longus | | |
| **6** | Interosseous ligament | **12** | Tibialis posterior |
| **7** | Interosseous membrane | | |

# Bones of the left foot

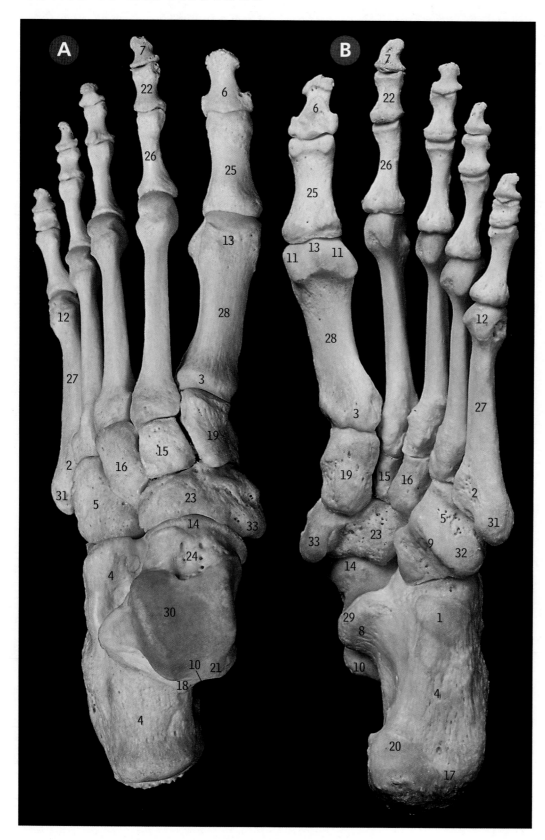

**A** from above (dorsum)

**B** from below (plantar surface)

1 Anterior tubercle of calcaneus
2 Base of fifth metatarsal
3 Base of first metatarsal
4 Calcaneus
5 Cuboid
6 Distal phalanx of great toe
7 Distal phalanx of second toe
8 Groove on calcaneus for flexor hallucis longus
9 Groove on cuboid for peroneus (fibularis) longus
10 Groove on talus for flexor hallucis longus
11 Grooves for sesamoid bones in flexor hallucis brevis
12 Head of fifth metatarsal
13 Head of first metatarsal
14 Head of talus
15 Intermediate cuneiform
16 Lateral cuneiform
17 Lateral process of calcaneus
18 Lateral tubercle of talus
19 Medial cuneiform
20 Medial process of calcaneus
21 Medial tubercle of talus
22 Middle phalanx of second toe
23 Navicular
24 Neck of talus
25 Proximal phalanx of great toe
26 Proximal phalanx of second toe
27 Shaft of fifth metatarsal
28 Shaft of first metatarsal
29 Sustentaculum tali of calcaneus
30 Trochlear surface of body of talus
31 Tuberosity of base of fifth metatarsal
32 Tuberosity of cuboid
33 Tuberosity of navicular

*Dislocation of the toe, hallux valgus, see page 355.*

# Bones of the left foot *attachments*

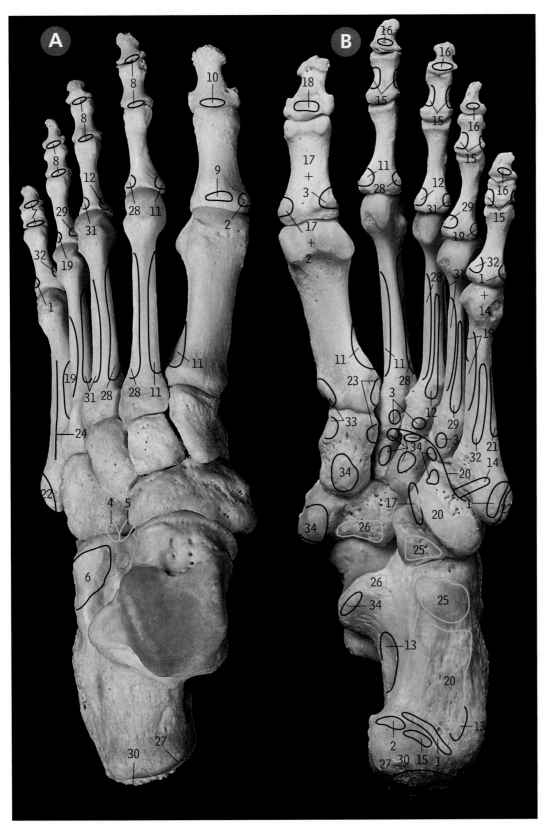

Metatarsal fractures, see page 356.

**A** from above

**B** from below

**Joint capsules and minor ligaments have been omitted.**

Pale green lines, ligament attachments.

1 Abductor digiti minimi
2 Abductor hallucis
3 Adductor hallucis
4 Calcaneocuboid part of bifurcate ligament
5 Calcaneonavicular part of bifurcate ligament
6 Extensor digitorum brevis
7 Extensor digitorum longus
8 Extensor digitorum longus and brevis
9 Extensor hallucis brevis
10 Extensor hallucis longus
11 First dorsal interosseous
12 First plantar interosseous
13 Flexor accessorius
14 Flexor digiti minimi brevis
15 Flexor digitorum brevis
16 Flexor digitorum longus
17 Flexor hallucis brevis
18 Flexor hallucis longus
19 Fourth dorsal interosseous
20 Long plantar ligament
21 Opponens digiti minimi (part of 14)
22 Peroneus (fibularis) brevis
23 Peroneus (fibularis) longus
24 Peroneus (fibularis) tertius
25 Plantar calcaneocuboid (short plantar) ligament
26 Plantar calcaneonavicular (spring) ligament
27 Plantaris
28 Second dorsal interosseous
29 Second plantar interosseous
30 Tendo calcaneus (Achilles tendon)
31 Third dorsal interosseous
32 Third plantar interosseous
33 Tibialis anterior
34 Tibialis posterior

# Bones of the left foot

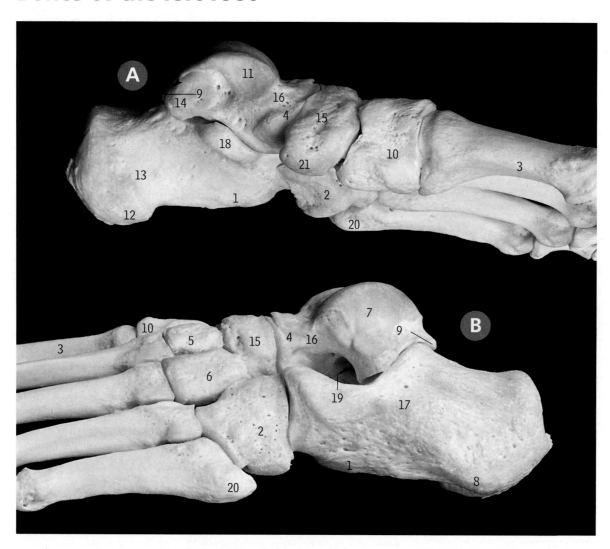

**A** from the medial side    **B** from the lateral side

1 Anterior tubercle of calcaneus
2 Cuboid
3 First metatarsal
4 Head of talus
5 Intermediate cuneiform
6 Lateral cuneiform
7 Lateral malleolar surface of talus
8 Lateral process of calcaneus

9 Lateral tubercle of talus
10 Medial cuneiform
11 Medial malleolar surface of talus
12 Medial process of calcaneus
13 Medial surface of calcaneus
14 Medial tubercle of talus
15 Navicular
16 Neck of talus

17 Peroneal (fibular) trochlea of calcaneus
18 Sustentaculum tali of calcaneus
19 Tarsal sinus
20 Tuberosity of base of fifth metatarsal
21 Tuberosity of navicular

*Hammer toe, see page 355.*

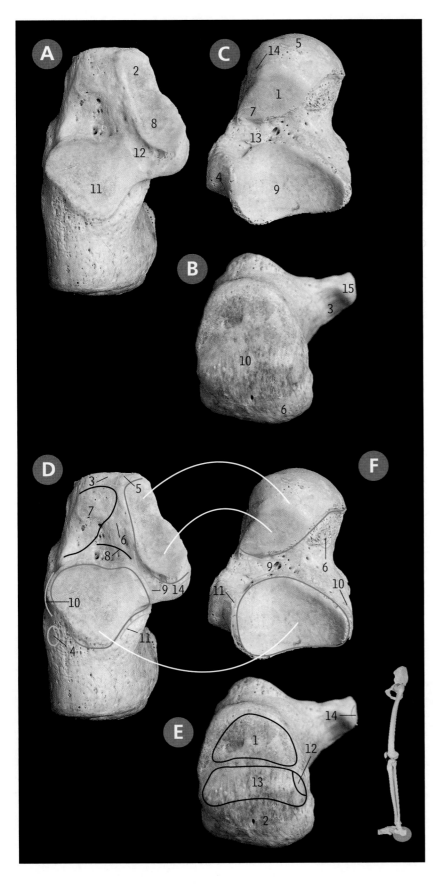

# Bones of the left foot
## *Left calcaneus*

**A** from above        **B** from behind

## *Left talus*

**C** from below

1  Anterior calcanean articular surface of talus
2  Anterior talar articular surface of calcaneus
3  Groove of calcaneus for flexor hallucis longus
4  Groove of talus for flexor hallucis longus
5  Head of talus
6  Medial process of calcaneus
7  Middle calcanean articular surface of talus
8  Middle talar articular surface of calcaneus
9  Posterior calcanean articular surface of talus
10  Posterior surface of calcaneus
11  Posterior talar articular surface of calcaneus
12  Sulcus of calcaneus
13  Sulcus of talus
14  Surface of talus for plantar calcaneonavicular (spring) ligament
15  Sustentaculum tali of calcaneus

# *Left calcaneus, attachments*

**D** from above        **E** from behind

# *Left talus, attachments*

**F** from below

Curved lines indicate corresponding articular surfaces: green, capsular attachment of talocalcanean (subtalar) and talocalcaneonavicular joints; pale green lines, ligament attachments.

1  Area for bursa
2  Area for fibrofatty tissue
3  Calcaneocuboid part of bifurcate ligament
4  Calcaneofibular ligament
5  Calcaneonavicular part of bifurcate ligament
6  Cervical ligament
7  Extensor digitorum brevis
8  Inferior extensor retinaculum
9  Interosseous talocalcanean ligament
10  Lateral talocalcanean ligament
11  Medial talocalcanean ligament
12  Plantaris
13  Tendo calcaneus (Achilles tendon)
14  Tibiocalcanean part of deltoid ligament

The interosseous talocalcanean ligament (cervical) (9) is formed by thickening of the adjacent capsules of the talocalcanean and talocalcaneonavicular joints.

For different interpretations of the term 'subtalar joint' see the notes on page 348.

# Left lower limb bones *secondary centres of ossification*

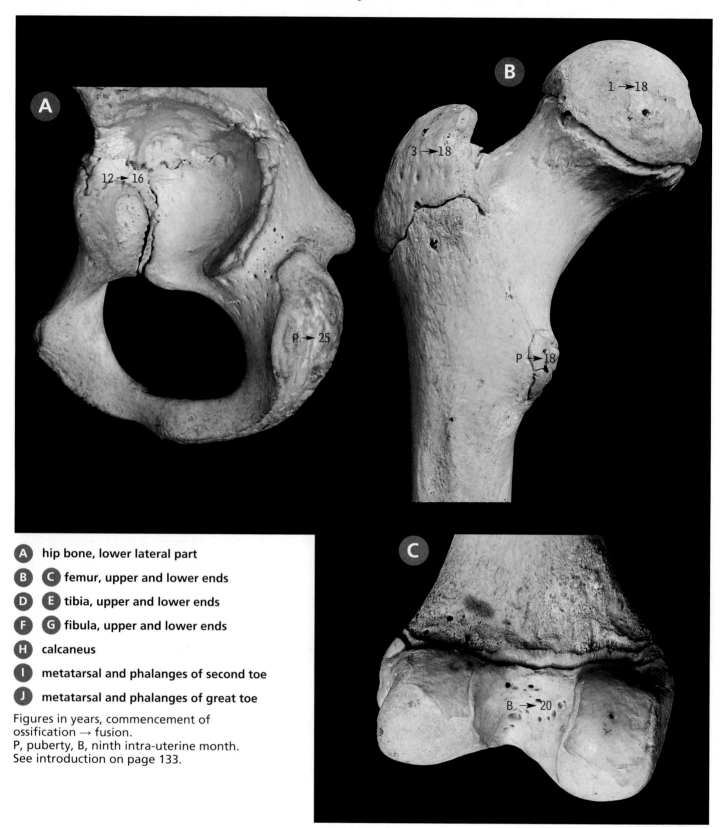

A    hip bone, lower lateral part

B    C    femur, upper and lower ends

D    E    tibia, upper and lower ends

F    G    fibula, upper and lower ends

H    calcaneus

I    metatarsal and phalanges of second toe

J    metatarsal and phalanges of great toe

Figures in years, commencement of
ossification → fusion.
P, puberty, B, ninth intra-uterine month.
See introduction on page 133.

*Slipped upper femoral epiphysis, see page 356.*

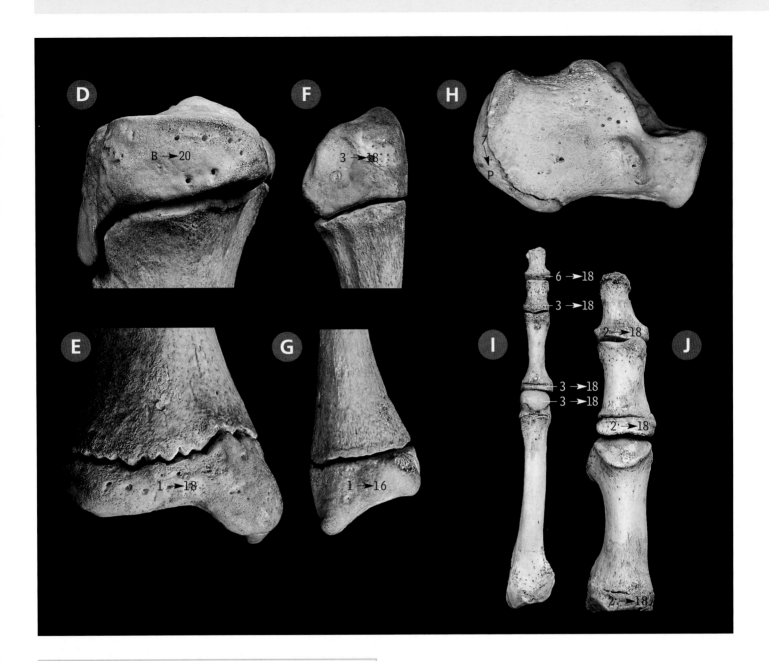

In the hip bone (A) one or more secondary centres appear in the Y-shaped cartilage between ilium, ischium and pubis. Other centres (not illustrated) are usually present for the iliac crest, anterior inferior iliac spine, and (possibly) the pubic tubercle and pubic crest (all P → 25).

The patella (not illustrated) begins to ossify from one or more centres between the third and sixth year.

All the phalanges, and the first metatarsal, have a secondary centre at their proximal ends; the other metatarsals have one at their distal ends.

Of the tarsal bones, the largest, the calcaneus, begins to ossify in the third intra-uterine month and the talus about three months later. The cuboid may begin to ossify either just before or just after birth, with the lateral cuneiform in the first year, medial cuneiform at two years and the intermediate cuneiform and navicular at three years.

The calcaneus (H) is the only tarsal bone to have a secondary centre.

## 🅐 Right gluteal region *surface features*

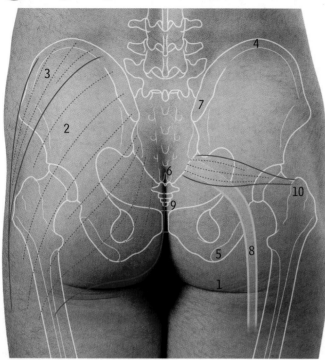

The iliac crest (4) with the posterior superior iliac spine (7), the tip of the coccyx (9), the ischial tuberosity (5) and the tip of the greater trochanter of the femur (10) are palpable landmarks. A line drawn from a point midway between the posterior superior iliac spine (7) and the tip of the coccyx (9) to the tip of the greater trochanter (10) marks the lower border of piriformis (illustrated on right buttock), which is a key feature of the gluteal region, where the most important structure is the sciatic nerve (indicated here in yellow, 8; see dissections and notes opposite).

**1**   Fold of buttock
**2**   Gluteus maximus
**3**   Gluteus medius
**4**   Iliac crest
**5**   Ischial tuberosity
**6**   Natal cleft
**7**   Posterior superior iliac spine
**8**   Sciatic nerve
**9**   Tip of coccyx
**10**   Tip of greater trochanter of femur

## 🅑 Right gluteal region *superficial nerves*

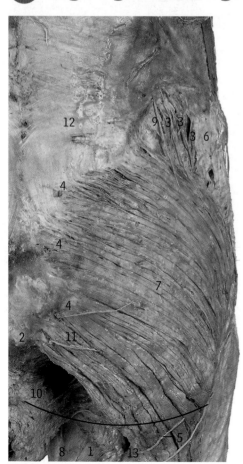

Skin and subcutaneous tissue have been removed, preserving cutaneous branches from the first three lumbar (3) and first three sacral (4) nerves, the cutaneous branches of the posterior femoral cutaneous nerve (5) and the perforating cutaneous nerve (11). The curved line near the bottom of the picture indicates the position of the gluteal fold (fold of the buttock). The muscle fibres of gluteus maximus (7) run downwards and laterally, and its lower border does not correspond to the gluteal fold.

**1**   Adductor magnus
**2**   Coccyx
**3**   Cutaneous branches of dorsal rami of first three lumbar nerves
**4**   Gluteal branches of dorsal rami of first three sacral nerves
**5**   Gluteal branches of the posterior femoral cutaneous nerve
**6**   Gluteal fascia overlying gluteus medius
**7**   Gluteus maximus
**8**   Gracilis
**9**   Iliac crest
**10**   Ischio-anal fossa and levator ani
**11**   Perforating cutaneous nerve
**12**   Posterior layer of lumbar fascia overlying erector spinae
**13**   Semitendinosus

---

The gluteal region or buttock is sometimes used as a site for intramuscular injections. The correct site is in the upper outer quadrant of the buttock, and for delimiting this quadrant, it is essential to remember that the upper boundary of the buttock is the uppermost part of the iliac crest. The lower boundary is the fold of the buttock. Dividing the area between these two boundaries by a vertical line midway between the midline and the lateral side of the body indicates that the upper outer quadrant is well above and to the right of the label 7 in B, and this is the safe site for injection – well above and to the right of the sciatic nerve which is displayed in the dissections opposite.

*Intramuscular injection – gluteal region, see page 355.*

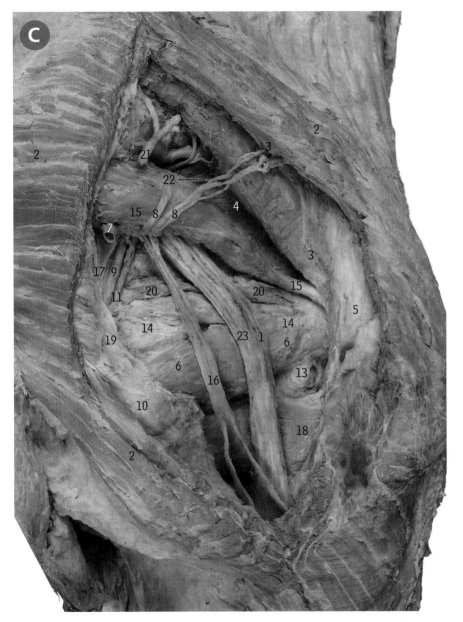

# Right gluteal region

**C** with most of gluteus maximus removed

**D** with the sciatic trunk displaced

**1** Common peroneal (fibular) part of sciatic nerve
**2** Gluteus maximus
**3** Gluteus medius
**4** Gluteus minimus
**5** Greater trochanter of femur
**6** Inferior gemellus
**7** Inferior gluteal artery
**8** Inferior gluteal nerve
**9** Internal pudendal artery
**10** Ischial tuberosity
**11** Nerve to obturator internus
**12** Nerve to quadratus femoris
**13** Obturator externus
**14** Obturator internus
**15** Piriformis
**16** Posterior femoral cutaneous nerve
**17** Pudendal nerve
**18** Quadratus femoris
**19** Sacrotuberous ligament
**20** Superior gemellus
**21** Superior gluteal artery
**22** Superior gluteal nerve
**23** Tibial part of sciatic nerve

The two parts of the sciatic trunk (common peroneal (fibular) and tibial, 1 and 23) usually divide from one another at the top of the popliteal fossa (page 330B) but are sometimes separate as they emerge beneath piriformis, and the common peroneal (fibular) may even perforate piriformis.

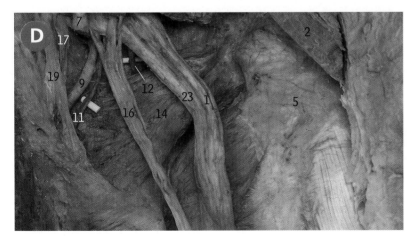

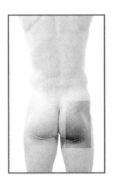

# Right thigh *posterior view*

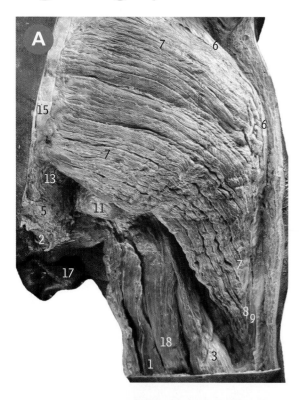

**A** Gluteal region and proximal hamstrings

**B** Deeper dissection revealing ischio-anal fossa

| | |
|---|---|
| **1** | Adductor magnus, hamstring part |
| **2** | Anus |
| **3** | Biceps femoris |
| **4** | Biceps femoris, tendon of long head |
| **5** | External anal sphincter |
| **6** | Gluteal fascia |
| **7** | Gluteus maximus |
| **8** | Gluteus maximus, attachment to iliotibial tract |
| **9** | Iliotibial tract (thickened fascia lata) |
| **10** | Inferior rectal vessels |
| **11** | Ischial tuberosity |
| **12** | Ischio-anal fossa |
| **13** | Levator ani |
| **14** | Pudendal vessels and pudendal nerve |
| **15** | Sacrum, dorsal fascia |
| **16** | Sciatic nerve within fascial sheath |
| **17** | Scrotal skin |
| **18** | Semitendinosus |
| **19** | Superior gluteal vessels |

*Torn hamstrings, see page 357.*

## C Right upper thigh *posterior view*

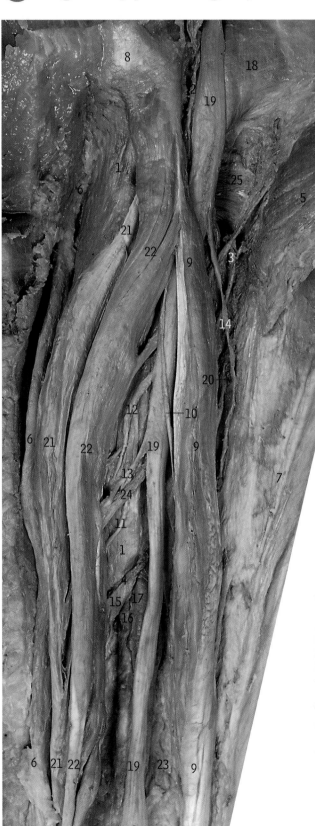

Gluteus maximus (5) has been reflected laterally and the gap between semitendinosus (22) and biceps (9) has been opened up to show the sciatic trunk (19) and its muscular branches.

| | |
|---|---|
| **1** Adductor magnus | **13** Nerve to semitendinosus |
| **2** Anastomotic branch of inferior gluteal artery | **14** Nerve to short head of biceps |
| | **15** Opening in adductor magnus |
| **3** First perforating artery | **16** Popliteal artery |
| **4** Fourth perforating artery | **17** Popliteal vein |
| **5** Gluteus maximus | **18** Quadratus femoris |
| **6** Gracilis | **19** Sciatic trunk |
| **7** Iliotibial tract overlying vastus lateralis | **20** Second perforating artery |
| | **21** Semimembranosus |
| **8** Ischial tuberosity | **22** Semitendinosus |
| **9** Long head of biceps | **23** Short head of biceps |
| **10** Nerve to long head of biceps | **24** Third perforating artery |
| **11** Nerve to semimembranosus | **25** Upper part of adductor magnus ('adductor minimus') |
| **12** Nerve to semimembranosus and adductor magnus | |

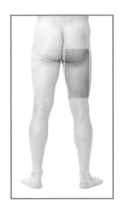

The only muscular branch to arise from the lateral side of the sciatic trunk (i.e. from the common peroneal (fibular) part of the nerve (19), uppermost 19, near the top of the picture), is the nerve to the short head of biceps (14). All the other muscular branches – to the long head of biceps (10), semi-membranosus (11), semimembranosus and adductor magnus (12) and semi-tendinosus (13) – arise from the medial side of the sciatic trunk (19, near the centre of the picture) (i.e. from the tibial part of the nerve).

## D Femoral arteriogram

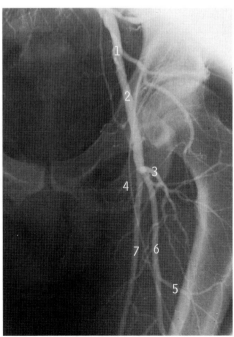

**1** Catheter introduced into distal abdominal aorta via right femoral artery
**2** Common femoral artery
**3** Lateral circumflex femoral artery
**4** Medial circumflex femoral artery
**5** Perforating artery
**6** Profunda femoris artery
**7** Superficial femoral artery

# Anterior thigh and lower abdomen

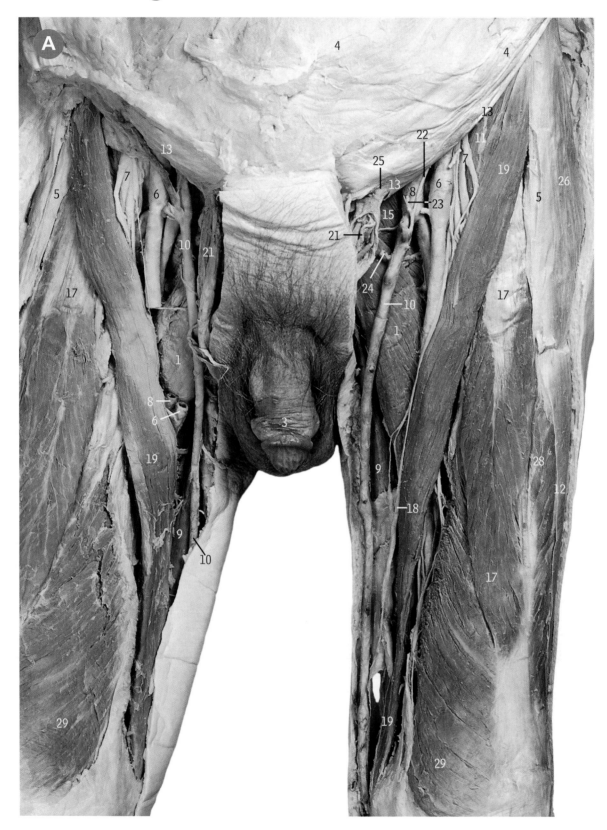

*Lumbar plexus block, varicella zoster virus, see pages 356, 357.*

# Upper anterior thigh　*Sartorius retracted medially to show subsartorial canal*

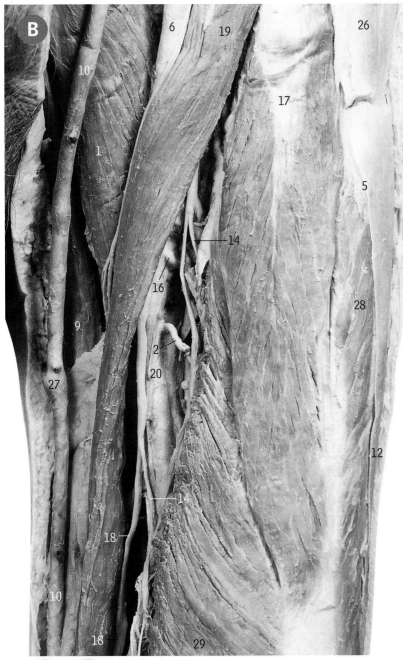

The boundaries of the femoral triangle are the inguinal ligament (13), the medial border of sartorius (19) and the medial border of adductor longus (1).

The femoral canal is the medial compartment of the femoral sheath (removed) which contains in its middle compartment the femoral vein (8), and in the lateral compartment the femoral artery (6). The femoral nerve (7) is lateral to the sheath, not within it.

| | | |
|---|---|---|
| **1** Adductor longus | **11** Iliacus | **21** Spermatic cord |
| **2** Arterial branch to vastus medialis | **12** Iliotibial tract | **22** Superficial circumflex iliac vein |
| **3** Corona of glans penis | **13** Inguinal ligament | **23** Superficial epigastric vein |
| **4** External oblique aponeurosis | **14** Nerve to vastus medialis | **24** Superficial external pudendal vein |
| **5** Fascia lata (cut edge) | **15** Pectineus | **25** Superficial inguinal ring |
| **6** Femoral artery | **16** Perforating branch of profunda femoris artery | **26** Tensor fasciae latae deep to fascia lata |
| **7** Femoral nerve | **17** Rectus femoris | **27** Valvular bulge in vein |
| **8** Femoral vein | **18** Saphenous nerve | **28** Vastus lateralis |
| **9** Gracilis | **19** Sartorius | **29** Vastus medialis |
| **10** Great saphenous vein | **20** Subsartorial fascia (thickened aponeurosis) | |

*Femoral nerve paralysis, obturator nerve paralysis, see pages 355, 356.*

# A Right femoral artery

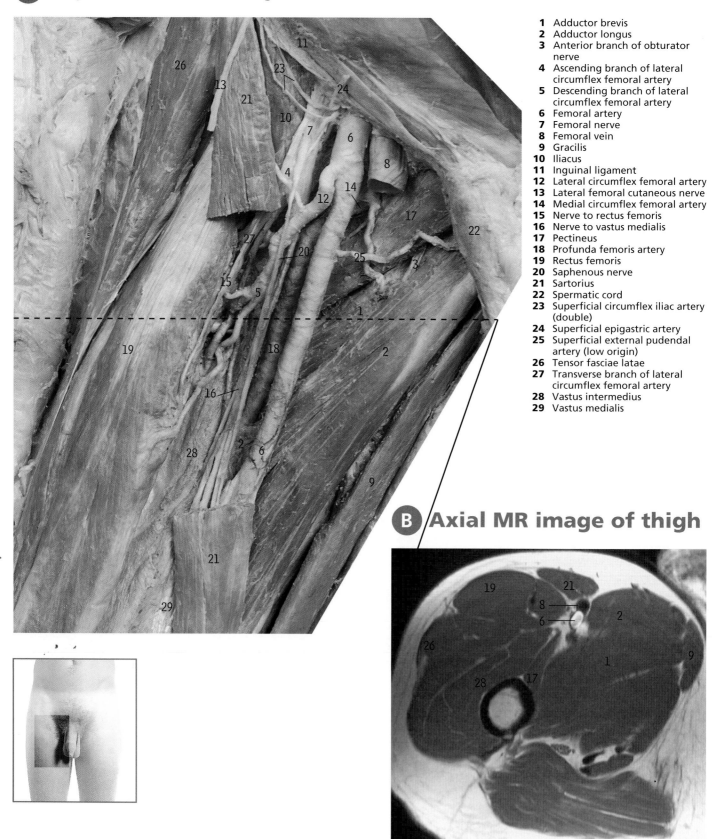

1 Adductor brevis
2 Adductor longus
3 Anterior branch of obturator nerve
4 Ascending branch of lateral circumflex femoral artery
5 Descending branch of lateral circumflex femoral artery
6 Femoral artery
7 Femoral nerve
8 Femoral vein
9 Gracilis
10 Iliacus
11 Inguinal ligament
12 Lateral circumflex femoral artery
13 Lateral femoral cutaneous nerve
14 Medial circumflex femoral artery
15 Nerve to rectus femoris
16 Nerve to vastus medialis
17 Pectineus
18 Profunda femoris artery
19 Rectus femoris
20 Saphenous nerve
21 Sartorius
22 Spermatic cord
23 Superficial circumflex iliac artery (double)
24 Superficial epigastric artery
25 Superficial external pudendal artery (low origin)
26 Tensor fasciae latae
27 Transverse branch of lateral circumflex femoral artery
28 Vastus intermedius
29 Vastus medialis

# B Axial MR image of thigh

*Femoral artery puncture, meralgia paraesthetica, see pages 355, 356.*

## C Right lower thigh

### from the front and medial side

The lower part of sartorius (13) has been displaced medially to open up the lower part of the adductor canal and expose the femoral artery (2) passing through the opening in adductor magnus (7) to enter the popliteal fossa behind the knee and become the popliteal artery (page 330).

1  Adductor magnus
2  Femoral artery
3  Gracilis
4  Iliotibial tract
5  Lowest (horizontal) fibres of vastus medialis
6  Medial patellar retinaculum
7  Opening in adductor magnus
8  Patella
9  Quadriceps tendon
10 Rectus femoris
11 Saphenous branch of descending genicular artery
12 Saphenous nerve
13 Sartorius
14 Vastus medialis and nerve

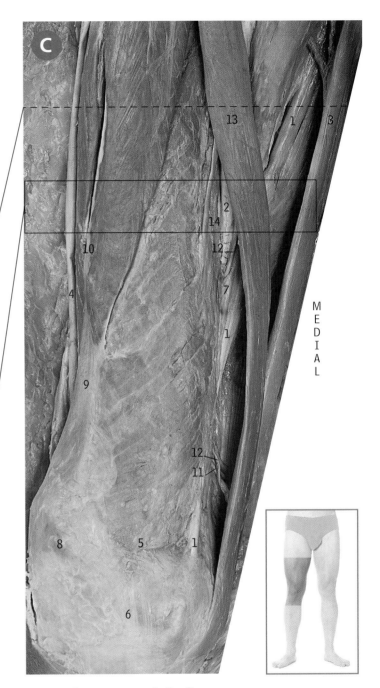

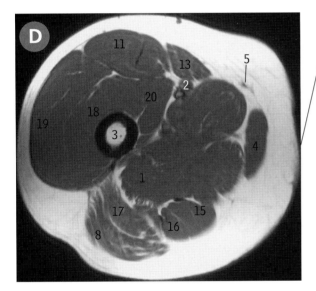

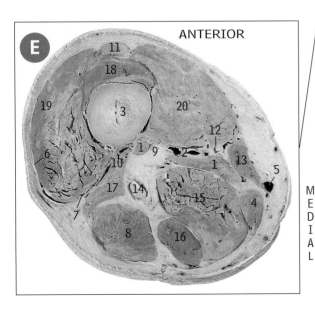

## Right lower thigh

### D axial MR image  E cross-section

1  Adductor magnus
2  Femoral vessels
3  Femur
4  Gracilis
5  Great saphenous vein
6  Iliotibial tract of fascia lata
7  Lateral intermuscular septum
8  Long head of biceps
9  Opening in adductor magnus
10 Profunda femoris vessels
11 Rectus femoris
12 Saphenous nerve
13 Sartorius
14 Sciatic nerve
15 Semimembranosus
16 Semitendinosus
17 Short head of biceps
18 Vastus intermedius
19 Vastus lateralis
20 Vastus medialis

*Femoropopliteal bypass, intermittent claudication, rupture of the quadriceps tendon, see pages 355, 356.*

# Right hip joint

**A** *from the front and below*   **B** *from the front and above*

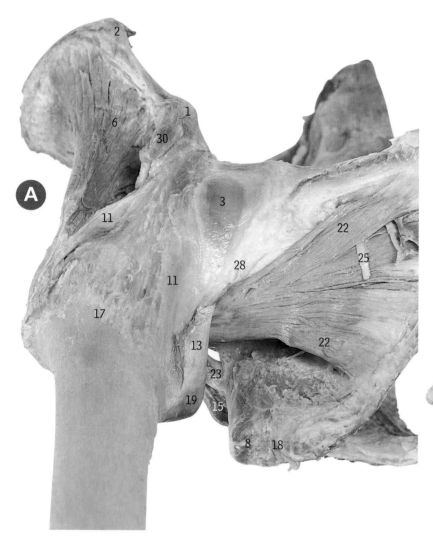

Some of the fibres of the ischiofemoral ligament help to form the zona orbicularis – circular fibres of the capsule that form a collar around the neck of the femur.

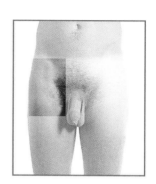

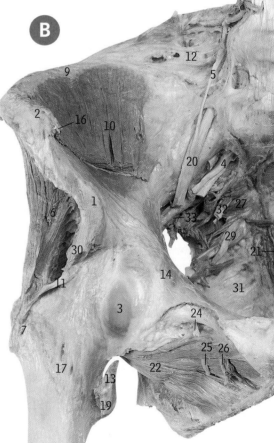

| | |
|---|---|
| **1** Anterior inferior iliac spine | **18** Ischial tuberosity |
| **2** Anterior superior iliac spine | **19** Lesser trochanter |
| **3** Bursa for psoas tendon | **20** Lumbosacral trunk |
| **4** First sacral nerve root | **21** Median sacral artery |
| **5** Fourth lumbar nerve root | **22** Obturator externus |
| **6** Gluteus minimus muscle | **23** Obturator internus tendon |
| **7** Greater trochanter | **24** Obturator nerve, anterior branch |
| **8** Hamstring origin | **25** Obturator nerve, posterior branch |
| **9** Iliac crest | **26** Obturator vessels |
| **10** Iliacus muscle | **27** Piriformis muscle |
| **11** Iliofemoral ligament | **28** Pubofemoral ligament |
| **12** Iliolumbar ligament | **29** Pudendal nerve |
| **13** Iliopsoas tendon | **30** Rectus femoris muscle |
| **14** Iliopubic eminence | **31** Sacrospinous ligament |
| **15** Inferior gemellus muscle | **32** Second sacral nerve root |
| **16** Inguinal ligament | **33** Superior gluteal artery |
| **17** Intertrochanteric line and capsule attachment | |

*Trendelenburg's sign, see page 357.*

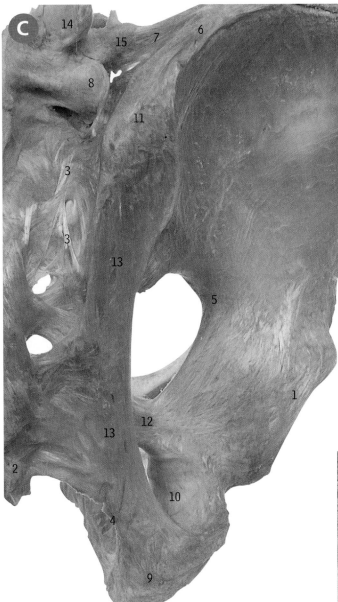

## C Right vertebropelvic and sacro-iliac ligaments
### *from behind*

1  Acetabular labrum
2  Coccyx
3  Dorsal sacro-iliac ligaments
4  Falciform process of sacrotuberous ligament
5  Greater sciatic notch
6  Iliac crest
7  Iliolumbar ligament
8  Inferior articular process of fifth lumbar vertebra
9  Ischial tuberosity
10  Lesser sciatic notch
11  Posterior superior iliac spine
12  Sacrospinous ligament and ischial spine
13  Sacrotuberous ligament
14  Superior articular process of fifth lumbar vertebra
15  Transverse process of fifth lumbar vertebra

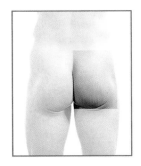

## D Right hip joint with femur removed *from the right*

The femur has been disarticulated from the acetabulum and removed, leaving the acetabular labrum (2), transverse ligament (10) and the ligament teres (5).

1  Acetabular fossa
   (non-articular)
2  Acetabular labrum
3  Adductor longus
4  Articular surface
5  Ligament teres femoris
6  Obturator externus
7  Pectineus
8  Reflected head of rectus femoris
9  Straight head of rectus femoris
10  Transverse ligament

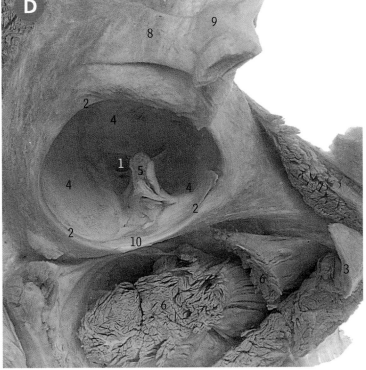

*Avascular necrosis of the head of the femur, see page 355.*

# Left hip joint Ⓐ *coronal section, from the front* Ⓑ *coronal MR image*

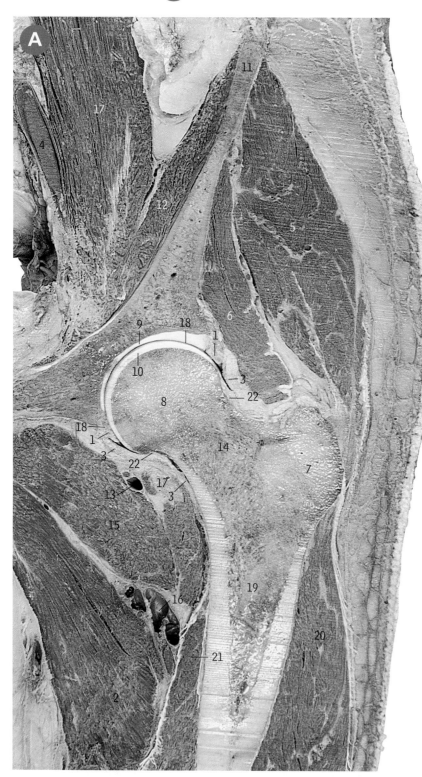

The section has almost passed through the centre of the head (8) of the femur and the centre of the greater trochanter (7). Above the neck of the femur (14), gluteus minimus (6) with gluteus medius (5) above it run down to their attachments to the greater trochanter (7), while below the neck the tendon of psoas major (17) and muscle fibres of iliacus (12) pass backwards towards the lesser trochanter. The circular fibres of the zona orbicularis (22) constrict the capsule (3) around the intracapsular part of the neck of the femur.

1 Acetabular labrum
2 Adductor longus
3 Capsule of hip joint
4 External iliac artery
5 Gluteus medius
6 Gluteus minimus
7 Greater trochanter
8 Head of femur
9 Hyaline cartilage of acetabulum
10 Hyaline cartilage of head
11 Iliac crest
12 Iliacus
13 Medial circumflex femoral vessels
14 Neck of femur
15 Pectineus
16 Profunda femoris vessels
17 Psoas major
18 Rim of acetabulum
19 Shaft of femur
20 Vastus lateralis
21 Vastus medialis
22 Zona orbicularis of capsule

\* Contrast outlines the joint cavity
\*\* Ligamentum teres

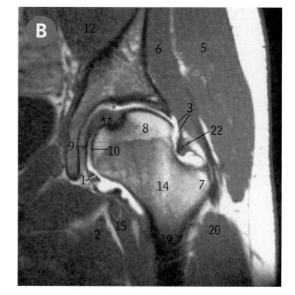

The convergence of gluteus medius and minimus (5 and 6) on to the greater trochanter is well displayed in this section. These muscles are classified as abductors of the femur at the hip joint, but their more important action is in walking, where they act to prevent adduction – preventing the pelvis from tilting to the opposite side when the opposite limb is off the ground (see Trendelenburg's sign, page 357).

*Total hip replacement surgery, see page 357.*

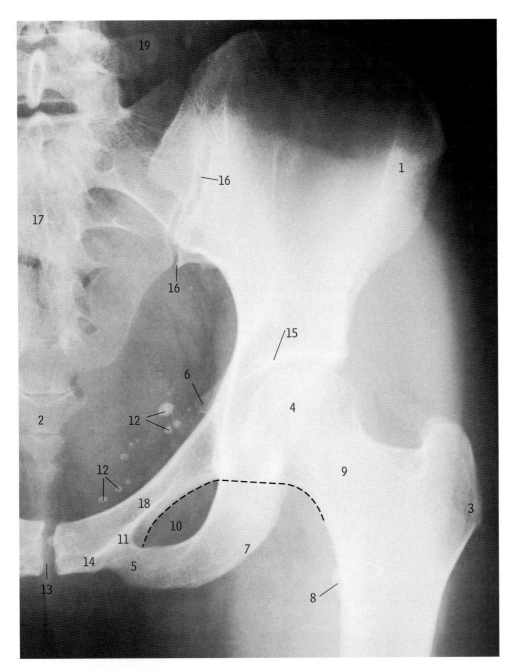

## C Left hip and sacro-iliac joint

### radiograph

In this standard anteroposterior view of the hip joint (15 and 4), much of the joint line of the sacro-iliac joint can also be seen (16). The dashed line on C is Shenton's line, a guide to diagnosing femoral neck fractures.

1 Anterior superior iliac spine
2 First coccygeal vertebra
3 Greater trochanter of femur
4 Head of femur
5 Inferior pubic ramus
6 Ischial spine
7 Ischial tuberosity
8 Lesser trochanter of femur
9 Neck of femur
10 Obturator foramen
11 Pectineal line
12 Phleboliths in pelvic veins
13 Pubic symphysis
14 Pubic tubercle
15 Rim of acetabulum
16 Sacro-iliac joint
17 Sacrum
18 Superior pubic ramus
19 Transverse process of fifth lumbar vertebra

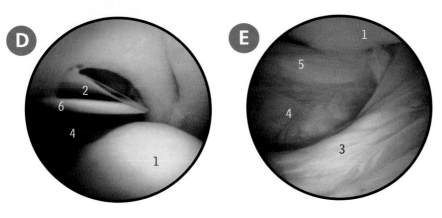

## Hip joint

## D E arthroscopic views

1 Femoral head
2 Irrigation needle
3 Ligamentum teres
4 Synovium
5 Transverse ligament
6 Zona orbicularis

*Posterior hip dislocation, see page 356.*

# Right knee
## *partially flexed*

**A** from the lateral side

**B** from the medial side

1 Biceps femoris
2 Common peroneal (fibular) nerve
3 Head of fibula
4 Iliotibial tract
5 Lateral head of gastrocnemius
6 Margin of condyle of femur
7 Margin of condyle of tibia
8 Patella
9 Patellar ligament
10 Popliteal fossa
11 Semimembranosus
12 Semitendinosus
13 Tuberosity of tibia
14 Vastus medialis

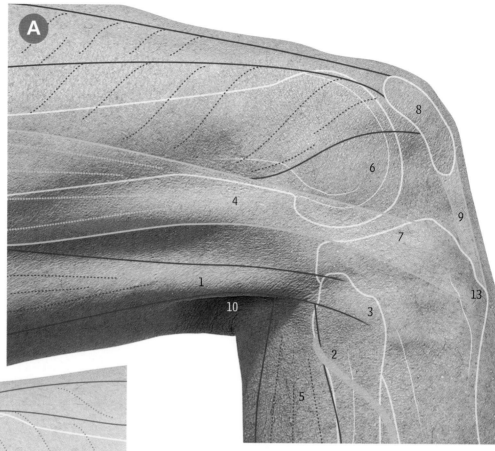

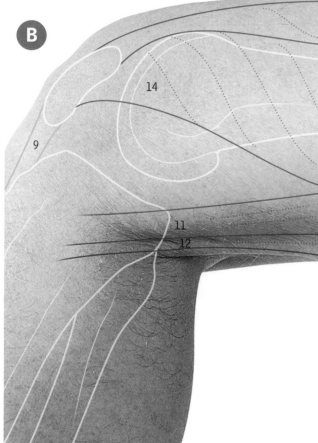

Behind the knee on the lateral side, the rounded tendon of biceps (1) can be felt easily, with the broad strap-like iliotibial tract (4) in front of it, with a furrow between them. On the medial side, two tendons can be felt – the narrow rounded semitendinosus (12) just behind the broader semimembranosus (11). At the front, the patellar ligament (9) keeps the patella (8) at a constant distance from the tibial tuberosity (13), while at the side the adjacent margins of the femoral and tibial condyles (6 and 7) can be palpated.

*Patellar tendon reflex, see page 356.*

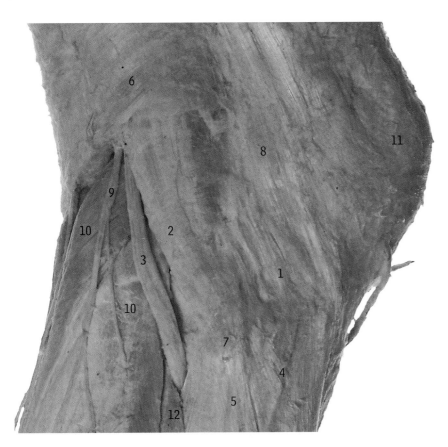

## C Right knee
### superficial dissection, from the lateral side

The fascia behind biceps (2) has been removed to show the common peroneal (fibular) nerve (3) passing downwards immediately behind the tendon, and then running between the adjacent borders of soleus (12) and peroneus (fibularis) longus (5), under cover of which it lies against the neck of the fibula. Minor superficial vessels and nerves have been removed.

1 Attachment of iliotibial tract to tibia
2 Biceps
3 Common peroneal (fibular) nerve
4 Deep fascia overlying extensor muscles
5 Deep fascia overlying peroneus (fibularis) longus
6 Fascia lata
7 Head of fibula
8 Iliotibial tract
9 Lateral cutaneous nerve of calf
10 Lateral head of gastrocnemius
11 Patella
12 Soleus

The iliotibial tract (8) is the thickened lateral part of the fascia lata (6). At its upper part, the tensor fasciae latae and most of gluteus maximus are inserted into it.

Its subcutaneous position and contact with the neck of the fibula make the common peroneal (fibular) nerve (3) the most commonly injured nerve in the lower limb.

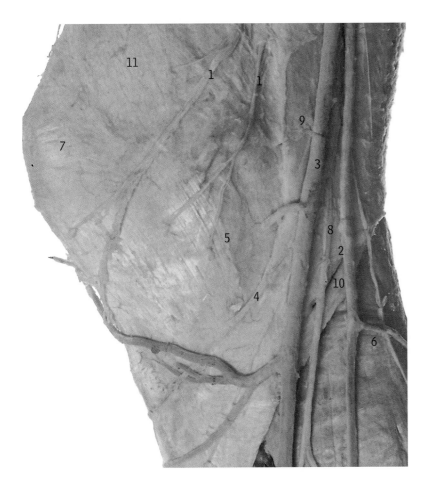

## D Right knee
### superficial dissection, from the medial side

The great saphenous vein (3) runs upwards about a hand's breadth behind the medial border of the patella (7). The saphenous nerve (8) becomes superficial between the tendons of sartorius (9) and gracilis (2), and its infrapatellar branch (4) curls forwards a little below the upper margin of the tibial condyle.

1 Branches of medial femoral cutaneous nerve
2 Gracilis
3 Great saphenous vein
4 Infrapatellar branch of saphenous nerve
5 Level of margin of medial condyle of tibia
6 Medial head of gastrocnemius
7 Patella
8 Saphenous nerve
9 Sartorius
10 Semitendinosus
11 Vastus medialis

# Right popliteal fossa *superficial dissections*

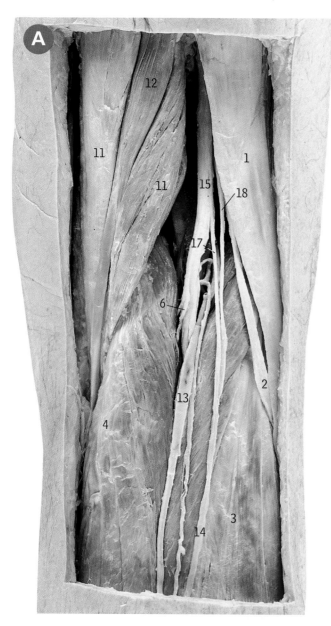

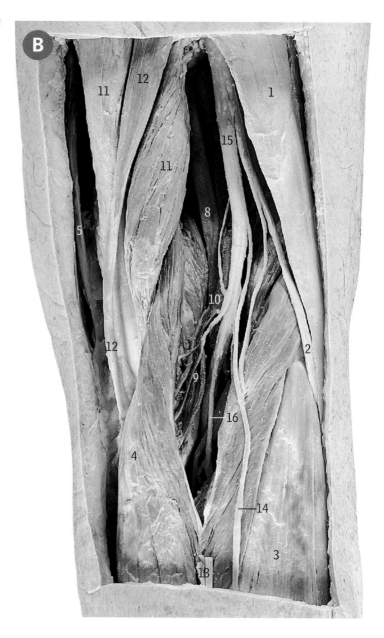

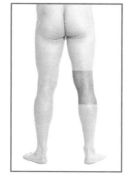

**A** Skin and fascia forming the roof of the diamond-shaped popliteal fossa and the fat within it have been removed but the small saphenous vein which pierces the fascia has been preserved. A high (proximal) union of the lateral and medial sural cutaneous nerves places the sural nerve in this field.

**B** Heads of gastrocnemius have been separated to show deeper structures.

1 Biceps femoris
2 Common peroneal (fibular) nerve
3 Gastrocnemius, lateral head
4 Gastrocnemius, medial head
5 Gracilis
6 Nerve to medial head of gastrocnemius
7 Plantaris
8 Popliteal artery
9 Popliteal vascular branches to gastrocnemius
10 Popliteal vein
11 Semimembranosus
12 Semitendinosus
13 Small saphenous vein
14 Sural nerve
15 Tibial nerve
16 Tibial nerve, muscular branches
17 Sural nerve, branch from tibial
18 Sural nerve, branch from common peroneal (fibular)

# Popliteal fossa *progressive dissections*

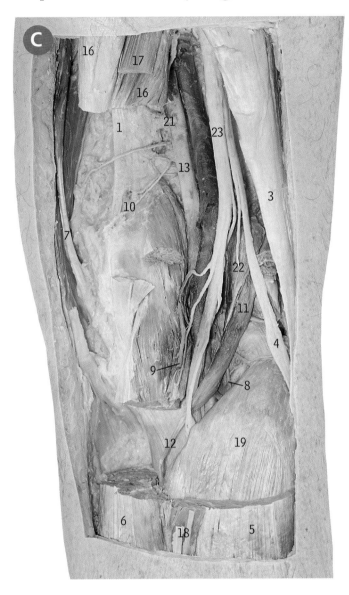

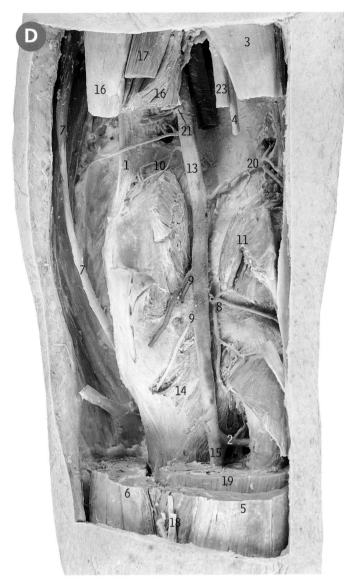

**C** Removal of the semitendinosus, semimembranosus and most of the origins of the gastrocnemius reveals the plantaris and branches of the deeply situated popliteal artery and soleus.

**D** Removal of the muscular boundaries of the popliteal fossa shows the popliteal artery, its genicular anastomoses and its terminal branches, the anterior and posterior tibial arteries.

| | |
|---|---|
| **1** Adductor magnus | **12** Plantaris tendon |
| **2** Anterior tibial artery | **13** Popliteal artery |
| **3** Biceps femoris | **14** Popliteus |
| **4** Common peroneal (fibular) nerve | **15** Posterior tibial artery |
| **5** Gastrocnemius, lateral head | **16** Semimembranosus |
| **6** Gastrocnemius, medial head | **17** Semitendinosus |
| **7** Gracilis | **18** Short saphenous vein |
| **8** Inferior lateral genicular artery | **19** Soleus |
| **9** Inferior medial genicular artery | **20** Superior lateral genicular artery |
| **10** Middle genicular artery | **21** Superior medial genicular artery |
| **11** Plantaris muscle | **22** Sural nerve |
| | **23** Tibial nerve |

*Popliteal (Baker's) cyst, popliteal artery aneurysm, see page 356.*

# Left knee joint *ligaments*

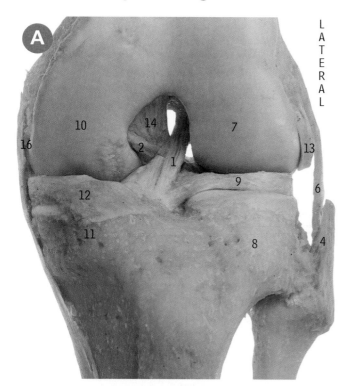

**B**   Coronal MR image    **D**   Coronal MR image

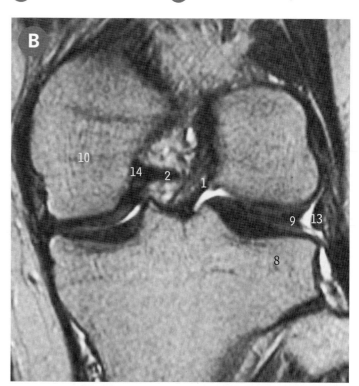

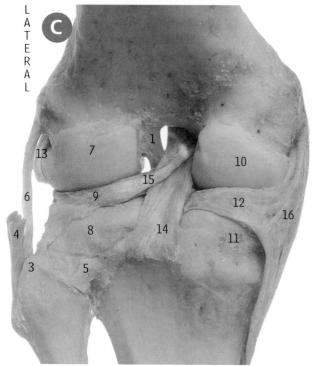

**A**   from the front    **C**   from behind

The capsule of the knee joint and all surrounding tissues have been removed, leaving only the ligaments of the joint, which is partially flexed.

**A–D** label key

| | |
|---|---|
| **1** Anterior cruciate ligament | **9** Lateral meniscus |
| **2** Anterior meniscofemoral ligament | **10** Medial condyle of femur |
| **3** Apex of head of fibula | **11** Medial condyle of tibia |
| **4** Biceps tendon | **12** Medial meniscus |
| **5** Capsule of superior tibiofibular joint | **13** Popliteus tendon |
| **6** Fibular collateral ligament (lateral) | **14** Posterior cruciate ligament |
| **7** Lateral condyle of femur | **15** Posterior meniscofemoral ligament |
| **8** Lateral condyle of tibia | **16** Tibial collateral ligament (medial) |

The fibular collateral (lateral) ligament (A6) is a rounded cord about 5 cm long, passing from the lateral epicondyle of the femur to the head of the fibula just in front of its apex (C3), largely under cover of the tendon of biceps (C4).

The medial meniscus (E12 and F12) is attached to the deep part of the tibial collateral ligament (E19 and F20). This helps to anchor the meniscus but makes it liable to become trapped and torn by rotatory movements between the tibia and femur.

The lateral meniscus (A9) is not attached to the fibular collateral ligament (A6), but is attached posteriorly to the popliteus muscle (F5).

The tibial collateral (medial) ligament (E19) is a broad flat band about 12 cm long, passing from the medial epicondyle of the femur (E11) to the medial condyle of the tibia (E10) and an extensive area of the medial surface of the tibia below the condyle (as in the lower part of E).

The cruciate ligaments are named from their attachments to the tibia.

The anterior cruciate ligament (A1 and F1) passes upwards, backwards and laterally to be attached to the medial side of the lateral condyle of the femur (C7).

The posterior cruciate ligament (C14 and F13) passes upwards, forwards and medially to be attached to the lateral surface of the medial condyle of the femur (A10).

# Left knee joint *ligaments*

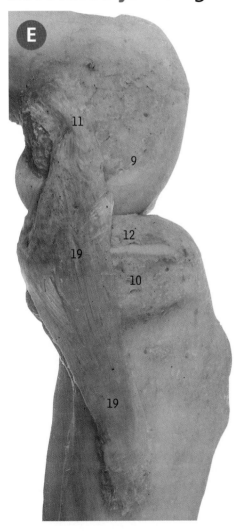

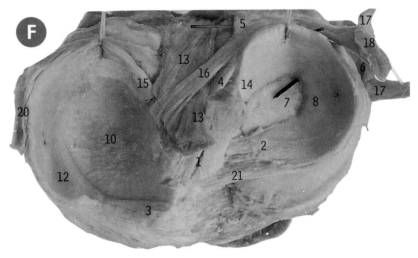

**E** from the medial side     **F** from above

The same specimen as in A and C is seen from the medial side in E, to show the broad tibial collateral ligament (19). F is the view looking down on the upper surface of the tibia after removing the femur by cutting through the capsule, the collateral ligaments, and the cruciate ligaments. The medial and lateral menisci (12 and 8) remain at the periphery of the articular surfaces of the tibial condyles. The horns of the menisci (3 and 15; 2 and 14) and the cruciate ligaments (1 and 13) are attached to the non-articular intercondylar area of the tibia. Compare with C on page 305.

| | |
|---|---|
| **1** Anterior cruciate ligament | **12** Medial meniscus |
| **2** Anterior horn of lateral meniscus | **13** Posterior cruciate ligament |
| **3** Anterior horn of medial meniscus | **14** Posterior horn of lateral meniscus |
| **4** Anterior meniscofemoral ligament | **15** Posterior horn of medial meniscus |
| **5** Attachment of lateral meniscus to popliteus (with underlying marker) | **16** Posterior meniscofemoral ligament |
| **6** Fibular collateral ligament | **17** Tendon of biceps |
| **7** Lateral condyle of tibia | **18** Tendon of popliteus |
| **8** Lateral meniscus | **19** Tibial collateral ligament |
| **9** Medial condyle of femur | **20** Tibial collateral ligament attached to medial meniscus |
| **10** Medial condyle of tibia | **21** Transverse ligament |
| **11** Medial epicondyle of femur | |

*Meniscal tears, rupture of the anterior cruciate ligament, see page 356.*

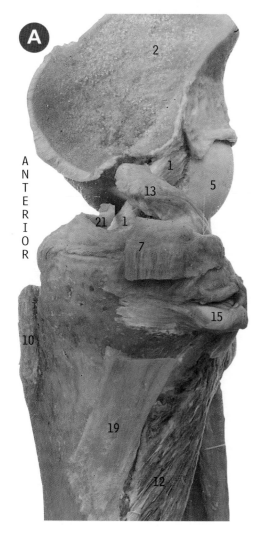

# Right knee joint

**A** from the medial side with the medial femoral condyle removed

**B** sagittal MR image

Removal of the medial half of the lower end of the femur enables the X-shaped crossover of the cruciate ligaments to be seen; the anterior cruciate (1) is passing backwards and laterally, while the posterior cruciate (13) passes forwards and medially. The MR image in B shows the infrapatellar fat pad (3).

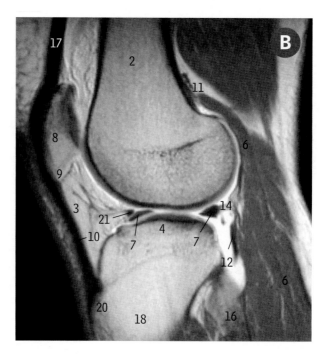

| | | |
|---|---|---|
| **1** Anterior cruciate ligament | **8** Patella | **15** Semimembranosus |
| **2** Femur | **9** Patellar apex | **16** Soleus |
| **3** Infrapatellar fat pad | **10** Patellar ligament (tendon) | **17** Tendon of quadriceps |
| **4** Intercondylar notch | **11** Popliteal artery and vein | **18** Tibia |
| **5** Lateral condyle of femur | **12** Popliteus | **19** Tibial collateral ligament |
| **6** Lateral head of gastrocnemius muscle | **13** Posterior cruciate ligament | **20** Tibial tubercle |
| **7** Meniscus | **14** Posterior meniscofemoral ligament | **21** Transverse (intermeniscal) ligament |

# Left knee *arthroscopic views*

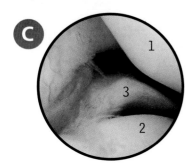

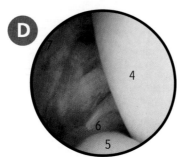

**C** anterolateral approach

**D** posteromedial approach

| | |
|---|---|
| **1** Lateral condyle of femur | **5** Medial meniscus |
| **2** Lateral condyle of tibia | **6** Posterior cruciate ligament |
| **3** Lateral meniscus | **7** Posterior part of capsule |
| **4** Medial condyle of femur | |

*Rupture of the posterior cruciate ligament, suprapatellar bursitis, see page 356.*

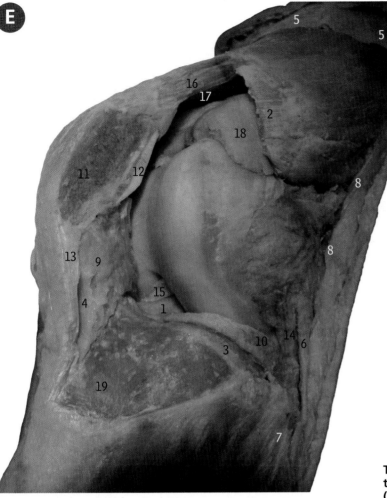

# E Left knee joint

## opened from the lateral side to reveal internal structures

1 Anterior cruciate ligament
2 Aponeurosis of vastus lateralis (cut edge)
3 Articular cartilage, tibial plateau
4 Deep infrapatellar bursa
5 Fascia lata (deep fascia)
6 Fibular collateral ligament
7 Head of fibula
8 Iliotibial tract (cut edge)
9 Infrapatellar fat pad
10 Lateral meniscus
11 Patella
12 Patellar articular cartilage
13 Patellar ligament (tendon)
14 Popliteus tendon, attachment to lateral tibial epicondyle
15 Posterior cruciate ligament
16 Quadriceps tendon
17 Suprapatellar bursa
18 Suprapatellar fat pad
19 Tibial tuberosity

# F Left knee joint

## from the medial side, with synovial and bursal cavities injected

The resin injection has distended the synovial cavity of the joint (3) and extends into the suprapatellar bursa (10), the bursa round the popliteus tendon (2) and the semimembranosus bursa (9).

1 Articularis genu
2 Bursa of popliteus tendon
3 Capsule
4 Medial meniscus
5 Patella
6 Patellar ligament
7 Quadriceps tendon
8 Semimembranosus
9 Semimembranosus bursa
10 Suprapatellar bursa
11 Tibial collateral ligament

> The suprapatellar bursa (F10) always communicates with the joint cavity. The bursa around the popliteus tendon (F2) usually does so. The semimembranosus bursa (F9) may do so.

# G Anterior cruciate ligament

## anterior arthroscopic view

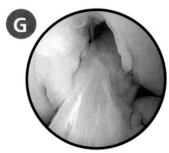

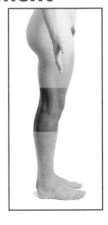

*Knee joint aspiration and injection, prepatellar bursitis, see page 356.*

# Knee *radiographs and arthroscopic views*

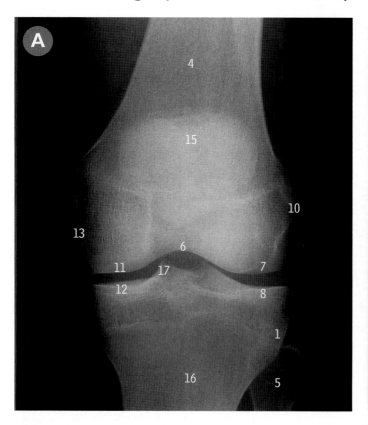

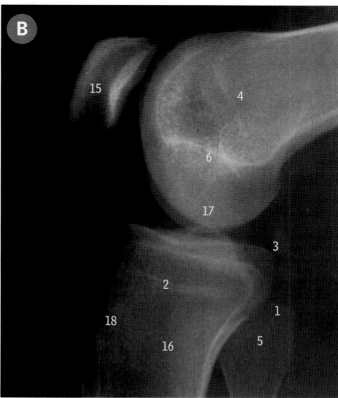

**A** from the front

**B** from the lateral side in partial flexion

**C** skyline view projection

**D** anterolateral approach

**E** lateral view of patella

In A, the shadow of the patella (15) is superimposed on that of the femur. The regular space between the condyles of the femur and tibia (7 and 8, 11 and 12) is due to the thickness of the hyaline cartilage on the articulating surface, with the menisci at the periphery. In C, with the knee flexed, the view should be compared with the bones seen on page 299, E, and the lateral edge of the patella (9) is seen in the arthroscopic view in E.

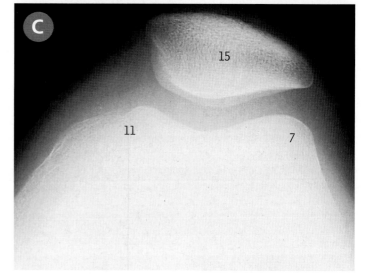

1 Apex (styloid process) of fibula
2 Epiphysial line
3 Fabella
4 Femur
5 Head of fibula
6 Intercondylar fossa
7 Lateral condyle of femur
8 Lateral condyle of tibia
9 Lateral edge of patella
10 Lateral epicondyle of femur
11 Medial condyle of femur
12 Medial condyle of tibia
13 Medial epicondyle of femur
14 Medial meniscus
15 Patella
16 Tibia
17 Tubercles of intercondylar eminence
18 Tuberosity of tibia

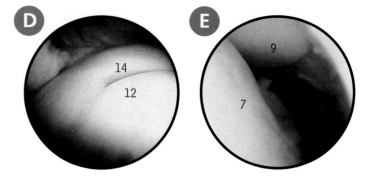

*Knee joint replacements surgeries, see page 356.*

## A Left leg *from the front and lateral side*

1 Anterior tibial artery overlying interosseous membrane
2 Branch of deep peroneal (fibular) nerve to tibialis anterior
3 Deep peroneal (fibular) nerve
4 Extensor digitorum longus
5 Extensor hallucis longus
6 Head of fibula
7 Lateral branch of superficial peroneal (fibular) nerve

8 Medial branch of superficial peroneal (fibular) nerve
9 Peroneus (fibularis) longus
10 Recurrent branch of common peroneal (fibular) nerve
11 Superficial peroneal (fibular) nerve
12 Tibialis anterior and overlying fascia
13 Tuberosity of tibia and patellar ligament

## B Left knee *from the lateral side to show common peroneal (fibular) nerve and articular branches*

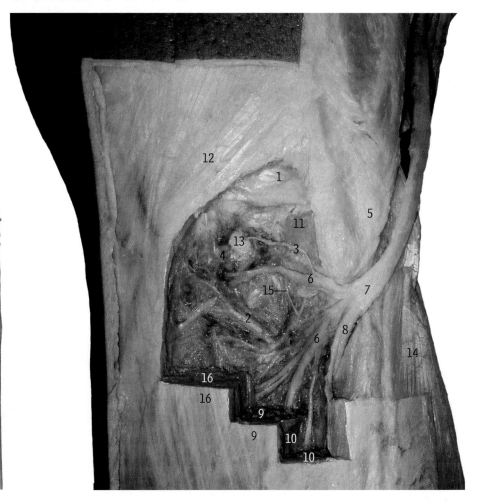

1 Anterior ligament of fibular head
2 Anterior tibial recurrent artery and vein
3 Articular branch from deep common peroneal (fibular) nerve
4 Articular vessels
5 Biceps femoris tendon
6 Common peroneal (fibular) nerve, deep branches
7 Common peroneal (fibular) nerve, overlying neck of fibula
8 Common peroneal (fibular) nerve, superficial branch

9 Extensor digitorum longus
10 Peroneus (fibularis) longus
11 Head of fibula
12 Iliotibial tract
13 Interosseous membrane
14 Lateral head, gastrocnemius muscle
15 Recurrent branch of deep peroneal (fibular) nerve
16 Tibialis anterior

*Common peroneal (fibular) nerve paralysis, see page 355.*

# Left knee and leg

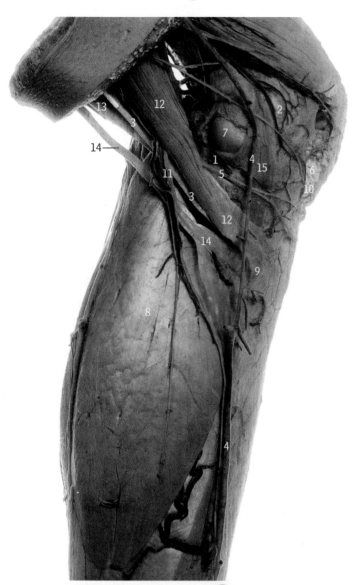

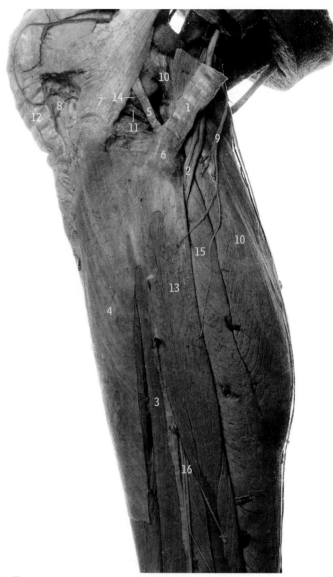

## Left knee and leg Ⓐ *from the medial side and behind*

A small window has been cut in the capsule of the knee joint to show part of the medial condyle of the femur (7) and the medial meniscus (1).

1 Branch of saphenous artery overlying medial meniscus
2 Branches of superior medial genicular artery
3 Gracilis
4 Great saphenous vein
5 Infrapatellar branch of saphenous nerve
6 Infrapatellar fat pad
7 Medial condyle of femur (part of capsule removed)
8 Medial head of gastrocnemius
9 Medial surface of tibia
10 Patellar ligament
11 Saphenous nerve and artery
12 Sartorius
13 Semimembranosus
14 Semitendinosus
15 Tibial collateral ligament

## Ⓑ *from the lateral side*

A small window has been cut in the capsule of the knee joint to show the tendon of popliteus (14) passing deep to the fibular collateral ligament (5). The common peroneal (fibular) nerve (2) runs down behind biceps (1) to pass through the gap between peroneus (fibularis) longus (13) and soleus (15). The superficial peroneal (fibular) nerve becomes superficial between peroneus (fibularis) longus (13) and extensor digitorum longus (3).

1 Biceps
2 Common peroneal (fibular) nerve
3 Extensor digitorum longus
4 Fascia overlying tibialis anterior
5 Fibular collateral ligament
6 Head of fibula
7 Iliotibial tract
8 Infrapatellar fat pad
9 Lateral cutaneous nerve of calf
10 Lateral head of gastrocnemius
11 Lateral meniscus
12 Patellar ligament
13 Peroneus (fibularis) longus
14 Popliteus
15 Soleus
16 Superficial peroneal (fibular) nerve

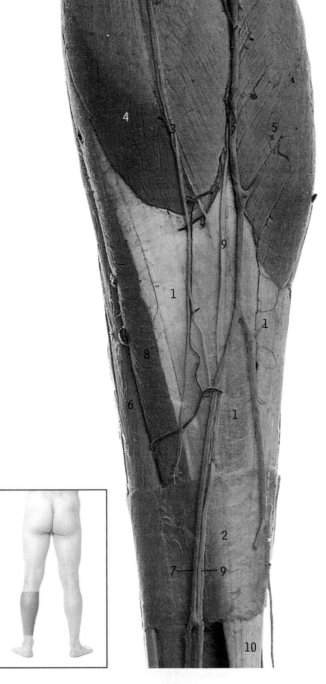

In the calf, the small saphenous vein (C7) is accompanied by the sural nerve (C9).

Below knee level, the great saphenous vein (A4) is accompanied by the saphenous nerve (A11).

## C Left calf
### *superficial dissection, from behind*

| | |
|---|---|
| **1** Aponeurosis of gastrocnemius | **7** Small saphenous vein |
| **2** Deep fascia | **8** Soleus |
| **3** Lateral cutaneous nerve of calf | **9** Sural nerve |
| **4** Lateral head of gastrocnemius | **10** Tendocalcaneus |
| **5** Medial head of gastrocnemius | (Achilles tendon) |
| **6** Peroneus (fibularis) longus | |

*Vein harvest for coronary artery bypass grafting (CABG), see page 357.*

# Left leg and ankle *superficial veins and nerves*

**A** *from the medial side* **B** *from behind*

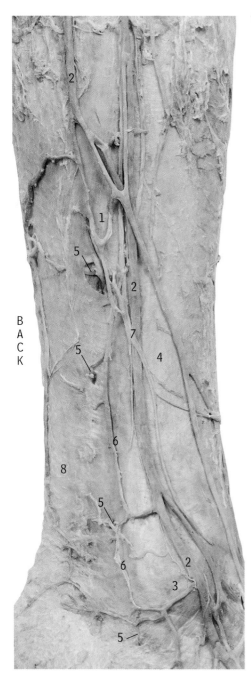

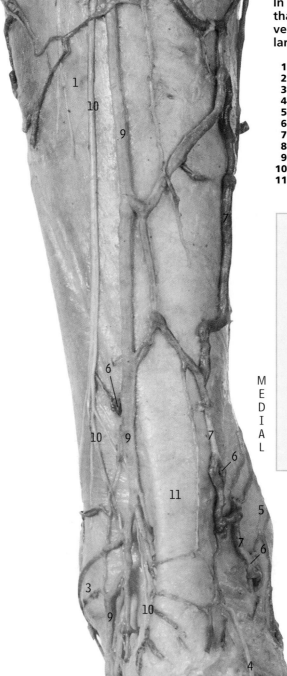

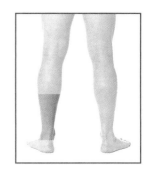

**In B (a different specimen from that in A), the posterior arch vein (7) on the medial side is large and becoming varicose.**

1 Deep fascia
2 Fibrofatty tissue of heel
3 Lateral malleolus
4 Medial calcanean nerve
5 Medial malleolus
6 Perforating vein
7 Posterior arch vein
8 Posterior surface of calcaneus
9 Small saphenous vein
10 Sural nerve
11 Tendocalcaneus (under fascia)

The perforating veins are communications between the superficial veins (outside the deep fascia) and the deep veins (inside the fascia). The commonest sites for them are just behind the tibia, behind the fibula and in the adductor canal. These communicating vessels possess valves which direct the blood flow from superficial to deep; venous return from the limb is then brought about by the pumping action of the deep muscles (which are all below the deep fascia). If the valves become incompetent or the deep veins blocked, pressure in the superficial veins increases and they become varicose (dilated and tortuous).

1 Deep fascia over soleus
2 Great saphenous vein
3 Medial malleolus
4 Medial (subcutaneous) surface of tibia
5 Perforating veins
6 Posterior arch vein
7 Saphenous nerve
8 Tendocalcaneus (Achilles tendon)

*Ankle ulceration from varicose veins, deep vein thrombosis, see page 355.*

## A Left popliteal fossa and upper calf   ## B Left lower calf and ankle

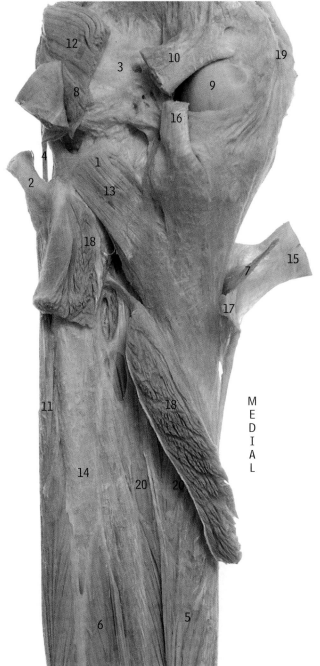

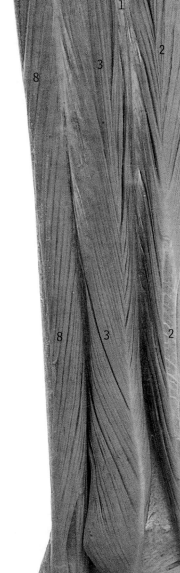

1 Fascia overlying tibialis posterior
2 Flexor digitorum longus
3 Flexor hallucis longus
4 Lateral malleolus
5 Medial malleolus
6 Part of flexor retinaculum
7 Peroneus (fibularis) brevis
8 Peroneus (fibularis) longus
9 Position of posterior tibial vessels and tibial nerve
10 Posterior talofibular ligament
11 Superior peroneal (fibular) retinaculum
12 Tendocalcaneus (Achilles tendon)
13 Tibialis posterior

1 Attachment of popliteus to lateral meniscus
2 Biceps
3 Capsule of knee joint
4 Fibular collateral ligament
5 Flexor digitorum longus
6 Flexor hallucis longus
7 Gracilis
8 Lateral head of gastrocnemius
9 Medial condyle of femur
10 Medial head of gastrocnemius
11 Peroneus (fibularis) longus
12 Plantaris
13 Popliteus
14 Posterior surface of fibula (soleus removed)
15 Sartorius
16 Semimembranosus
17 Semitendinosus
18 Soleus
19 Tibial collateral ligament
20 Tibialis posterior

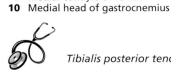
*Tibialis posterior tendonitis, see page 356.*

**A** **Right leg**
*posterior view, popliteal fossa*

**B** **Right calf**
*deep dissection right calf including muscles, nerves and vessels*

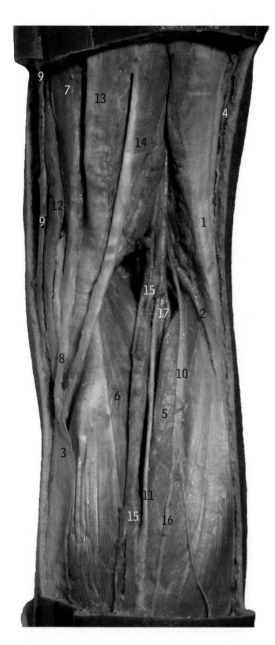

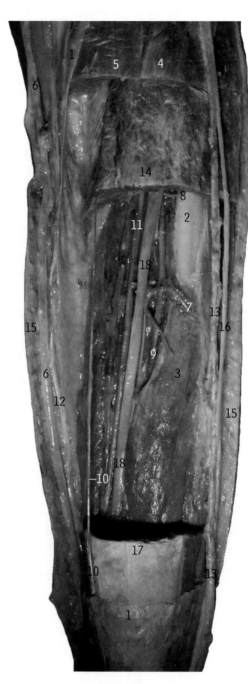

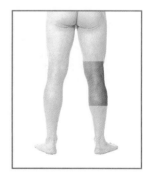

1  Deep fascia of calf, posterior compartment
2  Fibula, posterior surface
3  Flexor hallucis longus
4  Gastrocnemius, lateral head
5  Gastrocnemius, medial head
6  Great saphenous vein
7  Peroneal (fibular) artery, flexor hallucis longus branches
8  Peroneal (fibular) artery, fibula nutrient branch
9  Peroneal (fibular) artery, soleal branches
10  Plantaris tendon
11  Posterior tibial artery
12  Saphenous nerve
13  Small saphenous vein, displaced laterally
14  Soleus
15  Superficial fascia, subcutaneous fat
16  Sural nerve
17  Tendocalcaneus, formation
18  Tibial nerve

| | | | |
|---|---|---|---|
| 1 | Biceps femoris | 6 | Gastrocnemius, medial head |
| 2 | Common peroneal (fibular) nerve | 7 | Gracilis |
| 3 | Fascia lata (deep fascia) | 8 | Gracilis tendon |
| 4 | Fascia lata of thigh | 9 | Great saphenous vein |
| 5 | Gastrocnemius, lateral head | 10 | Lateral sural cutaneous nerve |
| | | 11 | Medial sural cutaneous nerve |

| | |
|---|---|
| 12 | Sartorius |
| 13 | Semimembranosus |
| 14 | Semitendinosus |
| 15 | Small saphenous vein |
| 16 | Sural communicating nerve |
| 17 | Tibial nerve |

*Compartment syndrome, see page 355.*

## C Right calf *deep dissection*

## D Popliteal angiogram

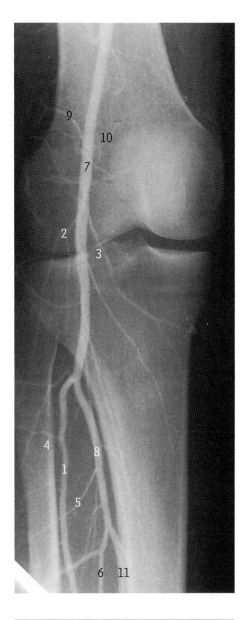

1 Anterior tibial artery
2 Inferior lateral genicular artery
3 Inferior medial genicular artery
4 Muscular branches of anterior tibial artery
5 Muscular branches of tibioperoneal trunk
6 Peroneal (fibular) artery
7 Popliteal artery
8 Tibioperoneal trunk
9 Superior lateral genicular artery
10 Superior medial genicular artery
11 Posterior tibial artery

The deep veins of the calf, deep to and within soleus, are sites for potentially dangerous venous thrombosis.

1 Fibula (posterior surface)
2 Flexor digitorum longus
3 Gastrocnemius
4 Peroneal (fibular) artery, fibula nutrient branch
5 Peroneal (fibular) artery, muscular branches
6 Peroneal (fibular) artery
7 Peroneal (fibular) vein
8 Peroneus (fibularis) longus
9 Plantaris tendon (reflected)
10 Posterior tibial artery
11 Small saphenous vein
12 Soleus
13 Sural nerve
14 Tendocalcaneus (Achilles tendon)
15 Tibial nerve
16 Tibialis posterior fascia

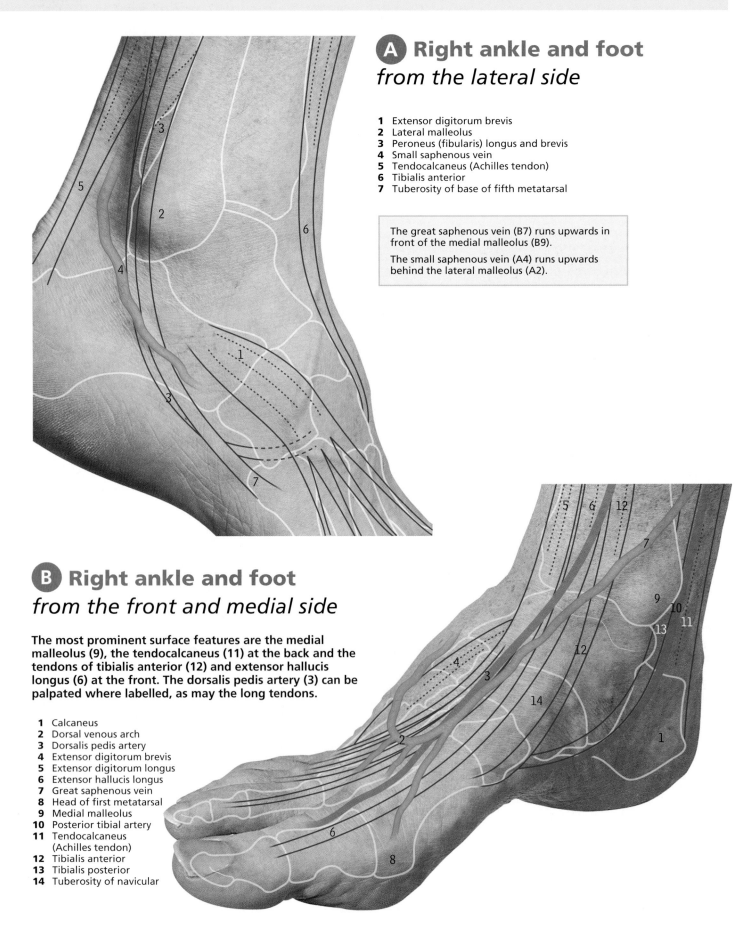

## A Right ankle and foot
*from the lateral side*

1 Extensor digitorum brevis
2 Lateral malleolus
3 Peroneus (fibularis) longus and brevis
4 Small saphenous vein
5 Tendocalcaneus (Achilles tendon)
6 Tibialis anterior
7 Tuberosity of base of fifth metatarsal

The great saphenous vein (B7) runs upwards in front of the medial malleolus (B9).

The small saphenous vein (A4) runs upwards behind the lateral malleolus (A2).

## B Right ankle and foot
*from the front and medial side*

The most prominent surface features are the medial malleolus (9), the tendocalcaneus (11) at the back and the tendons of tibialis anterior (12) and extensor hallucis longus (6) at the front. The dorsalis pedis artery (3) can be palpated where labelled, as may the long tendons.

1 Calcaneus
2 Dorsal venous arch
3 Dorsalis pedis artery
4 Extensor digitorum brevis
5 Extensor digitorum longus
6 Extensor hallucis longus
7 Great saphenous vein
8 Head of first metatarsal
9 Medial malleolus
10 Posterior tibial artery
11 Tendocalcaneus
   (Achilles tendon)
12 Tibialis anterior
13 Tibialis posterior
14 Tuberosity of navicular

*Achilles tendon reflex, Achilles tendon rupture, talipes equinovarus (club foot), venous cutdown, see pages 355, 356, 357.*

## C Right ankle and foot *from the lateral side*

Fascia has been removed but the thickenings that form the superior and inferior extensor retinacula (16 and 6) and the superior and inferior peroneal (fibular) retinacula (17 and 7) have been preserved. The synovial sheaths of tendons have been emphasised by blue tissue.

1 Abductor digiti minimi
2 Dorsal digital expansion
3 Extensor digitorum brevis
4 Extensor digitorum longus
5 Extensor hallucis longus
6 Inferior extensor retinaculum
7 Inferior peroneal (fibular) retinaculum
8 Lateral malleolus
9 Lateral surface of calcaneus
10 Medial and lateral branches of superficial peroneal (fibular) nerve

11 Peroneus (fibularis) brevis
12 Peroneus (fibularis) longus
13 Peroneus (fibularis) tertius
14 Soleus
15 Subcutaneous area of fibula
16 Superior extensor retinaculum
17 Superior peroneal (fibular) retinaculum
18 Sural nerve
19 Tendocalcaneus (Achilles tendon)
20 Tibialis anterior

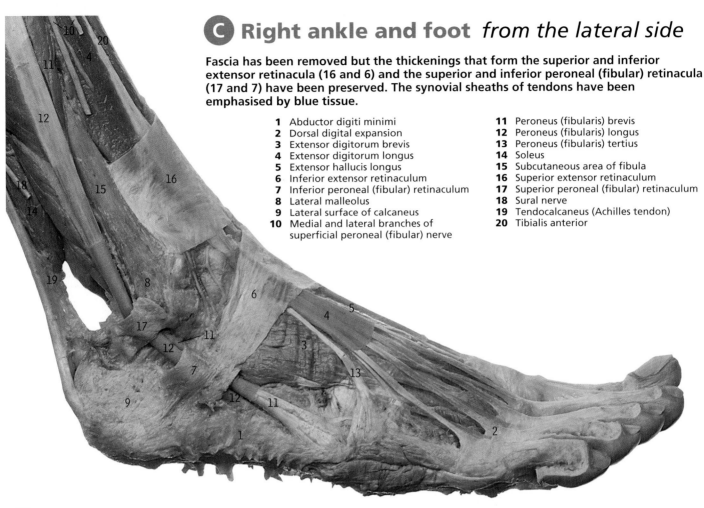

## D Right ankle and foot *from the medial side*

1 Abductor hallucis
2 Extensor hallucis longus
3 Flexor digitorum longus
4 Flexor hallucis longus
5 Flexor retinaculum
6 Inferior extensor retinaculum (lower band)
7 Inferior extensor retinaculum (upper band)
8 Medial calcanean nerve
9 Medial malleolus

10 Medial surface of tibia
11 Plantaris tendon
12 Posterior surface of calcaneus
13 Posterior tibial artery and venae comitantes
14 Soleus
15 Tendocalcaneus (Achilles tendon)
16 Tibial nerve
17 Tibialis anterior
18 Tibialis posterior

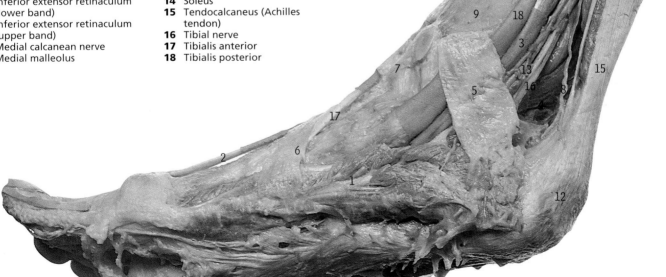

*Ankle arthroscopy, see page 355.*

## A Right lower leg and ankle

### *from the medial side and behind*

## B Right ankle

### *from the medial side*

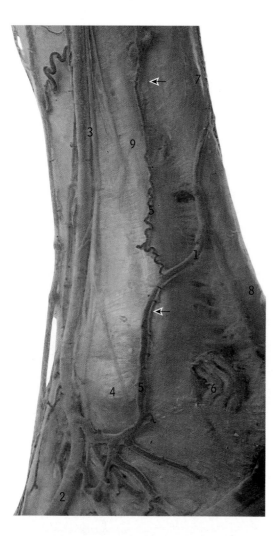

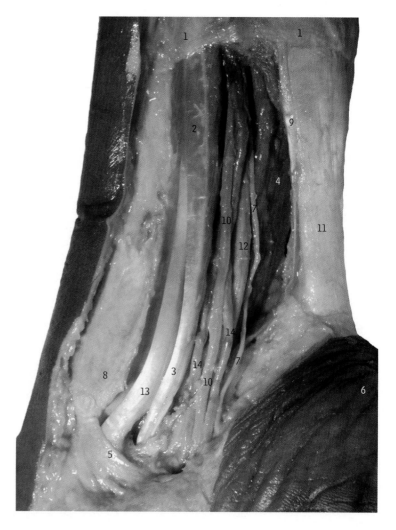

The deep fascia remains intact apart from a small window cut to show the position of the posterior tibial vessels and tibial nerve (6). The great saphenous vein (3) runs upwards in front of the medial malleolus (4) with the posterior arch vein (5) behind it. The arrows indicate common levels for perforating veins (page 340, A5 and B6).

1 Communication with small saphenous vein
2 Dorsal venous arch
3 Great saphenous vein and saphenous nerve
4 Medial malleolus
5 Posterior arch vein
6 Posterior tibial vessels and tibial nerve
7 Small saphenous vein
8 Tendocalcaneus (Achilles tendon)
9 Tibialis posterior and flexor digitorum longus underlying deep fascia

1 Deep fascia of calf
2 Flexor digitorum longus
3 Flexor digitorum longus, tendon
4 Flexor hallucis longus
5 Flexor retinaculum
6 Heel
7 Medial calcanean nerve
8 Medial malleolus, tibia
9 Plantaris tendon
10 Posterior tibial artery
11 Tendocalcaneus (Achilles tendon)
12 Tibial nerve
13 Tibialis posterior tendon
14 Vena comitantes of posterior tibial artery

*Ulceration of the foot, varicose veins, see page 357.*

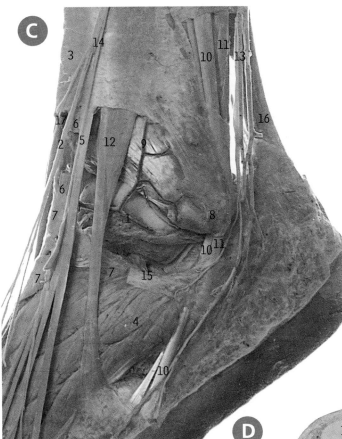

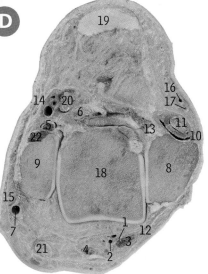

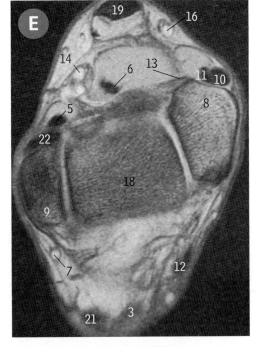

## C Left ankle and foot
### from the front and lateral side

The foot is plantar flexed and part of the capsule of the ankle joint has been removed to show the talus (1). The tendons of peroneus (fibularis) tertius (12) and extensor digitorum longus (5) lie superficial to extensor digitorum brevis (4). The sural nerve and small saphenous vein (13) pass behind the lateral malleolus (8).

1 Anterior lateral malleolar artery overlying talus (ankle joint capsule removed)
2 Anterior tibial vessels and deep peroneal (fibular) nerve
3 Deep fascia forming superior extensor retinaculum
4 Extensor digitorum brevis
5 Extensor digitorum longus
6 Extensor hallucis longus
7 Inferior extensor retinaculum (partly removed)
8 Lateral malleolus
9 Perforating branch of peroneal (fibular) artery
10 Peroneus (fibularis) brevis
11 Peroneus (fibularis) longus
12 Peroneus (fibularis) tertius
13 Small saphenous vein and sural nerve
14 Superficial peroneal (fibular) nerve
15 Tarsal sinus
16 Tendocalcaneus (Achilles tendon)
17 Tibialis anterior

## Left ankle

### D cross-section
### E axial MR image

This section, looking down from above, emphasizes the positions of tendons, vessels and nerves in the ankle region. The talus (18) is in the centre, with the medial malleolus (9) on the left of the picture and the lateral malleolus (8) on the right. The great saphenous vein (7) and saphenous nerve (15) are in front of the medial malleolus, with the tendon of tibialis posterior (22) immediately behind it. The small saphenous vein (16) and the sural nerve (17) are behind the lateral malleolus, with the tendons of peroneus (fibularis) longus (11) and peroneus (fibularis) brevis (10) intervening. At the front of the ankle, the dorsalis pedis vessels (2) and deep peroneal (fibular) nerve (1) are between the tendons of extensor hallucis longus (4) and extensor digitorum longus (3). Behind the medial malleolus (9) and tibialis posterior (22), the posterior tibial vessels (14) and tibial nerve (20) are between the tendons of flexor digitorum longus (5) and flexor hallucis longus (6).

1 Deep peroneal (fibular) nerve
2 Dorsalis pedis artery and venae comitantes
3 Extensor digitorum longus
4 Extensor hallucis longus
5 Flexor digitorum longus
6 Flexor hallucis longus
7 Great saphenous vein
8 Lateral malleolus of fibula
9 Medial malleolus of tibia
10 Peroneus (fibularis) brevis
11 Peroneus (fibularis) longus

12 Peroneus (fibularis) tertius
13 Posterior talofibular ligament
14 Posterior tibial artery and venae comitantes
15 Saphenous nerve
16 Small saphenous vein
17 Sural nerve
18 Talus
19 Tendocalcaneus (Achilles tendon)
20 Tibial nerve
21 Tibialis anterior
22 Tibialis posterior

*Charcot foot, see page 355.*

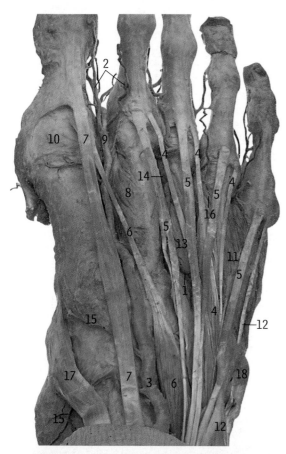

## A Dorsum of the right foot

| | | | |
|---|---|---|---|
| **1** | Arcuate artery | **11** | Fourth dorsal interosseous |
| **2** | Digital arteries | **12** | Peroneus (fibularis) tertius |
| **3** | Dorsalis pedis artery | **13** | Second dorsal interosseous |
| **4** | Extensor digitorum brevis | **14** | Second dorsal metatarsal artery |
| **5** | Extensor digitorum longus | **15** | Tarsal arteries |
| **6** | Extensor hallucis brevis | **16** | Third dorsal interosseous |
| **7** | Extensor hallucis longus | **17** | Tibialis anterior |
| **8** | First dorsal interosseous | **18** | Tuberosity of base of fifth |
| **9** | First dorsal metatarsal artery | | metatarsal and peroneus |
| **10** | First metatarsophalangeal joint | | (fibularis) brevis |

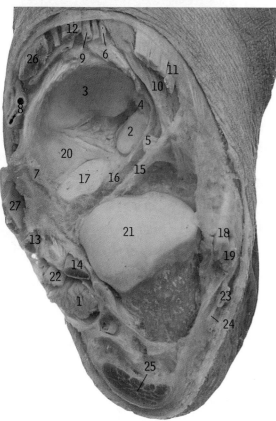

## B Right talocalcanean and talocalcaneonavicular joints

**The talus has been removed to show the articular surfaces of the calcaneus (21, 17 and 2), navicular (3) and plantar calcaneonavicular (spring) ligament (20).**

| | | | |
|---|---|---|---|
| **1** | Abductor hallucis | **16** | Interosseous talocalcanean ligament |
| **2** | Anterior articular surface on calcaneus for talus | **17** | Middle articular surface on calcaneus for talus |
| **3** | Articular surface on navicular for talus | **18** | Peroneus (fibularis) brevis |
| **4** | Calcaneonavicular part of bifurcate ligament | **19** | Peroneus (fibularis) longus |
| **5** | Cervical ligament | **20** | Plantar calcaneonavicular (spring) ligament |
| **6** | Deep peroneal (fibular) nerve | **21** | Posterior articular surface on calcaneus for talus |
| **7** | Deltoid ligament | **22** | Posterior tibial vessels and medial and lateral plantar nerves |
| **8** | Dorsal venous arch | |  |
| **9** | Dorsalis pedis artery and vena comitans | **23** | Small saphenous vein |
| **10** | Extensor digitorum brevis | **24** | Sural nerve |
| **11** | Extensor digitorum longus | **25** | Tendocalcaneus (Achilles tendon) |
| **12** | Extensor hallucis longus | **26** | Tibialis anterior |
| **13** | Flexor digitorum longus | **27** | Tibialis posterior |
| **14** | Flexor hallucis longus | | |
| **15** | Inferior extensor retinaculum | | |

Clinicians sometimes use the term subtalar joint as a combined name for both the talocalcanean joint and the talocalcanean part of the talocalcaneonavicular joint, because it is at both these joints beneath the talus that most of the movements of inversion and eversion of the foot occur, on the axis of the cervical ligament.

*Ankle block, see page 355.*

# Left ankle and foot *ligaments*

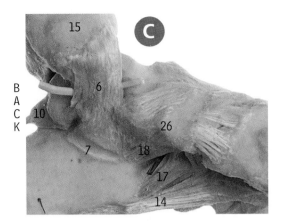

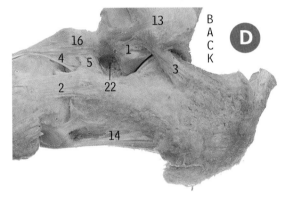

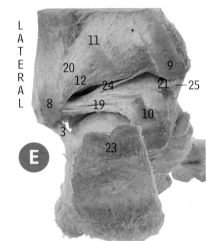

C  **from the medial side**

D  **from the lateral side**

E  **from behind**

**In C, the marker below the medial malleolus (15) passes between the superficial and deep parts of the deltoid ligament (6). The marker below the tuberosity of the navicular (26) passes between the plantar calcaneonavicular (spring) and calcaneocuboid (short plantar) ligaments (18 and 17).**

1 Anterior talofibular ligament
2 Calcaneocuboid part of bifurcate ligament
3 Calcaneofibular ligament
4 Calcaneonavicular part of bifurcate ligament
5 Cervical ligament
6 Deltoid ligament
7 Groove below sustentaculum tali for flexor hallucis longus
8 Groove on lateral malleolus for peroneus (fibularis) brevis
9 Groove on medial malleolus for tibialis posterior
10 Groove on talus for flexor hallucis longus
11 Groove on tibia for flexor hallucis longus
12 Inferior transverse ligament
13 Lateral malleolus
14 Long plantar ligament
15 Medial malleolus
16 Neck of talus
17 Plantar calcaneocuboid (short plantar) ligament
18 Plantar calcaneonavicular (spring) ligament
19 Posterior talofibular ligament
20 Posterior tibiofibular ligament
21 Posterior tibiotalar part of deltoid ligament
22 Tarsal sinus
23 Tendocalcaneus (Achilles tendon)
24 Tibial slip of posterior talofibular ligament
25 Tibiocalcanean part of deltoid ligament
26 Tuberosity of navicular

# F Left foot *sagittal section, from the right*

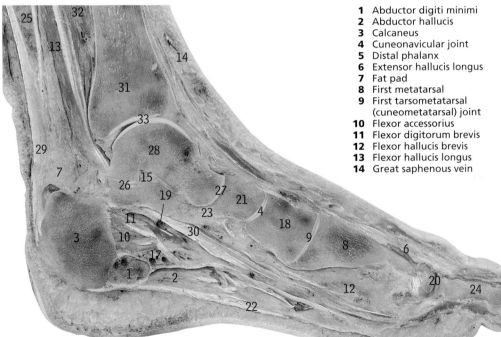

1 Abductor digiti minimi
2 Abductor hallucis
3 Calcaneus
4 Cuneonavicular joint
5 Distal phalanx
6 Extensor hallucis longus
7 Fat pad
8 First metatarsal
9 First tarsometatarsal (cuneometatarsal) joint
10 Flexor accessorius
11 Flexor digitorum brevis
12 Flexor hallucis brevis
13 Flexor hallucis longus
14 Great saphenous vein

15 Interosseous talocalcanean ligament
16 Interphalangeal joint
17 Lateral plantar nerve and vessels
18 Medial cuneiform
19 Medial plantar artery
20 Metatarsophalangeal joint of great toe
21 Navicular
22 Plantar aponeurosis
23 Plantar calcaneonavicular (spring) ligament
24 Proximal phalanx
25 Soleus muscle
26 Talocalcanean (subtalar) joint
27 Talonavicular part of talocalcaneonavicular joint
28 Talus
29 Tendocalcaneus (Achilles tendon)
30 Tendon of flexor hallucis
31 Tibia
32 Tibialis posterior muscle
33 Tibiotalar part of ankle joint

*Sprained ankle, see page 356.*

# Sole of the left foot

**A** *plantar aponeurosis*　　**B** *superficial neuromuscular layer*

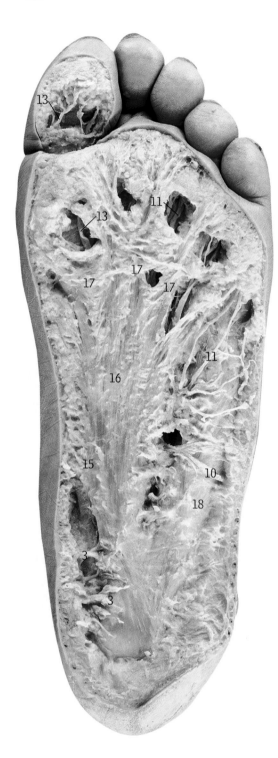

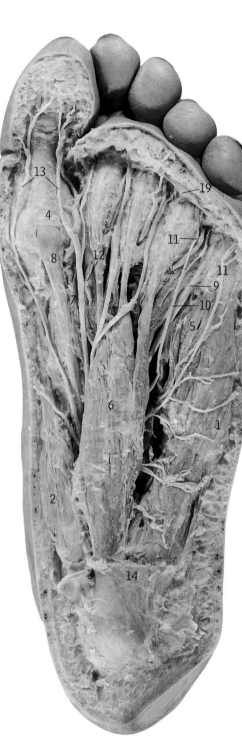

1　Abductor digiti minimi
2　Abductor hallucis
3　Calcaneal neurovascular bundle
4　Fibrous flexor sheath
5　Flexor digiti minimi brevis
6　Flexor digitorum brevis
7　Flexor hallucis brevis
8　Flexor hallucis longus
9　Lateral plantar artery
10　Lateral plantar nerve
11　Lateral plantar nerve, digital branches
12　Lumbrical
13　Medial plantar nerve, digital branches
14　Plantar aponeurosis
15　Plantar aponeurosis, overlying abductor hallucis
16　Plantar aponeurosis, overlying flexor digitorum brevis
17　Plantar aponeurosis, digital slips
18　Plantar aponeurosis, overlying abductor digiti minimi
19　Superficial transverse metatarsal ligament

**Removal of the plantar skin reveals the plantar aponeurosis with thick central and digital slips and thin lateral and medial parts.**

**Deep to the plantar aponeurosis lie the superficial plantar nerves, arteries and muscles.**

*Flat foot (pes planus), plantar fasciitis, see pages 355, 356.*

# Sole of the left foot

**C** *after removal of flexor digitorum brevis*
**D** *after removal of flexor digitorum longus*

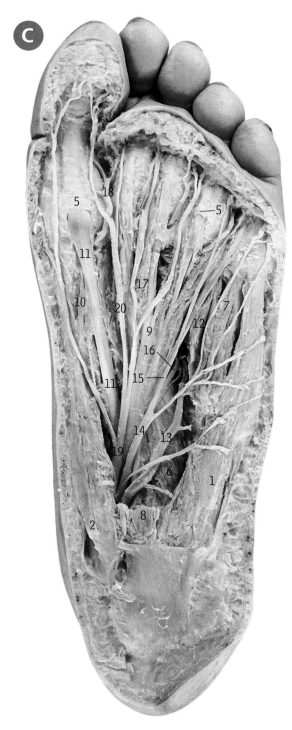

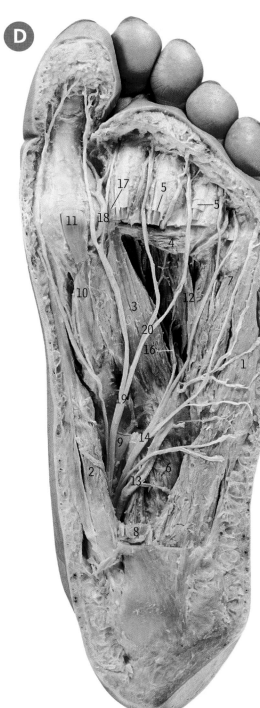

1  Abductor digiti minimi
2  Abductor hallucis
3  Adductor hallucis,
   oblique head
4  Adductor hallucis,
   transverse head
5  Fibrous sheath, flexors
6  Flexor accessorius
   (Quadratus plantae)
7  Flexor digiti minimi
   brevis
8  Flexor digitorum brevis
   (cut)
9  Flexor digitorum longus
10  Flexor hallucis brevis
11  Flexor hallucis longus
12  Interossei
13  Lateral plantar artery
14  Lateral plantar nerve
15  Lateral plantar nerve,
   common digital branch
16  Lateral plantar nerve,
   deep branch
17  Lumbrical
18  Medial plantar artery
19  Medial plantar nerve
20  Medial plantar nerve,
   common digital branch

*Extensor plantar response – Babinski sign, see page 355.*

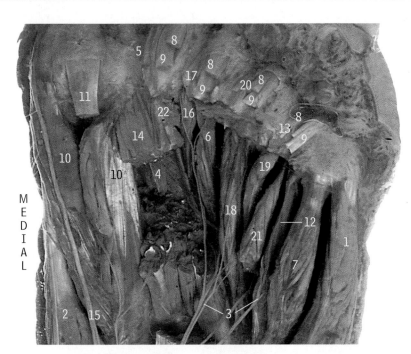

## A Sole of the left foot
### deep muscles, interossei

| | | | |
|---|---|---|---|
| **1** | Abductor digiti minimi | **13** | Fourth lumbrical |
| **2** | Abductor hallucis | **14** | Oblique head of adductor hallucis |
| **3** | Branches of deep branch of lateral plantar nerve | **15** | Plantar digital nerve of great toe |
| **4** | First dorsal interosseous | **16** | Second dorsal interosseous |
| **5** | First lumbrical | **17** | Second lumbrical |
| **6** | First plantar interosseous | **18** | Second plantar interosseous |
| **7** | Flexor digiti minimi brevis | **19** | Third dorsal interosseous |
| **8** | Flexor digitorum brevis | **20** | Third lumbrical |
| **9** | Flexor digitorum longus | **21** | Third plantar interosseous |
| **10** | Flexor hallucis brevis | **22** | Transverse head of adductor hallucis |
| **11** | Flexor hallucis longus | | |
| **12** | Fourth dorsal interosseous | | |

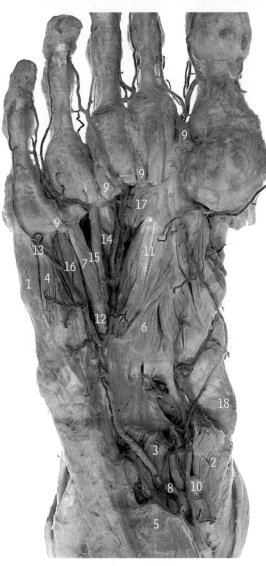

## B Sole of the right foot

### plantar arch

Most of the flexor muscles and tendons have been removed to show the lateral plantar artery (8) crossing flexor accessorius (quadratus plantae) (3) to become the plantar arch (12) which would lie deep to the flexor tendons.

| | | | |
|---|---|---|---|
| **1** | Abductor digiti minimi | **10** | Medial plantar artery and nerve |
| **2** | Abductor hallucis | **11** | Oblique head of adductor hallucis |
| **3** | Flexor accessorius (quadratus plantae) | **12** | Plantar arch |
| **4** | Flexor digiti minimi brevis | **13** | Plantar digital artery |
| **5** | Flexor digitorum brevis | **14** | Plantar metatarsal artery |
| **6** | Flexor hallucis brevis | **15** | Second plantar interosseous |
| **7** | Fourth dorsal interosseous | **16** | Third plantar interosseous |
| **8** | Lateral plantar artery | **17** | Transverse head of adductor hallucis |
| **9** | Lumbrical | **18** | Tuberosity of navicular |

# Sole of the left foot C *ligaments and tendons* D *ligaments*

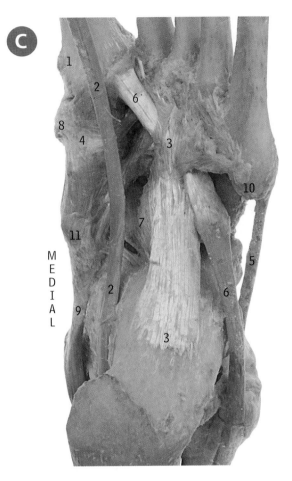

The anterior end of the long plantar ligament (3) forms with the groove of the cuboid (D6) a tunnel for the peroneus (fibularis) longus tendon (6) which runs to the medial cuneiform (4) and the base of the first metatarsal (1).

 1 Base of first metatarsal
 2 Flexor hallucis longus
 3 Long plantar ligament
 4 Medial cuneiform
 5 Peroneus (fibularis) brevis
 6 Peroneus (fibularis) longus
 7 Plantar calcaneocuboid (short plantar) ligament
 8 Tibialis anterior
 9 Tibialis posterior
10 Tuberosity of base of fifth metatarsal
11 Tuberosity of navicular

The plantar calcaneonavicular ligament (D9), commonly called the spring ligament, is one of the most important in the foot. It stretches between the sustentaculum tali (D7) and the tuberosity of the navicular (D16), blending on its medial side with the deltoid ligament of the ankle joint and supporting on the upper surface part of the head of the talus.

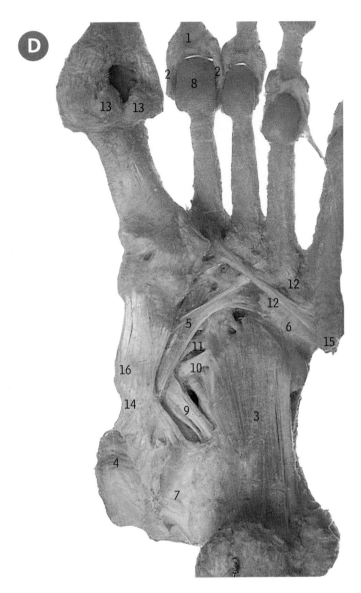

The anterior end of the long plantar ligament (3) has been removed to show the groove for peroneus (fibularis) longus on the cuboid (6).

 1 Base of proximal phalanx
 2 Collateral ligament of metatarsophalangeal joint
 3 Deep fibres of long plantar ligament
 4 Deltoid ligament
 5 Fibrous slip from tibialis posterior
 6 Groove on cuboid for peroneus (fibularis) longus
 7 Groove on sustentaculum tali for flexor hallucis longus
 8 Head of second metatarsal
 9 Plantar calcaneonavicular (spring) ligament
10 Plantar cuboideonavicular ligament
11 Plantar cuneonavicular ligament
12 Plantar metatarsal ligament
13 Sesamoid bone
14 Tibialis posterior
15 Tuberosity of base of fifth metatarsal
16 Tuberosity of navicular

# Ankle  *anteroposterior projection* **B** *calcaneus, lateral projection*

1 Calcaneus
2 Cuboid
3 Fibula
4 Head of talus
5 Lateral cuneiform
6 Lateral malleolus of fibula
7 Lateral tubercle of talus
8 Medial malleolus of tibia
9 Medial tubercle of talus
10 Navicular
11 Region of inferior tibiofibular joint
12 Sustentaculum tali of calcaneus
13 Talus
14 Tibia
15 Tuberosity of base of fifth metatarsal

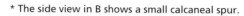
* The side view in B shows a small calcaneal spur.

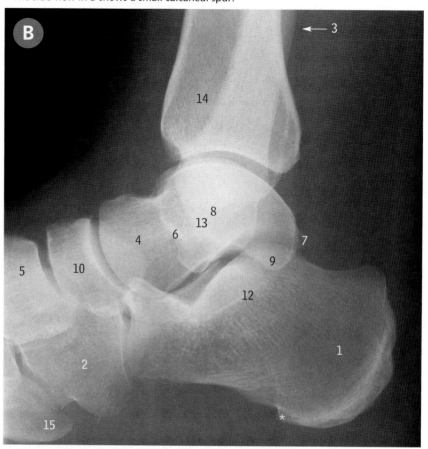

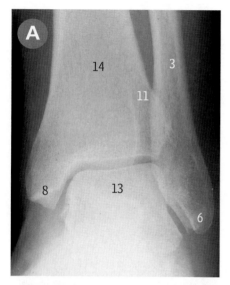

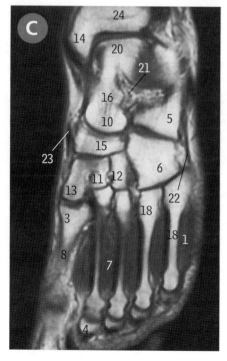

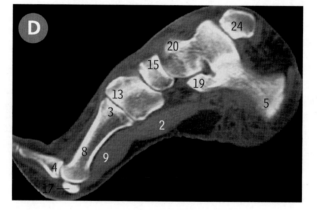

## Foot

**C** *oblique axial MR image*

**D** *sagittal CT through hallux*

1 Abductor digiti minimi muscle
2 Abductor hallucis
3 Base of metatarsal
4 Base of proximal phalanx
5 Calcaneus
6 Cuboid
7 Dorsal interossei muscle
8 First metatarsal
9 Flexor digitorum brevis
10 Head of talus
11 Intermediate cuneiform
12 Lateral cuneiform
13 Medial cuneiform
14 Medial malleolus
15 Navicular
16 Neck of talus
17 Sesamoid bone in flexor hallucis brevis
18 Shaft of metatarsal
19 Sustentaculum tali of calcaneus
20 Talus
21 Tarsal sinus
22 Tendon of peroneus (fibularis) brevis muscle
23 Tendon of tibialis anterior muscle
24 Tibia

*Pott's fracture (ankle), see page 356.*

# Lower limb

Clinical thumbnails, see DVD Lower limb for details and further clinical images

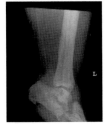

Achilles tendon tendocalcaneus reflex (ankle jerk)

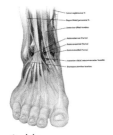

Ankle arthroscopy

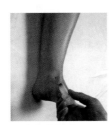

Ankle block

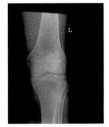

Ankle ulceration from varicose veins

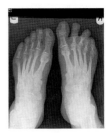

Avascular necrosis of the head of the femur

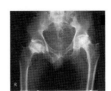

Bipartite patella

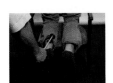

Charcot foot

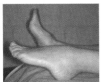

Common peroneal (fibular) nerve paralysis

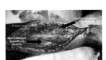

Compartment syndrome

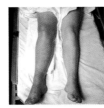

Deep vein thrombosis (DVT)

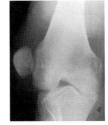

Dislocation of the knee joint and dislocation of the patella

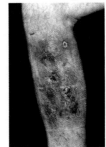

Dislocation of the toe

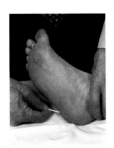

Extensor plantar response – Babinski sign

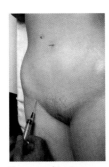

Femoral artery puncture

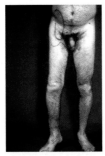

Femoral nerve paralysis

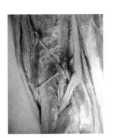

Femoropopliteal bypass

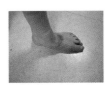

Flat foot (pes planus)

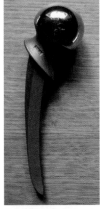

Fracture of the femoral neck

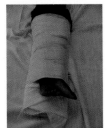

Fracture of the femoral shaft

Hallux valgus

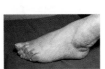

Hammer toe

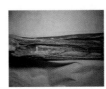

Intermittent claudication

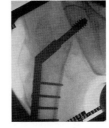

Intertrochanteric fracture of the femur

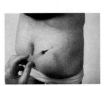

Intramuscular injection – gluteal region

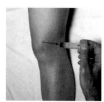
Knee joint aspiration and injection

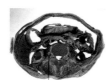
Knee joint replacement surgeries

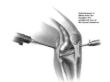
Lumbar plexus block

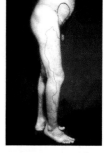
Meniscal tears

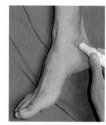
Meralgia paraesthetica

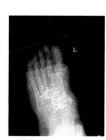
Metatarsal fractures

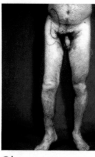
Obturator nerve paralysis

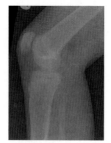
Osgood–Schlatter's disease

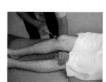
Patellar tendon reflex

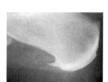
Plantar fasciitis

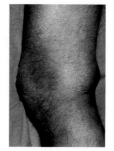
Popliteal (Baker's) cyst

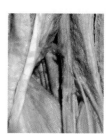
Popliteal artery aneurysm

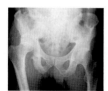
Posterior hip dislocation

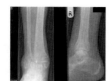
Pott's fracture and other fractures of the ankle

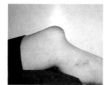
Prepatellar bursitis

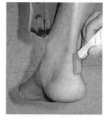
Rupture of the Achilles tendon

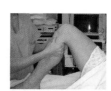
Rupture of the anterior cruciate ligament

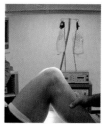
Rupture of the posterior cruciate ligament

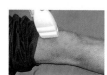
Rupture of the quadriceps tendon

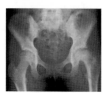
Slipped upper femoral epiphysis

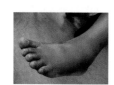
Sprained ankle

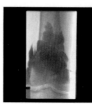
Suprapatellar bursa

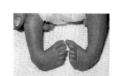
Talipes equinovarus (club foot)

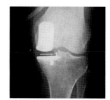
Tibialis posterior tendonitis

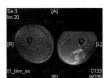

Torn hamstrings

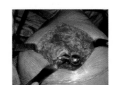

Total hip
replacement
surgery

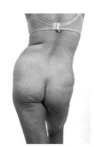

Trendelen-
burg's sign

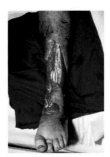

Ulceration of the
foot

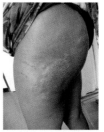

Varicella-zoster
virus infection –
lower limb

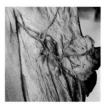

Varicose veins

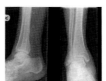

Vein harvest for
coronary artery
bypass grafting

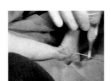

Venous cutdown

# Lymphatics

## Lymphatic system

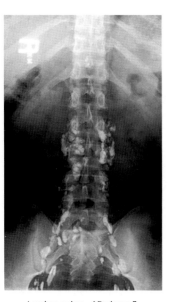

Lumbar spine - AP phase 2

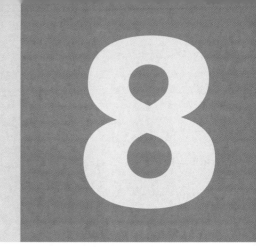

Thoracic duct termination in neck

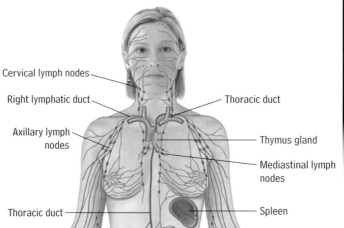

- Cervical lymph nodes
- Right lymphatic duct
- Thoracic duct
- Axillary lymph nodes
- Thymus gland
- Mediastinal lymph nodes
- Thoracic duct
- Spleen
- Cisterna chyli
- Lymphoid nodules of intestine
- Lumbar lymph nodes
- Iliac lymph nodes
- Inguinal lymph nodes
- Bone marrow

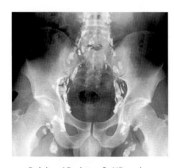

Pelvis - AP phase 2, NB nodes

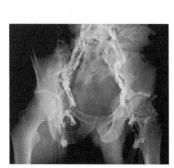

Pelvis - AP phase 1, NB vessels

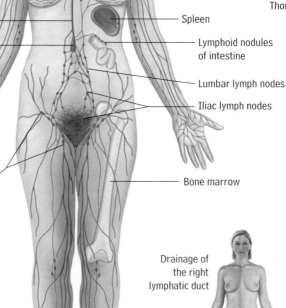

Drainage of the right lymphatic duct

Drainage of the thoracic duct

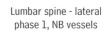

Lumbar spine - lateral phase 1, NB vessels

*Lymphatic system, see page 366.*

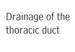

Phase one images are taken on day one and best show the vessels whereas phase two are taken at about 48 hours and best image the lymph nodes.

## A Thymus *lying in the superior and anterior mediastinum as seen through a split-sternal approach*

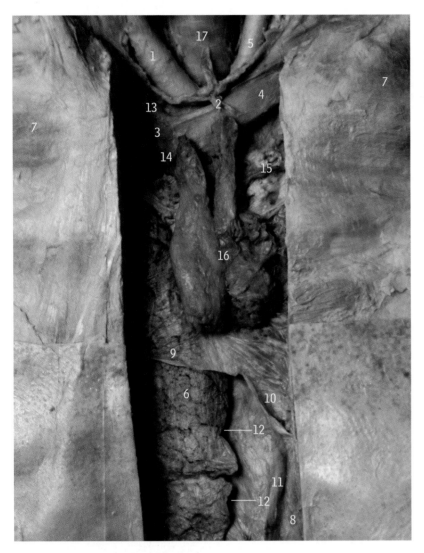

## B Chest radiograph of a child

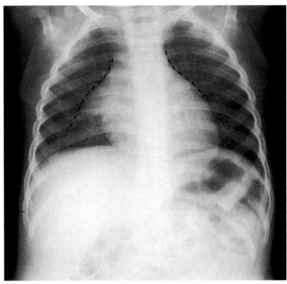

The child's thymus can be seen on a plain chest radiograph, appearing as a spinnaker sail (sail sign), as outlined by the interrupted line.

## C Palatine tonsils

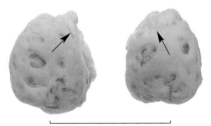

2 cm

The pits on the medial surfaces of these operation specimens from a child aged 14 years are the openings of the tonsillar crypts. The arrows indicate the intratonsillar clefts (the remains of the embryonic second pharyngeal pouch).

The palatine tonsils (commonly called 'the tonsils') are masses of lymphoid tissue that are frequently enlarged in childhood but become much reduced in size in later life. Together with the lymphoid tissue in the posterior part of the tongue (lingual tonsil) and in the posterior wall of the nasopharynx (pharyngeal tonsil) and the tubal tonsil they form a protective 'ring' of lymphoid tissue (Waldeyer's ring) at the upper end of the respiratory and alimentary tracts.

1 Brachiocephalic trunk (artery)
2 Inferior thyroid vein
3 Internal thoracic vein, right
4 Left brachiocephalic vein
5 Left common carotid artery
6 Lung, upper lobe right
7 Pectoralis major
8 Pericardium, fibrous
9 Pleura
10 Pleura (cut edge of left sac)
11 Pleura (cut edge of right sac)
12 Pleural cavity
13 Right brachiocephalic vein
14 Superior vena cava
15 Thymic vein draining into internal thoracic vein
16 Thymus gland (bilobed)
17 Trachea

*Thymus, Tonsillitis, see page 366.*

**Ⓐ Neck dissection** *termination of the thoracic duct into the left subclavian vein in the root of neck – as seen over left shoulder*

INFERIOR

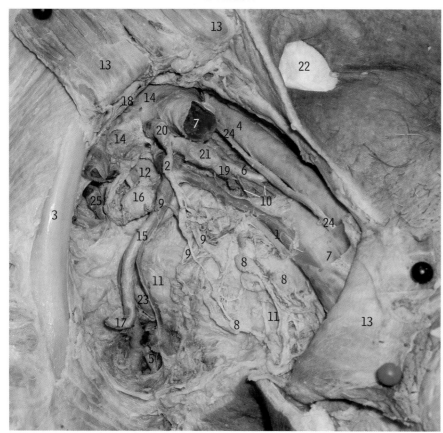

LATERAL

MEDIAL

SUPERIOR

1 Ascending cervical artery and vein
2 Cervical lymphatic trunk
3 Clavicle (left)
4 Common carotid artery
5 Dorsal scapular artery
6 Inferior thyroid artery
7 Internal jugular vein
8 Lymph nodes, deep cervical chain
9 Lymph vessel from node to cervical trunk
10 Muscular branches to longus colli
11 Prevertebral fascia
12 Scalenus anterior muscle
13 Sternocleidomastoid (reflected and pinned)
14 Subclavian vein
15 Superficial cervical artery
16 Supraclavicular node (Virchow – enlarged)
17 Suprascapular artery
18 Thoraco-acromial artery, clavicular branch
19 Thoracic duct
20 Thoracic duct, termination
21 Thoracic duct, ampulla
22 Tracheostomy site (midline)
23 Transverse cervical artery and vein
24 Vagus nerve
25 Vertebral vein

**Ⓑ Thoracic duct** *cervical part*

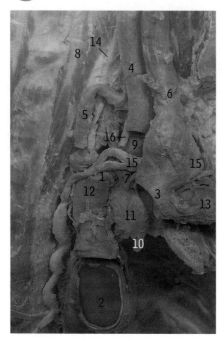

In this deep dissection of the left side of the root of the neck and upper thorax, the internal jugular vein (6) joins the subclavian vein (13) to form the left brachiocephalic vein (3). The thoracic duct (15) is double for a short distance just before passing in front of the vertebral artery (9) and behind the common carotid artery (4, whose lower end has been cut away to show the duct). The duct then runs behind the internal jugular vein (6) before draining into the junction of that vein with the subclavian vein (13).

1 Ansa subclavia
2 Arch of aorta
3 Brachiocephalic vein
4 Common carotid artery
5 Inferior thyroid artery
6 Internal jugular vein
7 Internal thoracic artery
8 Longus colli
9 Origin of vertebral artery
10 Phrenic nerve
11 Pleura
12 Subclavian artery
13 Subclavian vein
14 Sympathetic trunk
15 Thoracic duct
16 Vagus nerve

**Ⓒ First day lymphangiogram**

1 Common iliac vessels
2 Cisterna chyli
3 Lumbar crossover
4 Para-aortic vessels
5 Pre-aortic vessels
6 Thoracic duct

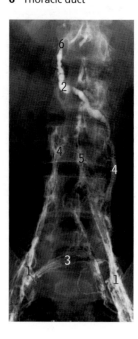

*Virchow's node, central venous catheterisation, see page 366, see also pages 209, 212.*

# Right axilla with moderate lymphadenopathy

SUPERIOR

LATERAL

MEDIAL

| | | |
|---|---|---|
| **1** | Apical node (infraclavicular – enlarged) | |
| **2** | Axillary fascial sheath | |
| **3** | Axillary fat | |
| **4** | Axillary nodes, anterior or pectoral group | |
| **5** | Axillary nodes, central group | |
| **6** | Axillary nodes, lateral group (normal) | |
| **7** | Axillary nodes, posterior group (enlarged) | |
| **8** | Axillary skin | |
| **9** | Axillary vein | |
| **10** | Brachial plexus within axillary sheath | |
| **11** | Cephalic vein | |
| **12** | Clavicle | |
| **13** | Clavipectoral fascia (cut) | |
| **14** | Coracobrachialis | |
| **15** | Deltoid | |

**16** Intercostobrachial nerve
**17** Lateral thoracic artery
**18** Lateral thoracic, axillary skin and sweat gland branches
**19** Lateral thoracic, nodal arterial branch
**20** Lymphatic vessels
**21** Pectoralis major (reflected)
**22** Pectoralis minor
**23** Subclavius muscle
**24** Subscapular artery
**25** Subscapular vein
**26** Thoraco-acromial artery
**27** Thoraco-acromial artery, deltoid branch
**28** Thoraco-acromial artery, clavicular branch
**29** Thoraco-acromial artery, pectoral branch

\* Quill placed to lift vessels and nerves

*Axillary lymph node (sentinal node) dissection, lymphangitis, lymphoedema, see page 366.*

# Cisterna chyli and thoracic duct in posterior mediastinum

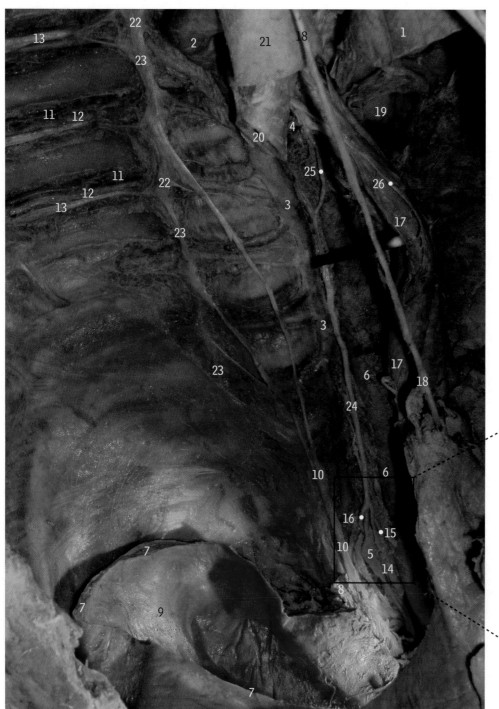

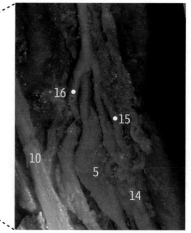

1 Ascending aorta
2 Azygos arch
3 Azygos venous system
4 Carinal node
5 Cisterna chyli
6 Descending thoracic aorta
7 Diaphragm, cut edge, light from abdomen inferiorly
8 Diaphragm, right crus
9 Diaphragmatic visceral peritoneum
10 Greater splanchnic nerve
11 Intercostal vein
12 Intercostal artery
13 Intercostal nerve
14 Intestinal lymphatic trunk
15 Lumbar lymphatic trunk, left
16 Lumbar lymphatic trunk, right
17 Oesophagus, displaced anteriorly by marker
18 Phrenic nerve, right
19 Pulmonary vein, left
20 Right lower lobe bronchus
21 Superior vena cava
22 Sympathetic ganglion
23 Sympathetic trunk
24 Thoracic duct
25 Thoracic duct, crossover
26 Vagus nerve, anterior oesophageal plexus

# Female pelvis *left half of midline sagittal section with lymphadenopathy*

**NB: retroverted uterus – a normal variant.**

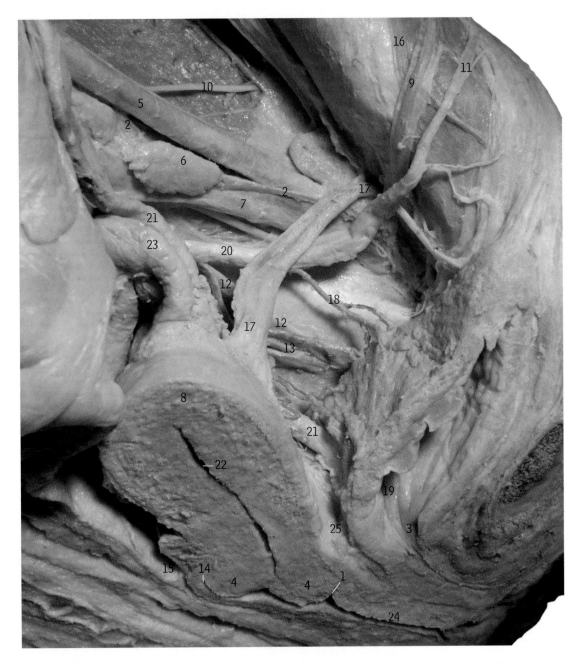

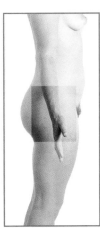

| | | | |
|---|---|---|---|
| **1** | Anterior vaginal fornix | **10** | Lateral cutaneous nerve of the thigh |
| **2** | Arterial supply to lymph node | **11** | Medial umbilical ligament |
| **3** | Bladder neck | **12** | Obturator nerve |
| **4** | Cervix | **13** | Obturator vessels |
| **5** | External iliac artery | **14** | Posterior vaginal fornix |
| **6** | External iliac lymph node (enlarged) | **15** | Rectouterine peritoneal pouch |
| **7** | External iliac vein | **16** | Rectus abdominis |
| **8** | Fundus of uterus | **17** | Round ligament of uterus |
| **9** | Inferior epigastric vessels | **18** | Superior vesical artery |

| | |
|---|---|
| **19** | Trigone of bladder |
| **20** | Umbilical artery (remnant) |
| **21** | Ureter |
| **22** | Uterine cavity |
| **23** | Uterine tube (Fallopian) |
| **24** | Vagina |
| **25** | Vesicouterine peritoneal pouch |

*Carcinoma of uterus lend cervix, see page 366, see also pages 275–277.*

# Gross lymphadenopathy of the pelvis *relationship of nodal groups*

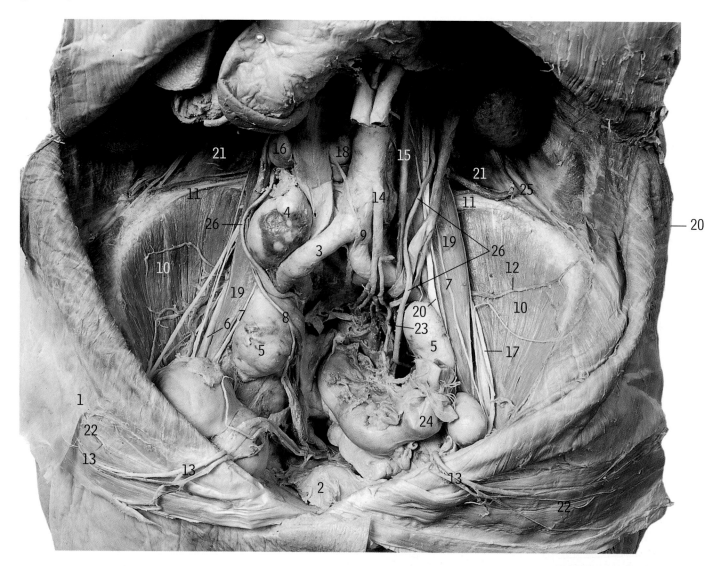

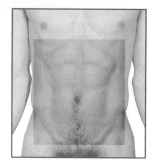

| | |
|---|---|
| **1** Arcuate line of posterior rectus sheath | **14** Inferior mesenteric artery |
| **2** Bladder | **15** Inferior mesenteric vein |
| **3** Common iliac artery | **16** Lateral aortic (right chain) node (enlarged) |
| **4** Common iliac node (grossly enlarged) | **17** Lateral cutaneous nerve of thigh |
| **5** External iliac node (grossly enlarged) | **18** Pre-aortic (aortocaval) node (enlarged) |
| **6** Femoral nerve | **19** Psoas major |
| **7** Genitofemoral nerve | **20** Psoas minor |
| **8** Gonadal vein | **21** Quadratus lumborum |
| **9** Hypogastric plexus, superior | **22** Rectus abdominis |
| **10** Iliacus | **23** Sigmoid branches of left colic artery |
| **11** Iliolumbar ligament | **24** Sigmoid colon |
| **12** Iliolumbar vein | **25** Subcostal nerve |
| **13** Inferior epigastric vessels | **26** Ureter |

*Lymphadenopathy, lymphoma, see page 366.*

# Lymphatics of thigh and superficial inguinal lymph nodes

## B moderate lymph adenopathy

* Marker quill is in the right anterior superior iliac spine

## A minor lymphadenopathy

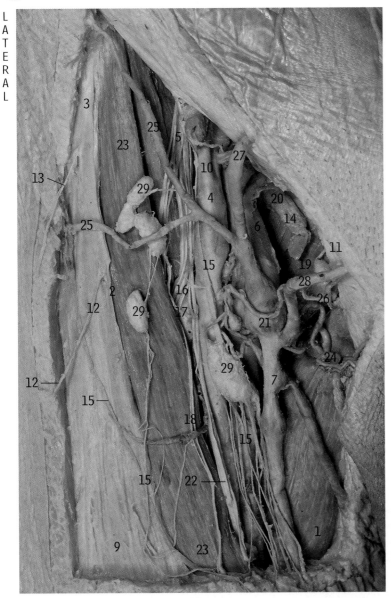

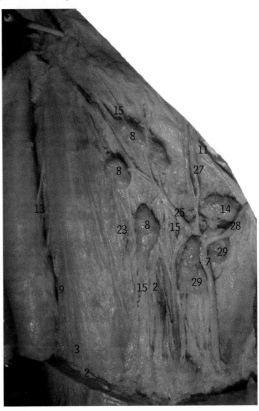

1 Adductor longus
2 Fascia lata, cut edge
3 Fascia lata overlying tensor fasciae latae
4 Femoral artery
5 Femoral nerve
6 Femoral vein
7 Great saphenous vein
8 Horizontal chain of superficial inguinal nodes
9 Iliotibial tract overlying vastus lateralis
10 Inferior epigastric vessels
11 Inguinal ligament
12 Intermediate cutaneous nerve of the thigh
13 Lateral cutaneous nerve of the thigh
14 Lymph node (Cloquet)
15 Lymph vessels
16 Muscular branches of femoral nerve overlying lateral circumflex femoral vessels
17 Nerve to sartorius
18 Nerve to vastus lateralis
19 Pectineus
20 Position of femoral canal
21 Saphena varix
22 Saphenous nerve
23 Sartorius
24 Scrotal veins
25 Superficial circumflex iliac vein
26 Superficial external pudendal artery
27 Superficial epigastric vein
28 Superficial external pudendal vein
29 Vertical chain of superficial inguinal lymph nodes

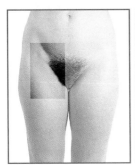

The boundaries of the femoral triangle are the inguinal ligament (11), the medial border of sartorius (23) and the medial border of adductor longus (1).

The femoral canal (20) is the medial compartment of the femoral sheath (removed) which contains in its middle compartment the femoral vein (6) and in the lateral compartment the femoral artery (4). The femoral nerve (5) is lateral to the sheath, not within it.

*Milroy's disease, lymphangioma circumscriptum, lymphogranuloma venereum (LGV), elephantiasis, see page 366.*

# Lymphatics

Clinical thumbnails, see DVD Lymphatics for details and futher clinical images

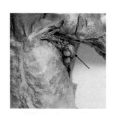

Axillary lymph node dissection for breast cancer

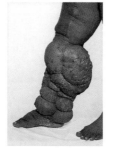

Elephantiasis

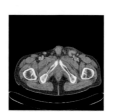

Lymphadenopathy

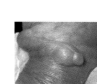

Lymphangioma circumscriptum

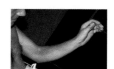

Lymphangitis

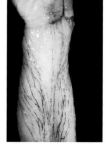

Lymphatic system

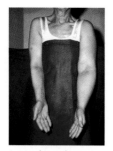

Lymphoedema

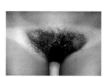

Lympho-granuloma venereum

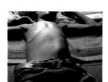

Lymphoma

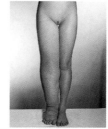

Milroy's disease

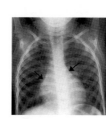

Thymus

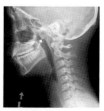

Tonsillitis

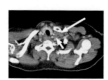

Virchow's node

# Index